Handbook of Geriatric Care Management

Cathy Cress, MSW
President
Cresscare, Case Management for Elders
Pacific Grove, California

AN ASPEN PUBLICATION®
Aspen Publishers, Inc.
Gaithersburg, Maryland
2001

The authors have made every effort to ensure the accuracy of the information herein. However, appropriate information sources should be consulted, especially for new or unfamiliar procedures. It is the responsibility of every practitioner to evaluate the appropriateness of a particular opinion in the context of actual clinical situations and with due considerations to new developments. The authors, editors, and the publisher cannot be held responsible for any typographical or other errors found in this book.

Library of Congress Cataloging-in-Publication Data

Handbook of geriatric care management/[edited by] Cathy Cress.
p. ; cm.
Includes bibliographical references and index.
IBSN 0-8342-1667-1
1. Geriatrics—Handbooks, manuals, etc.
2. Aged—Medical care—Management—Handbooks, manuals, etc.
I. Cress, Cathy.
[DNLM: 1. Health Services for the Aged—organization & administration.
2. Geriatrics.   3. Practice Management—organization & administration.
WT 31 H236 2000]
RC952.55.H386 2000
362.1'9897—dc21
00-048088

Orders: (800) 638-8437
Customer Service: (800) 234-1660

About Aspen Publishers • For more than 40 years, Aspen has been a leading professional publisher in a variety of disciplines. Aspen's vast information resources are available in both print and electronic formats. We are committed to providing the highest quality information available in the most appropriate format for our customers. Visit Aspen's Internet site for more information resources, directories, articles, and a searchable version of Aspen's full catalog, including the most recent publications:
www.aspenpublishers.com
Aspen Publishers, Inc. • The hallmark of quality in publishing
Member of the worldwide Wolters Kluwer group.

Editorial Services: Nora McElfish
Library of Congress Catalog Card Number: 00-048088
ISBN: 0-8342-1667-1

Printed in the United States of America

1 2 3 4 5

Contents

Contributors

Miriam K. Aronson, EdD
Professional Geriatric Care Manager
Hillsdale, New Jersey
Vice President Geriatric Services
Bergen Regional Medical Center
Paramus, New Jersey

Carolyn Barber, MSN, PHN, CMC
Geriatric Case Manager
Cresscare, Case Management for Elders
Pacific Grove, California

Rona S. Bartelstone, MSW, LCSW, CMC
President/CEO
Rona Bartelstone Associates, Inc.
Ft. Lauderdale, Florida

Cathy Cress, MSW
President
Cresscare, Case Management for Elders
Pacific Grove, California

Robyn L. Golden, MA, LCSW
Clinical Director
Council for Jewish Elderly
Chicago, Illinois

Laura Spitler Hansen, MSW
Chief Executive Officer
Age Concerns, Inc.
San Diego, California

Karen Knutson, MSN, MBA, RN
President and Founder
Open Care
Past President of the Board of Directors
The National Association of Professional
    Geriatric Care Managers
Charlotte, North Carolina

Leonie Nowitz, MSW
Director
Center for Lifelong Growth
Faculty
Brookdale Center on Aging
Hunter College
New York, New York

Merrily Orsini, MSSW
President
My Virtual Corp.
Past President, Chairman, and Founder
Elder Care Solutions
Louisville, Kentucky

Robert E. O'Toole, MSW, BCD
President
Informed Decisions, Inc.
Dedham, Massachusetts

Anne Rosenthal, PhD, MFT, CMC
Director of Community Services
Esther & Jacques Reutlinger
    Community for Jewish Living
Danville, California

B.J. Curry Spitler, LCSW, PhD
Founder/Chairman of the Board
Age Concerns, Inc.
San Diego, California

Monika White, PhD
President/CEO
Center for Healthy Aging
Santa Monica, California

Michael Zawadski, JD
Vice President of Operations
Getcare.com
Oakland, California

Rick Zawadski, PhD
Senior Partner
RTZ Associates
Oakland, California

Foreword

Geriatric care management is a profession that has been developing for the past 10 years. It is now on the verge of exploding. The latest statistics show that baby boomers currently have more parents than children, live farther away from their parents, and often are dual career couples with little time for caregiving activities. While time is usually at a premium in our busy lives, so is the desire to be sure our parents are well taken care of.

Finally, we have a book that expounds on the important aspects of this growing profession. The *Handbook of Geriatric Care Management* is the first of its kind. It is the only book available that offers an accurate history of the profession and how it continues to evolve. It raises the important issues of ethics, standards of care, qualifications, and decision making. It is a how-to guide written by the leaders of the profession for the profession. From the personal aspects of the profession to the business aspects of the practice, this book covers it all.

Dealing with the elderly often leaves one to address the issues of family dynamics, health care decisionmaking, housing options, financial decisions, competency, end of life, and personal interests. All are complicated issues. Many of them can be emotional issues. However, knowing that the elderly person is the client (not the person who happens to pay the bill) allows a care manager to focus on that person's quality of life. Statistics have shown that people live longer, happier, and more productive lives when they are in their own surroundings. Thus, the role of the care manager is important in promoting the quality, comfort, and longevity of a loved one's life.

This book correctly portrays the care manager as a problem solver who works with clients and their families to optimize resources and ensure his or her quality of life. Being able to supplement or replace (in the absence of family) those functions that traditionally were taken care of by the extended family is extremely important in an era of independence, self-reliance, and smaller or detached families.

Most care managers will work in a small for-profit company or in a not-for-profit agency. For those who venture out on their own, this *is* the resource for developing a solid care management business. The concepts of marketing and practice management are new for many in the professional service field who never took a business course in college. Nowhere else is there a how-to book that addresses all the aspects of building and maintaining a profitable care management business.

Congratulations to Cathy Cress and the contributing authors of this book. It will serve as one of the leading books in care management for many years to come.

Laury Adsit Gelardi, MBA
Executive Director
National Association of Professional
Geriatric Care Managers
Tucson, Arizona

Dianne Boazman, MSW, LCSW, CMC
2000 President
National Association of Professional
Geriatric Care Managers
Tucson, Arizona

Acknowledgments

Through their assistance with editing, constructive comments and suggestions, and professional perspective, I would like to acknowledge and express sincere thanks to the many individuals who made this book possible.

I would like to thank Marcie Parker, who was an invaluable guide. Her excellent editing skills, broad overview, and impeccable historical perspective on the development of the field of geriatric care management were of great assistance. I would also like to thank Monika White for references and friendly support whenever I called upon her. Her wide world of contacts in the geriatric care management and aging fields gave me invaluable assistance in creating this book. I would like to acknowledge Casey Milne, Nancy Alexander, and Lenard Kaye for their help in editing for content, accuracy, and perspective. I greatly appreciate the time these individuals took out of their busy academic and professional lives to lend me a hand.

I would like to thank Mary Anne Langdon, Senior Developmental Editor at Aspen Publishers, Inc., for her superb editing. I could not have been more lucky to have Mary Anne as the editor of my first book. Her acuity, faith, patience, relaxed manner, and wonderful sense of humor were a catalyst to both the caliber and excellence of the book, and my creativity in drawing the information together into a readable whole. I can't thank her enough for the excellent job she did in helping me do the most creative work possible. I would also like to thank Nora McElfish, Associate Editor, for her editing skills, kind support, and assistance. She, too, made my first book an enjoyable experience and greatly enhanced the quality of the contents through her editing.

I would like to thank the authors who contributed to this book: Monika White, Laura Spitler Hansen, B.J. Curry Spitler, Robyn L. Golden, Merrily Orsini, Karen Knutson, Miriam K. Aronson, Rona S. Bartelstone, Rick Zawadski, Michael Zawadski, Robert E. O'Toole, Carolyn Barber, Anne Rosenthal, and Leonie Nowitz. Their unflagging humor, perseverance, hard work, and professional expertise made the book possible. In this new field, they are all founding mothers and fathers, and I am especially grateful they shared their pioneering work and perspectives in their excellent chapters.

I would like to dedicate this book to my late mother, Kathleen Marie Cress. Her brilliance, deep social concern, and will to stand up and fight for what she believed in are reflected in everything I have done in my life and in this book. Her supreme sacrifice—to support me when I moved 3,000 miles away to attend graduate school at University of California Berkeley in the new field of aging—occurred at a time when she really needed me herself. This book is the fruit of that sacrifice, and hopefully, some compensation for her loss. There is not a day in my life when I do not miss her.

I would like to thank my husband Pete Peterson, whose belief in me and my writing has been with me for the 24 years we have been together. His gift of faith and love has sustained me each moment of our relationship.

I would also like to offer my love and thanks to my two daughters, Kali Peterson and Jill Gallo. We are a family of compassionate, intelligent women, who work hard for our beliefs and values and labor assiduously to actualize our vision. I want to thank them for carrying on that tradition.

Introduction

Geriatric care management addresses a vital need for seniors in the American health care system. In recent years, the number of older persons has grown in record numbers and we have witnessed the evolution of myriad senior services, including housing services, health care services, and home care services. Geriatric care management came on the scene at the end of the 20th century to oversee this continuum of care. Geriatric care managers (GCMs) can look at this complex and fragmented web of senior services and come up with the right care plan for each older person. GCMs ensure that care is geared toward the individual and well coordinated.

The *Handbook of Geriatric Care Management* is being published at a time when geriatric care management is evolving rapidly. Although the field has existed for more than 25 years, it is really just coming into its own. Geriatric care management originated as a cutting-edge addition to case management. But as the profession has grown, it has become relatively mainstream and separate from case management. Geriatric care management issues cross over into larger domains such as elder law, banking trusts, accounting, and managed care. The profession's growth is also reflected in its increasing inclusion in the portfolios of very large health care businesses (e.g., managed care providers, national health care corporations).

Why has this new field grown so quickly and spread so far? What created it in the first place? Quite simply, the field evolved out of a genuine gap in services. There was a burgeoning popula-

tion of middle- and upper-income older persons who needed community and health care services to remain at home and independent. Their needs were not met. And the adult children of these older persons, nicknamed the "sandwich generation" because they had responsibilities to care for both their children and their parents, were at times too overwhelmed with family and work to fully address the problems of their aging parents. In addition, many adult children had moved far away from their aging parents just when those aging parents needed them most. All of these factors converged to launch the field of geriatric care management in U.S. health care.

What has not evolved is a training program for GCMs, a large gap that is addressed by this book. Since there are few schools and universities nationally that offer geriatric care management training programs, schools of social welfare and nursing and many programs in gerontology and human services are the front line of training for geriatric care management. Therefore, this book can be a useful tool in making geriatric care management a part of the curriculum in undergraduate and graduate courses. The book can be an addition to courses taken by future GCMs or individuals in related fields who want to learn more about geriatric care management.

As the profession of geriatric care management has grown, so has a much-needed credentialing process. There are now multiple GCM credentials. This book discusses these many credentialing choices and the credentialing process in general. Why is the credentialing process important? It is a guide for persons seeking a skilled and professionally trained GCM. The credentialing process is also helpful to GCMs because it gives them credibility with the public, thus helping them build their practice. This book will help aspiring and experienced GCMs alike to choose which credentials to pursue.

This handbook will help beginning GCMs get their footing and experienced GCMs grow as professionals. The handbook discusses many aspects of operating a GCM practice, including getting the business started, promoting the business, expanding the business, understanding geriatric assessment, and knowing how to work with dementia clients and their families. A bevy of "how to" information is included in the handbook.

This handbook will also serve as a tool for persons in the business world. Persons seeking to integrate geriatric care management into their business or portfolio of businesses (e.g., accountants, elder-law attorneys, persons who work in a trust department or large national health care corporation) will learn all they need to know.

Because the definition of geriatric care management is still somewhat fuzzy, marketing geriatric care management services can be difficult. This book offers clear guidance on defining geriatric care management as a business product in order to sell it. This information will be helpful to beginning GCMs, experienced GCMs, nonprofit agencies offering geriatric care management services, and health care corporations that already integrate geriatric care management into their menu of services or wish to do so.

This handbook also offers an entire chapter on the ethics of geriatric care management. GCMs try to ensure that senior services are not only highly individualized, appropriate, and coordinated but also ethical. GCM providers help seniors and their families make very difficult decisions. GCMs have also developed a code of ethics for all practitioners to follow. Consumers should know to choose only GCMs who abide by this code of ethics.

Because this handbook is intended as a practical guide, it includes sample forms and letters. These tools are intended to both be used as-is and be modified. And because the handbook is intended as a teaching tool, it contains many case examples in each chapter. Instructors working with this handbook in classes can use the examples to explain some of the how-to techniques mentioned and give students a good sense of the problems likely to arise and how they can be solved. Some contact information for organizations mentioned in the book is listed in Appendix A.

Geriatric care management in the year 2025 may be completely different from geriatric care management today. This handbook gives a sense of the metamorphosis that the field is likely to undergo in the next few decades.

The book is meant as a rich resource discussing an incredibly complex and interesting field. I hope that it will serve you well, helping you become a better GCM or integrate geriatric care management into your business.

PART I

Introduction to Geriatric Care Management

CHAPTER 1

Overview and History of Geriatric Care Management

Cathy Cress

What is geriatric care management? It is a series of steps taken by a geriatric care manager (GCM) to help solve older people's problems. A GCM, who may be a social worker, a nurse, or another human service professional, serves older people and their families. The GCM usually steps in when the older person or family is in crisis. Geriatric care management is also a preventative service rendered on demand, increasing the quality of an older person's life, managing all the players rendering services to the older person, and offering assurance and peace of mind to the adult children of the older individual. How does the GCM solve these problems and render these services? The GCM uses classic social work and nursing tools, including client assessment, care planning, service coordination, and referral and monitoring.

What is a GCM? GCMs' jobs are similar to case managers' jobs, and GCMs use all the classic tools of case management. But unlike other case managers, GCMs specialize in serving adults ages 65 and up and offer very personalized services. GCMs have historically had much smaller caseloads than case managers (especially those in public case management settings), giving GCMs great flexibility in delivering highly personalized services to their older clients. And unlike many case managers in public case management settings, GCMs are generally available 24 hours a day, 7 days a week, 365 days a year. They respond to client needs at the convenience of the client, allowing the GCM to cross the line from public sector human services into the for-profit service business. The GCM's product is service, and that product must be available at all times to be useful to older people, their families, and third parties such as trust departments and conservators, who are willing to buy the product if it is offered in this manner.[1]

The GCM is not just the classic anonymous public-sector case manager delivering nonindividualized services. In fact, the GCM is a kind of surrogate family member with special expertise in the phases and tasks of care management and a long-standing and personal relationship with clients. GCMs deliver the kind of "old-fashioned" good service that many older clients remember nostalgically. GCMs both respond to clients' demands and are proactive, always maintaining a positive attitude.

In addition, GCMs deliver the level of service that clients' adult children expect. These children are usually baby boomers from two-income families accustomed to purchasing services (housecleaning, day care, after-school transportation, tax assistance) to make their busy lives easier. Purchasing geriatric care management services to assist with the problems of their older family members, who frequently live far away, seems logical to these adult children. The GCM is providing time and expertise, neither of which the adult child has. The GCM also sells peace of mind. Most baby boomers do not want to get up in the middle of the night to respond to an older person's crisis, but the GCM will. The adult child may not have enough vacation time to fly to the parent's home to arrange services once the older person gets out of hospital, but the GCM will. Most adult children want the assurance that the older family member is cared for and safe, without having to solve the problem themselves. So the personalized services of the GCM, a surrogate family member, appeal to adult children.[2]

In addition to handling client assessment, care planning, service coordination, and referral and monitoring, the GCM keeps track of a giant web of senior services, the continuum of care. GCMs are like Charlotte, the friendly spider in *Charlotte's Web*. They run back and forth across the web, linking services, repairing gaps, spinning new solutions to problems, and coordinating answers. GCMs are at their root problem solvers.

This chapter offers an overview of what a GCM does, then discusses the history of the profession.

OVERVIEW OF A GCM's RESPONSIBILITIES

Geriatric care management involves a series of problem-solving steps. This section gives an overview of some of the most important steps in the process: assessing clients, planning care, coordinating and implementing the solution, and monitoring the care plan.

Assessing Clients

The process starts with assessment, which is discovering what health-related and psychosocial, financial, and legal problems an older person may be experiencing, by using an assessment tool (see Chapter 11). The assessment should be comprehensive and systematic and assess the person's functional and cognitive capacity and limitations. It also should look at other needs, strengths, abilities, and existing resources and supports.

Consider the following case. Harry Brown has dementia and his wife is exhausted from the care she renders at home. The Brown adult children call a GCM to come in and do an assessment because Mr. Brown is losing weight and his wife is not sleeping. Harry recently wandered out of the house and down the street. Agnes called the po-

lice, and Harry was found in a neighbor's home, not sure where he was. Agnes called her daughter in another state, who contacted a GCM to help her sort out what to do to help her parents. The daughter is also exhausted because there have been many similar calls and she is not only trying to help her parents but raising two teenagers, working outside the home, and serving on several boards at her children's school. She is sandwiched between the needs of her parents and the needs of her children as well as trying to meet her own needs.

The GCM does an assessment of Harry. She uses her assessment tool to assess Harry's psychosocial and health problems. In addition, she assesses Harry's cognitive deficits through a tool that measures mental status. She does all this while gently interviewing Harry and Agnes and their daughter, who has flown in from out of state. In addition, she sends a signed release of information to Harry's physician along with a physician's report, supplied by the GCM, that assesses Harry's problems.

Planning Care

The next step is care planning, or taking the findings of the assessment and creating a plan of care. This care plan should solve the problems identified in the assessment (see Table 1–1). The care plan is also based on how much the older person is able to pay for services and what local community resources are available.

The GCM's suggested care plan identifies one of the Browns' problems as caregiver burnout and another as a need for a medication review by Harry's physician and a geriatric psychiatrist. To solve these problems, the GCM might suggest that the family get a part-time aide to offer respite, or the GCM might help the family enroll Harry into an adult day care program for people with dementia. In addition, the care plan suggests having Harry reassessed by his physician. The GCM will suggest that she work with Agnes so that Agnes can learn how to relieve stress. The GCM also will suggest long-term planning that may include a list of local Alzheimer's facilities, if Mr. Brown needs to be placed.

Table 1–1 Care Plan

Problem	Solution
1. **Knowledge deficit: Alzheimer's moderate stage**	**a.** Hire care provider for 4 hours a day, 3 afternoons a week **b.** Enroll Mr. Brown in Alzheimer's day care center 3 mornings a week **c.** Enroll Mr. Brown in a wanderers program **d.** Assess Mr. Brown by a geriatric psychiatrist
2. **Caregiver burnout: Mrs. Brown stressed by care of husband for several years**	**a.** Hire care provider 4 hours a day, 3 afternoons a week **b.** Enroll Mr. Brown in Alzheimer's day care center 3 mornings a week **c.** Enroll Mrs. Brown in exercise class **d.** Arrange for regular pedicures, facials, manicures, and massages for Mrs. Brown **e.** Enroll Mrs. Brown in an Alzheimer's support group
3. **Self-care deficit: cannot shower alone**	**a.** Hire provider to help Mr. Brown shower 3 times a week
4. **Impaired home management: cannot assist wife with any household tasks**	**a.** Hire care provider to prepare dinner before she leaves each day **b.** Hire care provider to clean bathroom and kitchen as needed **c.** Hire care provider to do laundry as needed
5. **Alteration in nutrition: Mr. Brown's appetite diminished and he consequently lost weight**	**a.** Hire care provider to encourage snacks **b.** Hire care provider to prepare dinner **c.** See physician to review weight loss
6. **Medications for dementia need to be reviewed**	**a.** See physician for a complete medication review **b.** Assess Mr. Brown by a geriatric psychiatrist for second opinion on medications
7. **Long-term planning needed for the Browns**	**a.** Provide daughter and wife with a list of Alzheimer's facilities if he needs to be placed in the future

Coordinating and Implementing the Solution

The GCM then coordinates and implements the solution. This means taking the services and actions indicated in the care plan and starting them in a cost-effective and timely manner. The implementation must also respect the client's and family's desires regarding services and providers. GCMs use formal and informal services, including home health agencies, volunteers, friends, and neighbors. The case manager will arrange the services and then coordinate them.

The GCM implements a solution for Harry and Agnes by arranging a home health agency to send a caregiver 4 hours a day, 3 days a week, offering care to Harry and giving Agnes respite. The GCM arranges for Harry to attend an adult day care center specializing in dementia 3 mornings a week. She sets up an appointment for Harry to be assessed by his physician and requests that the physician do a complete medication review. She also works with the wife to help her plan some ways for her to use her free time to relieve stress, including a light exercise class and a regular appointment to get her nails and hair done.

Monitoring the Care Plan

The GCM then monitors the plan of care to make sure it is working. Case management demands that services be monitored to make sure they are of the highest quality, match what is in the care plan, are implemented in a timely manner, and meet the client's needs. Services also must respond to changes in the client and the family. For example, if Harry improves, then services can be reduced or eliminated. If his situation deteriorates, then services need to be stepped up. In hospital programs, monitoring occurs weekly. In outpatient settings, services tend to be monitored bimonthly. In acute care settings, monitoring occurs across different care settings. For example, the GCM might see the client in the hospital one week and follow up with a visit in the rehab facility the next week. Some programs do telephone monitoring. GCMs monitor in different settings and at times negotiate with the client.

During the first month after the plan is implemented, the GCM working with Harry and Agnes goes to the Brown home once a week to talk to Agnes and see how things are going. She finds out during her first visit that Harry dislikes the caregiver sent from the home health agency. The GCM calls the home health agency and asks that another aide be sent, one who is gentler and more caring with Harry. The GCM comes the next week and finds that Harry has gone to the adult day care center and been rejected by the center, told that he cannot be there without an aide. So the GCM asks the family if she can extend the care of the aide through the home health agency and have the aide help Harry at the adult day care center. Although she finds that Agnes enrolled in teh Alzheimer's support group, she also finds that Agnes has not yet signed up for an exercise class or a weekly hair and nail appointment. The GCM then gently reminds the wife she agreed to do this and arranges for her to see a

social worker herself, paid by Medicare, to help her deal with some of her denial.

HISTORY OF GERIATRIC CARE MANAGEMENT

GCMs are now relatively familiar participants in the world of senior services and health care. But what conditions led to the rise of geriatric care management? This section will discuss the history of this important profession.

The Origins of Case Management

In a seminal study of geriatric care management, Secord and Parker note that case management itself, the root of geriatric care management, has its foundation in the emerging social services for new immigrants and other poor people in the late 1800s.[3] At that time, urbanization and industrialization had left so many people poor and homeless that churches and local communities were paralyzed and unable to care for everyone in need. Social service bureaucracies began to arise, which led to the beginning of case management. Secord and Parker hypothesize that the core elements of today's case management were born by "helping the client find the least costly, most appropriate services to meet his or her needs."[3(p4)] Since then, community agencies, social workers, hospital discharge planners, and case coordinators have provided what we now call case management.

No one group or movement was solely responsible for the emergence of case management. In the arena of early social services, Joseph Tuckerman organized a group of churches to help needy families in 1833. The Settlement House movement at the turn of the century is another example of early case management. The Settlement House movement established institutions called settlement houses that tried to improve living conditions in city neighborhoods. Most settlement houses had social workers on their staffs. Many charity organizations and societies coordinated assistance for children and families; a case management program was set up by the Massachusetts Board of Charities in the mid-1800s. The roots of case management can also be found in early workers' compensation programs of the 1940s.[4]

In the medical world, case management appeared in the treatment of chronically ill and long–term-care populations, including children, people with disabilities, substance abusers, and acquired immune deficiency syndrome victims. As acute care costs skyrocketed after World War II in the United States, case management techniques developed to lower costs. Case managers appeared in institutional settings to follow patients into the community and coordinate the care of high-cost, high-risk individuals. At the same time, private medical case managers appeared to respond to the needs of patients, insurers, and medical providers by helping them make difficult decisions (e.g., is a medical procedure appropriate, is there a less costly alternative, or can a patient spend recovery time at home). Today, the medical case manager makes a path for the patient through the maze of the health care delivery system, coordinates a plan of care, and offers support from family agencies and suppliers of health care or health care entities.[5]

Growth of Case Management for Older People

Case management for older people emerged because of two factors, according to Parker and Secord. The first was the rapid growth of the older population in the United States. The second was the increased cost of health care, especially Medicare, in the United States. At the time of their study in 1987, Secord and Parker reported that Medicare expenditures totaled $83 billion in 1981 and were projected to increase to $200 billion in the year 2000.[3]

With health care costs exploding in the 1950s and 1960s, and the number of older people growing, there was a national effort to stem the fiscal bloodletting. This was true especially with nursing home expenditures, which did and continued to eat up a large part of public funds, mostly through Medicaid payments for older people. In the 1970s and 80s, many states developed nursing home preadmission screening programs in an attempt to reduce nursing home placement. In other states there was a moratorium on nursing home bed construction. People realized that nursing home placement was not only costly but often unnecessary or inappropriate; many older Americans could be cared for in their own homes.

In addition, services for older people were expanding. This growth was driven (post World War II) by five major federal programs with mandates to finance gerontological services: Title VIII of the Social Security Act (Medicare), Title XIX of the Social Security Act (Medicaid), Title XX of the Social Security Act, the Older Americans Act, and the Department of Veterans Affairs.[6]

As a result of these developments, a plethora of senior programs blossomed in the United States in the 1960s and 1970s. These services included home care, homemaker services, chore services, housing alternatives, transportation services, adult day care, and in-home meals. These senior services, all of which helped keep seniors in their own homes, were not coordinated. Some services had emerged from states, some from the federal government, and some from the local community. Because this fragmented system was difficult to navigate, it did not serve older people well.

To help with this fragmentation and lack of a single point of entry to the web of senior programs, many public and private programs developed aspects of case management. In the 1970s, Medicare funded a number of Medicare waiver programs to find out if older people could remain more independent with community-based coordinated care. Case managers would guide older people through the complex web of senior services and decide which services would be appropriate for each individual.

A case manager might help in the following way: An older person who lives alone at home and is very lonely might become depressed enough to stop eating on a regular basis. The nutritional deficit leads to confusion, which leads to not taking needed medications. If these medications are for high blood pressure, the unmedicated older person may have a stroke and be hospitalized, then placed in a nursing home.

This eventual nursing home placement could be avoided if the older person had a case manager who knew that depression might lead to this outcome and who understood that a regular friendly visitor could allay the depression. The case manager might also suggest regular visits to a senior center as a way for this person to reenter the world. The case manager might talk to some of the older person's friends and encourage more frequent visiting or a weekly meal together so that the older person had company and something to look forward to each week. The case manager might also arrange for the older person to visit his or her physician for medication monitoring and for daily prepared meals to be dropped off by Meals on Wheels. Thus, the case manager could help avoid an unnecessary nursing home placement by navigating the older person through the very confusing continuum of care.

The emerging Medicare waiver programs of the 1970s also allowed for the purchase of items that people would not normally be able to buy through Medicare, such as medications and eyeglasses. This was done on an experimental basis to see what mix of services would help keep older people out of nursing homes and in the community.

Case management was seen as central to these Medicare waiver programs, including Connecticut Triage on the East Coast and the Multipurpose Senior Services Project on the West Coast, the National Long Term Care Channeling Project, the 2176 Medicaid Waiver Programs, and the Community Nursing and Home Health programs. Out of these very experimental programs of the 1970s and 1980s emerged the classic model of case management.[7]

The Emergence of Professional Geriatric Care Management

The frail elderly have historically been the prime consumers of case management services. They experience functional and cognitive impairments that demand a wide array of informal and formal services. Case managers are expert in brokering these services. The publicly funded case management programs of the 1970s and 1980s demonstrated that case management was an ideal tool in brokering these formal and informal services and in helping older people to remain in the community. Years of studies showed that older people wanted to stay at home and that they could remain at home with coordinated in-home and community-based services. The key was case management. Many factors came together to encourage the development of geriatric care management, at first a specialized form of case management.

One factor that contributed to the rise of geriatric care management was a new pool of qualified people interested in pursuing a slightly different type of work. Many case managers from public case management programs became burned out from working in the public system so long; they wanted more independence in their jobs while still doing good and working with older people. Others from the helping professions (nurses and social workers) had not worked in public case management programs but had experienced burnout and wanted a different, perhaps more exciting career path where they would still be helping others.

At the same time, the voluminous and very fragmented web of senior services continued to expand, tangle, and unravel, with no central point of entry and mind-boggling rules at the federal, state, and local levels. Contemporaneously, the number of older people was increasing. Many of these older people had large enough incomes and amounts of assets to be ineligible for publicly-funded and community-based programs. Seventy percent of the wealth in the United States is controlled by people 50 years old and older. Older people in this $800 billion market have at least $115 billion in discretionary income. Since long-term care management and chronic care management are not covered by Medicare, this care is a discretionary purchase. The over-65 cohort is much more affluent than all the age groups under 45. Households headed by persons over 65 have considerable purchasing power, with one-third of all the discretionary income in the country. Therefore, older people needed and could afford geriatric care management services.[6]

Two other factors contributed to the development of geriatric care management. First, more women were working out of the house. Although women remain the principal informal caregivers in the United States today, they have accounted for a significant percentage of the work force since the 1950s. Women entered the work force partly because of many societal changes, including the women's movement, and partly because families needed two incomes to stay afloat. Fifty-five percent of all women today work, leaving not only children but older adults in need of care. Despite the crushing emotional, physical, and financial burdens, the U.S. family has not abandoned its elders. A 1990s study by the U.S. House of Representatives showed that the average woman spends 17 years caring for her children and 18 years or more caring for her older parents. Piggybacked on this is another startling statistic, that for the first time in U.S. history, Americans today have more parents than children.[8]

Second, most Americans tend to live far from their older family members. The United States is an incredibly mobile society. Individuals no longer stay where they grew up. They may work in many different locations while their parents stay in the hometown. According to a study by the American Association of Retired Persons, one-third of all adult children in the United States live at least 30 minutes away from their aging parents.[9] This leaves vulnerable older people at risk if they have a crisis, because the main system of support is still the family. If the family lives far away, a crisis can turn into a mega-crisis if there is no one to offer assistance.

All of these factors have led to the need for geriatric care management. Public and private case managers as well as nurses and social workers who chose to leave the system saw a wonderful niche to fill. They understood how to provide care professionally. Many understood case management. And they saw the frustration of many older people, who had the money to purchase services but were not sure which services to choose, and of the families, usually the daughters, overworked and far away. Adult children realized they could do what they already did for

housecleaning and other services: they could purchase help for their parents.

THE BIRTH OF GERIATRIC CARE MANAGEMENT ORGANIZATIONS

Geriatric care management became a profession gradually, like all professions. Because the people who started the profession came from diverse fields, there was no central meeting ground for them in the beginning. Social workers belonged to the National Association of Social Workers, while nurses belonged to many different associations, including the American Nurses Association. To work on common goals and interests, the new GCMs started several organizations. The most important early ones were the National Association of Professional Geriatric Care Managers (NAPGCM) and the Case Management Society of America (CMSA).

NAPGCM

The first few GCMs, who were scattered throughout the country, were originally drawn together through a 1984 article in the *New York Times*.[10] GCMs from different areas were surprised to learn that other people were doing what they were doing. Social workers who were interviewed in the article were asked to join a coalition. The first meeting of what would be the NAPGCM was held in the home of Adele Elkind, a social worker who was the founding force of NAPGCM, in January 1985. Professionals who had expertise in this relatively new body of knowledge began to share information to help each other run better businesses. They agreed that if they could help each other, they could help the public. They put together a brochure to describe their services and moved on to develop criteria to decide who could be a member of the group. They formalized their network into the Greater New York Network on Aging (GNYNA) and began to refer cases to each other. Sara Cohen, a founding member, suggested the radical idea that the fledgling group have a national conference; in 1985, 100 human service professionals gathered in New York City to take part in the first National Conference of Private

Geriatric Care Managers. The gathering was hosted by GNYNA, which was by then a growing group of social workers, psychologists, nurses, and clinical gerontologists. This group had the vision of a national association dedicated to private geriatric care management.[11]

In 1986 this vision became a reality when the same group had a conference in Philadelphia, adopted membership standards, and unanimously voted to found the National Association of Private Geriatric Care Managers. In 1992 the association changed its name to the National Association of Professional Geriatric Care Managers, reflecting the fact that members might be from public, private for-profit, or private nonprofit backgrounds.

NAPGCM began with 30 members; now it has 1,200. The organization has been able to bring unity and consistency to geriatric care management by forming an information base for aspiring and practicing GCMs. In 16 years of meetings, its members have also been able to gather a body of research about the GCM field. This body of knowledge has been presented in yearly NAPGCM national and regional conferences and in the *GCM Journal*. This journal, in existence for 10 years, publishes research and other information about the field and addresses topics of interest to GCMs, including business and practice issues.

NAPGCM has many publications that are helpful in starting a geriatric care management business, including a business start-up manual, several years of workshop tapes from conferences covering business issues, and a forms book. These can be ordered by contacting NAPGCM (see Appendix A).[12]

CMSA

CMSA is another association that addresses the needs of budding GCMs. CMSA does not specifically focus on geriatric care management but addresses the entire field of case management. However, many of its members work in settings involving geriatric care management. CMSA has workshops and products that meet the needs of GCMs. CMSA also has an Elder Care Special Interest Group. This group offers a newsletter, peer networking directories, roundtable presentations, and specialized education programs.

The association was founded in 1990 to support and develop the profession of case management through education, networking, and legislation. It now has 100 affiliated and pending chapters.

CMSA merged with the Individual Case Management Association (ICMA) in 1996. ICMA was founded in 1988 to address the needs of medical case managers, case managers who addressed the needs of clients with catastrophic, high-cost medical care. Most of these case managers were registered nurses. This association started a magazine called *The Case Manager* and began holding conferences for medical case managers called Medical Case Management Conventions. ICMA initiated a national certification program for case managers called Certified Case Manager in 1990 and created the first certification in the field.[13]

Many CMSA case managers have knowledge relevant to GCMs. Almost 1,500 have expertise in long-term care, and about 2,100 have expertise in geriatrics. CMSA members are found in several work settings that involve the practice of geriatric care management. These include approximately 1,200 who work in home health, 650 who work in nursing homes, and 700 business owners. Appendix A has information on how to contact CMSA.[13]

Benefits of Membership

Joining an association is probably a very wise step for a budding GCM. Like any new professionals, new GCMs want to learn from those with experience, and associations are a good place to find knowledgeable people who may even become mentors. There is a rich body of information in the field of geriatric care management. However, because this profession is relatively new, the information is still mainly available in workshops and journals, both of which are produced by associations.

From time spent with other members of these associations, newcomers can learn what to avoid as they enter the field. GCMs who have practiced for any length of time have opinions in many areas, starting with whether becoming a GCM is a good idea. They can also provide tips about billing, setting up an office, hiring staff members, doing geriatric assessments, using prefabricated forms, dealing with the stress of running a small business, and developing that business in spite of the stress.

CONCLUSION

GCMs appeared in response to a societal needed: a wide array of fragmented senior services was available, but older people and their adult children were having trouble figuring out which senior services would be helpful. GCMs are caring problem solvers who match older people to the appropriate senior services and monitor the care. People who provide this very personalized service have organized into associations to help define and advance the geriatric care management profession.

NOTES

1. Parker M. Private care management: how families are served. *J Case Manage.* 1992;1:108–112.

2. Cress C. The business of for-profit case management. *J Case Manage.* 1992;1:113–116.

3. Secord L, Parker M. *Private Case Management for Older Persons and Their Families.* Excelsior, MN: Interstudy; 1987.

4. US Department of Health and Human Services. *A National Agenda for Geriatric Education.* Vol 1. Rockville, MD: Interdisciplinary Geriatrics and Allied Health Branch, Division of Associated Dental and Public Health Professions, Bureau of Health Professions; 1998.

5. Mullahay CM. *The Case Manager's Handbook.* Gaithersburg, MD: Aspen Publishers; 1998.

6. Kaye LW. The evolution of private care management. *J Case Manage.* 1992;1:103–107.

7. Cress C. Care management news takes hold in long term care. *Aging Int.* 1992;19.

8. Kilborn B. Eldercare: its impact on the workplace. *Update Aging.* 1990;16.

9. American Association of Retired Persons. *A Profile of Older Americans.* Washington, DC: AARP Fulfillment; 1998.

10. Collins G. Long distance care for the elderly. *New York Times.* January 1984.

11. Elkind A. Development and growth of a regional network. GNYNA: the first two years, joys and growing pains. *Geri Gazette.* 1986;1:1–4.

12. National Association of Professional Geriatric Care Managers. *GCM Directory of Members.* Tucson, AZ; 1999.

13. Case Management Society of America, National Office, 1999.

CHAPTER 2

Ethics and Geriatric Care Management

Cathy Cress

What is ethics? Ethics is a process of studying ourselves and our behavior, according to Nancy Alexander, a geriatric care manager (GCM), social worker, and attorney who has written much on ethics and geriatric care management.[1] According to John Banja, a noted writer on ethics and case management, the word ethics derives from the Greek ethikos. Banja says that the word ethikos means character; for people like Plato and Aristotle, an ethical person had a good character and many virtues. This idea of virtues has had a renaissance in William B. Bennett's best-selling book, *The Book of Virtues: A Treasury of Good Moral Stories*.[2] Banja notes that to the Greeks, being ethical was not difficult. The Greeks simply assumed that a person of good character would make ethical decisions because he or she knew right from wrong. When tough ethical decisions had to be made, Aristotle would simply suggest that a group of reasonable and upstanding people decide together. Banja notes that Aristotle believed this process was as good as any because deciding what is moral and traversing dilemmas along the way are so complex that there are no simple rules to follow.

Aristotle and the Greeks did not make discovering the ethical choice overly complex. There were no rigid formulas to give one the correct answer. In fact, even today, knowing the right behavior is pretty easy because this knowledge is so embedded in our societal understanding of the right path. We know the basics: We must pay our debts, be good parents, be honest, be respectful, and so forth. How do we know these basic

truths? Some would hold, as Banja points out, that God or another creator imprinted these truths on our soul. Banja then shows us another possible source.

Banja uses Edgar Schein's theories on organizational behavior to explain another way of learning basic truths.[2] Schein says that we first learn moral rules as young people because we are born into a system of ethics. We are taught this system by our parents and the institutions of which we are part (e.g., synagogues, churches, schools, communities). When we become a member of a group, we must then adapt to the external reality the group confronts. Groups then go through a second step, according to Schein's theory. That second step is to integrate their internal operations. This is done through role definition. In the family group, for example, one role would be that of a mother; in a university, a professor; in geriatric care management, a GCM.

Here is where morality comes in. Those who have a certain role within a group (e.g., a mother in the family group, a GCM in the Case Management Society of America [CMSA] or National Association of Professional Geriatric Care Managers [NAPGCM]) must act consistently in a manner that the group deems acceptable for a person in that role. Persons who have these roles must set aside their own beliefs to be socially responsible to the group and carry out their obligations to the group. Individuals who fail may be penalized by the group.

For instance, consider a young mother who gives in to her need to enjoy herself and leaves her children unattended while she goes out to a bar. She is reprimanded either by society or a group, perhaps by being arrested for child abandonment. She has exposed her children to harm and forfeited her obligation as a mother to her family. Even though she has a desire for pleasure and happiness, she does not act morally according to society's concept of harm and duty in the family. So being a mother means that one has to act in a socially responsible way as defined by the group, setting one's other needs aside.

A GCM must be socially responsible to the group of GCMs and carry out the obligations of the GCM group. In NAPGCM, that would mean following the GCM Pledge of Ethics (Exhibit 2–1).[3] That pledge means, among other things, that GCMs should always make referrals in the client's interest, not their own interest. For example, if a GCM has a relationship with an area physician and hopes to increase business by getting client referrals from that physician, the GCM might be tempted to refer all clients to that

---

Exhibit 2–1 Pledge of Ethics for Members of the National Association of Professional Geriatric Care Managers

Provisions of Service
I will provide ongoing service to you only after I have assessed your needs and you, or a person designated to act for you, understand and agree to a plan of service, the results that may be expected from it, and the cost of service.

Self-Determination
I will base my plan of service on goals you, or a person designated to act for you, have defined, and which enhance the decisions you have made concerning your life.

Cooperation
I will strive to ensure cooperation between all of the individuals involved in providing service and care to you.

Referrals/Disclosure
I will refer you only to services and organizations I believe to be appropriate and of good quality. I will fully explain to you any business relationship I have with any service I propose, and give you information on alternatives, if at all possible, so that you, or a person designated to act for you, can make an informed decision to accept or reject the services I recommend to you.

Termination of Service
I will end service to you only after reasonable notice. I will recommend a plan for you to continue to receive the services as needed.

Confidentiality
I will hold in trust any confidence you give me, disclosing information to others only with your permission, or if I am compelled to do so by a belief that you will be seriously harmed by my silence, or if the laws of this State require me to do so.

Substitute Judgment
I will not substitute my judgment for yours unless I am acting in the role of your guardian, appointed by a Court of Law, or with your approval, or the approval of someone designated to act for you.

Loyalty
My first duty is loyalty to you. I will always provide services based on your best interest, even if this conflicts with my interests or the interests of others.

Qualifications
I am fully qualified in my profession to provide the services I undertake. I continue to improve my skills and knowledge by participating in professional development programs and maintaining certification and licensing in my profession.

Discrimination
I will not promote or sanction any form of discrimination.

physician to gain reciprocal business from the physician, in spite of the fact that the physician is not appropriate for every client and that clients should be offered multiple health care choices. This GCM would not be setting personal interests aside and putting client interests first. He or she would also be ignoring his obligation to be fair and not do harm to his clients, an obligation codified by CMSA and NAPGCM. He or she would be violating the NAPGCM's Pledge of Ethics, which states:

> I will only refer you to services and organizations I believe to be appropriate and of good quality. I will fully explain to you any business relationship I have with any service I propose, and give you information on alternatives, if at all possible, so that you, or a person designated to act for you, can make an informed decision to accept or reject services recommended to you.[1]

Out of this theory of group ethics, we can see how concepts like goodness, harm, risk, and benefit emerge in a group. All groups develop an understanding of these ideas to help the group survive. We all have our own desires for pleasure or self-gain. However, to act morally in a group, we must go along with the group's understanding of concepts like harm, benefit, duty, justice, and fairness. These become the rules of the group, and belonging to a group means complying with the group's rules or code of morality. The rules also involve policies, vocabulary, and a system of enforcement within the group. Rules are learned not only in groups but in infancy.[2]

Banja points out that the case manager receives a code of moral concepts made up by his or her profession or group. As part of the field of case management, GCMs also follow a professional moral code. For example, as mentioned above, GCMs must avoid conflicts of interest. If a conflict exists, the GCM must disclose the conflict to the interested party.[1] GCMs who refer clients to home health agencies in which the GCMs have financial interests violate the GCM code of ethics. The GCM has to disclose that interest to the client.

A third construct of Schein's, basic assumptions, then comes up. Banja says that these basic assumptions both drive the system and explain its morality. He reasons that these assumptions tell people when they have to do certain things in a group and what justifies that behavior. Beauchamp and Childress, in their classic *Principles of Biomedical Ethics*, tell us that there are four accepted guides to ethical decisions: beneficence, nonmaleficence, justice, and autonomy (Exhibit 2–2).[4]

Basic assumptions begin to show us the group's policies, beliefs, and practices. These group tenets reveal the group's moral concepts. When we begin to look into this morality, we also look at whether the group's moral system is defensible or acceptable. We then enter the realm of ethics.[2]

Although Beauchamp and Childress's four principles are the moral principles accepted as guides in medicine, they can also be applied to geriatric care management. These are the basic assumptions referred to by Banja. These principles are in balance with each other, and no principle supersedes another. GCMs try to adhere to these principles. They sometimes have difficulty when they are unsure which principle applies or when one principle collides with another.[5] Here we are entering the world of ethical probing and ethical dilemmas.

WHAT IS AN ETHICAL DILEMMA?

What is an ethical dilemma? Banja tells us that morality is simply a group's moral code or

---

Exhibit 2–2 Principles of Biomedical Ethics

- Autonomy: Respecting the client's worth
- Nonmaleficence: Refraining from harm
- Beneficence: Advancing an individual's benefit
- Justice: Acting in fairness and equitably giving clients the services they need

fabric—its policies and its understanding of right and wrong. Ethics, as Banja says, is a major step beyond morals. Ethics queries whether a group's moral beliefs are defensible, coherent, factual, honorable, and fair.

If we are to accept Beauchamp and Childress's four tenets, how do we apply them to a society, where we have limited resources?[2] For instance, if beneficence, or doing the greatest good for all older people, is a goal, why does Medicare not cover home care? We know that one answer given by the federal government is that having Medicare fund home care might damage the federal budget. This is an ethical dilemma. How does one choose between preserving government funds and helping older people?

Another example of an ethical dilemma might be the conflict between a legal mandate and a basic GCM assumption like the autonomy of an older person. An older woman, for instance, might be having memory problems, forgetting to take medications, and burning pots. This may lead family members to believe that the woman can no longer care for herself and that a conservator may need to be appointed. Here an ethical dilemma concerning surrogate decision making might arise. GCMs believe in the basic assumption of autonomy, respecting a person's freedom. However, if the woman's safety or health is compromised by her poor decisions and unsafe actions, should her freedom be curtailed through conservatorship? Is she no longer legally competent—capable of making decisions, understanding, and acting reasonably? The GCM can take a step in solving this dilemma by getting the family and the woman's permission to do a mental competency exam.

In a survey of 251 case managers in 10 states, Rosalie Kane and Arthur Caplan uncovered other ethical dilemmas case managers regularly encounter.[6] Case managers were interviewed about their general attitudes. Case managers' dilemmas included the following:

- The case managers overwhelmingly agreed that case managers should make sure that clients receive all possible services. But at the same time the case managers almost as strongly agreed that they should be responsible for seeing that taxpayers' money is well spent. This creates an ongoing ethical dilemma: It is difficult to both restrict costs and provide all the services necessary.
- The case managers believed that family members should care for their older relatives. Yet at the same time, the case managers supported the idea that if older people want to keep family members out of their business, they have the right to do so.
- The case managers believed that a client should have the right to die at home. But at the same time, the case managers felt that if the agency could not arrange enough services for the client to be safe in the home, the agency should withdraw services altogether, perhaps resulting in the client being forced into an institution and not being able to die at home.

Other types of ethical dilemmas that Kane and Caplan discuss are taken up later in this chapter.

Case Study

Here is a more detailed account of one GCM's ethical dilemma. Mary, a GCM, contracts with a senior housing complex to do geriatric assessments. Her employer, Pleasant Gardens, wants her to do a geriatric assessment on a resident. Pleasant Gardens has a rule that if a resident scores a 7 or above on the mental status quotient (MSQ) exam section of the geriatric assessment, the resident is deemed too confused to live independently and is asked to move. Mary knows this. Mary also knows that when the unit is rented again, Pleasant Gardens will get triple the present rent because housing for older people is in great demand.

Eighty–eight-year-old resident Becca Virden's neighbors state that they have seen her putting silverware in the washing machine, that there is spoiled food in her refrigerator, and that they have sometimes seen her wearing two dresses. Mary does the geriatric assessment. Becca scores above a 7 on the MSQ section.

There is some spoiled food in the refrigerator, but Becca has limited vision and may not have been able to see the spoilage. She was not wearing two dresses during the assessment, but her clothes, although clean, are worn and shoddy compared to those of her neighbors, who are obviously more affluent than Becca. Becca says that she does not want to move out of her apartment, where she has lived for 10 years, and tells the GCM that she is terrified to go into a nursing home. She also says that the neighbors who have moved to the complex in the last few years are "hoity-toity" or above her class and don't like her because she uses common language and was never well-to-do or a "ladies luncheon" person.

Here an ethical dilemma arises. Should Mary tell the Pleasant Gardens staff that Becca has an MSQ score high enough for her to be evicted from Pleasant Gardens and almost surely end up in a nursing home? Mary has contracted with Pleasant Gardens as a consultant, so she is not obligated to report the MSQ score to the Pleasant Gardens staff. Is there anything the matter with a GCM's assessment causing an older person to move out of her residence, given that the move is certainly in the senior housing facility's fiscal interest? Does the fact that Mary is getting paid by Pleasant Gardens force her to disclose everything? If Pleasant Gardens finds out she did not reveal information, could the facility sue her?

Before doing the assessment, should Mary have told Becca that she could not promise confidentiality?

If she gives information that will result in Becca being moved, will she be violating her responsibility as a GCM to always safeguard the best interests of the client? After all, asks Mary, who is my client, the older person or Pleasant Gardens? Is Mary inherently unethical for not disclosing to Becca that she works for Pleasant Gardens? Mary now faces the ultimate conundrum. She has been hired, as Banja says, to serve two masters—her employer and her client.

A Collision of Moral Systems

Two different GCMs could easily make totally different decisions about Mary's ethical di-

lemma. Both individuals might believe that their analysis of the situation is objective and that they have found the ethical answer. Being ethical simply means considering a situation and deciding what response is correct.

This is why, Banja says, we run into ethical dilemmas. If a person's actions are called into question by multiple parties and the ethics of the person's decision is debated, each debating party can reach a different conclusion, with an excellent supporting argument. In ethical dilemmas about such charged issues as physician-assisted suicide and abortion, each side can give fine reasons to justify its position. Each side believes that it has the "most right position" as Banja says.[2(p45)] Each side is calling on its own moral system, which it believes to be superior. These types of unresolved dilemmas usually involve the collision of two moral systems.

For example, a young woman who is unmarried and pregnant might see both a counselor at a women's health clinic and a counselor at a Right to Life clinic to help her decide whether to terminate the pregnancy. Both counselors will give the young woman advice according to their own moral principles. The Right to Life counselor might advise the young woman to carry out the pregnancy, advice based on the counselor's highest religious principles. The woman's health counselor might give the young woman the option of carrying out the pregnancy and the option of a legal abortion, based on the counselor's belief in a woman's freedom of choice. Both counselors would believe that their advice was justified and moral.

ETHICAL CONFLICTS BETWEEN THE CLIENT'S NEEDS AND THE CLIENT'S WANTS

As this chapter has already made clear, GCMs encounter many ethical conflicts. Frequently, these revolve around the lack of harmony between what the client needs and what the client wants. In an analysis of the study done on the ethics of home care and case managers, Kane and Caplan refer to this tension.[6] In the study, case managers pointed out the ethical dilemma encountered when the client chose to do something that the case manager did not feel was healthy, given the client's condition. An example of this would be an older woman who is depressed and prescribed the drug Zoloft, with the specific instruction not to drink alcohol. In spite of the warning, the older woman drinks three glasses of wine a day, 2 before dinner and 1 with dinner. She never appears drunk or acts inappropriately. Her family hires a GCM to assess her for depression. The GCM knows that the excess alcohol might contribute to her depression. The GCM's assessment mentions the need to help the client stop consuming alcohol.

The woman is mentally clear and not under the care of a conservator. She states that she enjoys the wine and is not going to stop drinking it every night. The GCM is then caught between the client's assessed need and the client's right to choose what to do. This kind of tension often frustrates GCMs.

Case Studies

Here are two detailed examples of GCMs facing the conflict between client needs and client wants. John Powers is an 81–year-old colonel and a former aeronautical engineer who worked on many famous U.S. missile systems before retiring because he had Parkinson's. He is an attractive, dignified, and mentally competent older man who enjoys the company of his female caregivers, who are there 24 hours a day. He has reached a stage in his Parkinson's where he has several falls a month. Although the private caregivers use transfer belts and do standby assistance at all times, they occasionally must leave him to go to the bathroom or do something else outside the room. When the caregivers are out of the room, he often gets up by himself. He refuses to wear headgear to protect his head from the falls that result from his Parkinson's. He says that he is still in charge of his life and does not want to be restrained in any way or wear anything as unattractive as a helmet.

He is visited by a GCM (who is also a registered nurse [RN]) weekly, and she is quite frustrated. She has assessed his need to be protected from

falls but is sympathetic to his refusal to wear the headgear. She understands his desire to preserve his dignity and be independent. He has no appointed conservator, so he has the choice to refuse the restraints and helmet, and his family refuses to force the issue. The GCM is experiencing a dilemma because the client's desires conflict with her assessment of his physical needs.

Alice Manges is a 79–year-old woman who has a gastrointestinal tube inserted in her stomach. She had throat cancer and after the operation could not eat solid foods or drink liquids. She has 24-hour care, and the caregivers are monitored and supervised by both a GCM who is a social worker and a GCM who is an RN. Alice, the GCMs discover, is an alcoholic who had been very protected by her husband, a respected judge in the community. He recently died. They have no children, and her nephew is in charge of her care but lives far away. The RN GCM assesses Alice in the beginning of the case and creates a care plan that says to bring no alcohol into the home and not to let Alice drink. Alice has no conservator and when given an MSQ scores perfectly. The care providers start to report that Alice has a cleaning person bring wine into the house every week. In addition, they report that Alice is drinking the wine through her feeding tube. When the social worker GCM discovers this, she orders the care providers to discard the alcohol. Alice calls her attorney and her trust officer. The attorney reviews the situation and says that Alice is mentally clear, not in need of a conservator, and has the right to drink alcohol even if it may damage her health. The nephew reluctantly agrees, as does the trust officer. Both the RN GCM and the social worker GCM are caught between the client's choice of lifestyle and the client's health needs.

THE ETHICAL CONFLICT REGARDING CLIENT EXPLOITATION

Another dilemma mentioned in Kane and Caplan's study is the ethical conflict case managers experience if their clients are associating with individuals who could exploit the clients.[6] Older people who are lonely often end up in new relationships, frequently with members of the opposite sex, as older people are frequently widowed or divorced. However, these new relationships can alarm case managers and families if they feel that the new female or male companion might take advantage of the older person by getting cash or having themselves added to the older person's will. If the older person is competent, how can the case manager address this dilemma?

Case Study

Emily Jones is a 78–year-old woman who has been married to an alcoholic 82–year-old man for 20 years. This is her second marriage. She is a very attractive older woman who has retained her figure and loves to dress beautifully, and she always looks attractive. Harold Jones, her husband, was well-to-do when they first married, but Emily's extravagant lifestyle and Harold's alcoholism have severely diminished their finances. They have been friends with another couple, Tommy and Heidi Smith, for 15 years. Tommy always flirted with Emily, but it was socially acceptable among the couples and never led to anything more.

Heidi died after a long illness, and Tommy moved 50 miles away but always kept in touch with Emily and Harold, as he was very lonely and distraught over the death of his wife of 44 years. Over a 5-year period, a relationship started between Emily and Tommy. They have lunch together frequently, at Emily's instigation, without Harold's knowledge, and are obviously increasingly attracted to each other. Harold's alcoholism causes him to act inappropriately in social situations. Emily has been thinking of leaving Harold for Tommy. One night at a party following a bar mitzvah, Harold acts very inappropriately after drinking. Angry, Emily moves out to a friend's house that evening. However, her real reason for leaving is her attraction to Tommy.

Eventually, Emily moves in with Tommy. She is impoverished, as she and Harold had little money and now she only has her meager Social Security income. Tommy pays all the bills, and his adult children are angry, seeing Emily as a "money grubber." Eventually Emily talks

Tommy into letting her live in his house if he dies, although when she dies the house will go to his children. Tommy changes his will to this effect. Tommy's children are incensed and tell Tommy they do not approve. Tommy refuses to cooperate, saying he loves Emily and wants her to have a place to live until she dies. The children believe that Tommy is being exploited and want to force him to make Emily move out and change his will again. They want to move him to the home of one of his children who lives 500 miles away to get him away from Emily. As Tommy is in his eighties, they feel he will eventually give in to their wishes. They have also talked to Emily's children, who feel bad about the situation and are willing to take her in.

Tommy's children's attorney advises them to get an assessment from a GCM, and the children call in a local GCM. After assessing the situation, the GCM concludes that Emily has influenced Tommy to change his will. The GCM states in her assessment that Emily has been exploitive in this relationship and has influenced Tommy to change his will to her benefit. Tommy's loneliness after his wife's death made him more open to Emily's flirtations. However, the GCM assesses Tommy's mental status and finds him fully competent, with the right to make this choice, even if his children disapprove. She advises the children not to move him at this time. She, however, encourages further assessment if his will is changed again. So, as Kane and Caplan's study points out, the GCM is left in an ethical dilemma between the client's wants and the client's needs.[6] The client is associating with an exploitive person but, in this case at least, has the right to continue the association.

CONFLICT BETWEEN THE CLIENT'S SAFETY AND THE CLIENT'S AUTONOMY

Another type of ethical dilemma discussed by Kane and Caplan involves case managers with clients who live a life that involves high risk.[6] An example of this might be older men or women who insist on driving even though they have compromised eyesight, limited response times, or even confusion. Does a person's right to be independent supersede his or her need to be safe or the public's safety? If the person has passed a driver's test, what can a case manager do?

CONFLICTS AROUND CONFIDENTIALITY AND DISCLOSURE

Kane and Caplan's study also found that case managers had ethical conflicts around the issues of confidentiality and disclosure. The largest group of respondents (22%) reported having had conflicts over what to disclose to family members. The second-largest group (17%) reported having had conflicts over what to disclose to agency providers. More than 50% of those who reported having conflicts over confidentiality stated that they used their judgment to resolve what to disclose and to whom.[6] The conflict that the GCM Mary experienced with regard to her client Becca, discussed above, was partly a conflict involving confidentiality and disclosure. Another example of this type of conflict follows.

Case Study

The White family daughters hired a GCM to do a geriatric assessment of their mother, Blanche. Blanche lived with one son and his wife, whom the other family members suspected of physically abusing, overmedicating, and intimidating their mother. In doing the assessment the GCM found evidence of potential physical and medication abuse, which warranted turning the situation in to Adult Protective Services (APS). However, the GCM knew that APS was so underfunded and understaffed that it might not do anything about the situation immediately, although by law it would make an investigative visit, tipping off the son and his wife to the problems uncovered.

The geriatric assessment confirmed the children's fear that the son and his wife were physically abusing the mother and overmedicating her. They decided to send the mother to another sister in Atlanta. One local daughter planned to take Blanche out for a supposed day trip and actually put her on a plane to Atlanta to go live with another sister, who would implement all the GCM's suggestions. These suggestions included a medication review by a geriatric RN, a possible reduction of medication, and attendance at an adult day care program for additional socialization. The family members did not want to tell the brother with whom the mother lived, as they feared he would stop them and might harm the mother.

The GCM was in a ethical dilemma. The family members did not want her to report the case to APS until they got their mother on the plane to Atlanta. The GCM worked for the family. However, by law the GCM was obligated to report the case to APS, even though she knew it might stop the plans to get the mother away from the abusive son. The GCM had a conflict about confidentiality involving what to disclose to an agency.

ANALYZING ETHICAL DILEMMAS

Patricia Burbank provides one framework for analyzing ethical problems (Exhibit 2–3). Burbank suggests many avenues to help in ethical decisions and states that analysis does not have to be done in isolation. Among her suggestions is using ethics review boards in institutions because they are there to help health professionals resolve ethical dilemmas. If this option is not possible, she suggests team conferences including all the parties involved in the dilemma. She also suggests reaching out to other professionals, while always respecting the confidentiality of the client. Here the GCM could use NAPGCM, CMSA, the National Association of Social Workers, or any other professional association with a code of ethics and an ethics committee (see Appendix A for contact information).[5]

Another possible method of ethical dilemma analysis is suggested by E. Haavi Morreim.[7] He suggests that the first step is fact finding. The GCM should seek the primary sources of information, not rely on secondhand information. The GCM should not make unwarranted assumptions

Exhibit 2–3 Analyzing Ethical Problems

1. Review the situation.
   - What health problems exist?
   - What decisions need to be made?
   - Which components are ethical and which are based on scientific knowledge?
2. Gather additional information necessary to make a decision.
3. What are relevant ethical principles?
   - What are the historical, philosophical, and religious bases for each of the principles?
4. What are your values and beliefs?
   - From your family and other personal experience?
   - From your professional code of ethics?
5. What are the values and beliefs of others in the situation?
6. What are the value conflicts in the situation?
7. Who is the best person to make the decision?
8. What is the fullest range of possible decisions and actions?
   - What are the implications/consequences of possible decisions and actions?
   - Do the possible decisions and actions and your professional code of ethics agree?
9. Decide on a course of action and take steps to implement it.
10. Evaluate the outcomes of the decisions and use this information for future decision making.

or depend on other people's assumptions. Objectively gathering facts to discover basic problems is the first step in routine geriatric assessment. Therefore, it should be familiar to GCMs.

Morreim's second step is to identify all those whose interests and wishes might be affected by the results (e.g., family members, friends, other agencies, other professionals). The client is the GCM's most important responsibility, but Morreim says to uncover all the other players

and then uncover all the values that are at stake (e.g., autonomy, justice, freedom).

Lastly, Morreim says to take a third step: creative problem solving. Like the other steps in the process, creative problem solving is part of a GCM's basic skills in geriatric assessment and general geriatric care management. Morreim tells GCMs to respect the important moral values in the problem and to not only consider obvious options but try to come up with creative new options.

HOW TO RESOLVE ETHICAL DILEMMAS

Resolving ethical dilemmas is difficult at best. There are several different pathways suggested in the body of literature about ethics and case or care management—a body of literature that grew considerably in the late 1990s. As noted at the beginning of the chapter, Aristotle thought that solving ethical dilemmas was so complex that there was no simple set of rules to follow.

In Kane and Caplan's study, case managers who had ethical dilemmas with other case managers or agencies tended to resolve the conflict in various ways. Negotiation and compromise were used by 31% of the case managers responding to the survey. Ten percent mentioned overriding their providers and colleagues. Appealing to a higher authority, another 10% said they occasionally went over the head of the individual and caused difficulty. Winning the confidence of their providers and colleagues was used by only 6%. Kane and Caplan state that the case managers sometimes assisted the client in finding another agency or just refused to further refer to an organization or professional causing a conflict. However, Kane and Caplan state that most case managers had a difficult time with the concept of blackballing.[6]

Sixty-eight percent, the largest percentage of case managers in the study, used discussion with their supervisors to solve ethical dilemmas. As many GCMs operate as entrepreneurs and have no supervisors, GCMs might consider the second most common approach to resolve ethical dilemmas: discussion with colleagues. This method was utilized by 39% of case managers in Kane and Caplan's survey. Seventeen percent said they used care and case conferences, where professional care managers meet to discuss client problems and resolve ethical dilemmas. If a GCM works for an agency or has many other GCMs in his or her own agency, this is an excellent avenue to consider.

Banja says that the process of resolving ethical dilemmas may reveal not only what to do but also what not to do.[2] He makes another interesting point: when resolving an ethical dilemma, both sides can get very emotional. The average person gets defensive, making all kinds of excuses when there is an allegation of error. A prominent flaw in the majority of the poor reasons used to justify a type of conduct is that the poor reasons rarely address the problems at hand. Instead, these reasons avoid the real issue and involve justifications for disregarding the real issue, causing the ethical dilemma.

CONCLUSION

As geriatric care management and case management evolve as professions, GCMs have a great opportunity to learn how to think ethically. GCMs have the codes of ethics of both NAPGCM and CMSA to govern their ethics and help with ethical dilemmas. Both associations also offer ethics committees to help clarify and resolve problems. Membership in an association also gives GCMs colleagues with whom to discuss ethical problems—just as the Greeks would have done. Both associations have rules, disciplinary procedures, and penalties for breaking these codes. As Kane and Caplan's survey showed, professionals find many ways to resolve these interesting but painful ethical dilemmas.

NOTES

1. Alexander N. An international code of ethics for care/case managers. *GCM J.* 1999;4:6.

2. Banja J. Ethical decision making: origins, process, and applications to case management. *Case Manager.* 1999;9:41–42.

3. Brostoff PM. A short history of drafting the GCM Pledge of Ethics. *GCM J.* 1999;10:6.

4. Beauchamp T, Childress J. *Principles of Biomedical Ethics,* 4th ed. New York: Oxford University Press; 1994.

5. Burbank PM. Legal and ethical issues in health care of older adults. *GCM J.* 1999;27.

6. Kane R, Caplan AL. *Ethical Conflicts in the Management of Home Care: The Case Manager's Dilemma.* New York: Springer; 1993.

7. Morreim E. Ethical issues in care management: case studies in moral problem solving. *GCM J.* 1999;9.

PART II

Beginning, Expanding, or Adding a Geriatric Care Management Business

CHAPTER 3

How To Begin or Add a Geriatric Care Management Business

Cathy Cress

ENTREPRENEURIAL RISKS

There are several types of geriatric care management businesses. In 1999, the most common type was the owner-run business. However, new models are appearing, including practices pairing geriatric care managers (GCMs) with physicians, attorneys, and accountants. This chapter will focus on starting a geriatric care management business from scratch but will also discuss adding a geriatric care management practice onto a existing business or not-for-profit agency.

According to a survey done by the National Association of Professional Geriatric Care Managers (NAPGCM) in 1997, 80% of all geriatric care management businesses were owner run, with just 20% run by nonowners.[1] Entrepreneurial people who do not mind some risk usually start owner-run businesses. Starting a geriatric care management business is not for the faint of heart. Many new businesses are started every day, only to be boarded shut within a few years.

People thinking of beginning a geriatric care management business should first find out whether they are comfortable with this type of risk by doing a self-assessment (Exhibit 3–1). Entrepreneurs share many traits, including high energy, aggressiveness, a love of ambiguity, a zest for problem solving, and monumental self-discipline.

Having done this general self-assessment, people should consider whether they are cut out to be GCMs. In a presentation to the national NAPGCM 1998 conference in Chicago, Eliza-

beth Bodie Gross and Linda Fordini Johnson outlined some of the skills and personality traits GCMs should have.[2]

- Have they worked as care managers? Have they worked with older adults or had education or training in geriatrics or gerontology? These experiences help people know what to expect and whether they like the work.
- Do they have a business background? Do they know accounting, have they ever had to meet a payroll, and can they tolerate not being paid the first few years? Can they do another job while also being a GCM? Many budding GCMs have held another job for as many as a few years until their geriatric care management practice made enough money for them to quit.
- Do they have the energy to run a 24–hour-a-day, 7–day-a-week business? Can their family tolerate calls night and day? Can their family accept this invasion of privacy and family life? Will their children suffer from receiving less attention?

In the beginning, running a geriatric care management business can be lonely. The entrepreneur is practically the entire business, doing the billing, seeing the clients, marketing to get new clients, being on call 24 hours a day to solve client problems, and perhaps running to the bank to borrow more money. Often, the entrepreneurs see much less of their families because they are consumed by running their fledgling operation.

Exhibit 3–1 Are You Entrepreneur Material?

- Are you a leader?
- Are you a self-starter?
- Do you make decisions easily?
- Do you like competition?
- Do you get along well with different types of people?
- Are you good at planning and organizing?
- Do you have the physical and emotional strength to run a business?
- Do you have the drive to maintain your motivation in times of trouble and slowdowns?
- Can your family survive on a more limited income the first few years of your business?
- Do you have self-discipline?

And they often face initial criticism or rejection of their services (Chapter 7 discusses marketing in more detail). They must seek experienced professionals' advice about structuring the business, and they must change where necessary.

So what are the rewards of running a geriatric care management business? According to Kraus, the dividends are many.[3] GCM entrepreneurs

- find an outlet for their creativity
- work on a flexible schedule
- earn the respect of their community by offering a service that gives great support to older people and their families
- do a variety of tasks every day
- interact with many other professionals in a variety of disciplines, through assessment, marketing, and interacting with clients
- meet other people like them through joining NAPGCM and the Case Management Society of America (CMSA) and exchanging new and creative ideas about geriatric care management and running a geriatric care management business
- work in an up-and-coming discipline

Another way for people to find out whether they really want to start a geriatric care management business is to talk to working GCMs. Prospective GCMs can try one or more of the following options to learn from the experience of working GCMs:

- attend a NAPGCM or CMSA conference to meet GCMs and talk with them about their practice
- call NAPGCM or CMSA and ask for names of nearby GCMs, then make an appointment to meet with a GCM in person to discuss his or her business experience (see Appendix A for contact information)
- buy tapes and manuals that discuss starting a geriatric care management business (tapes and manuals are available at NAPGCM and CMSA conferences)

Prospective GCMs should try to learn from the experiences of others who have been down the path before.

TYPES OF GERIATRIC CARE MANAGEMENT BUSINESSES

This section will discuss three types of geriatric care management businesses: solo practices, partnerships, and corporations.

Solo Practices

Most GCMs begin their business as a solo practice. They choose a legal entity known as sole proprietorship, which means that the business is owned and controlled by a single party. In a sole proprietorship the proprietor is always responsible for any legal or financial liabilities that occur during the course of business. In a 1997 survey of GCMs, Knutson and Langer found that 45% of all GCMs were running sole proprietorships.[1]

A sole proprietorship is probably the easiest type of business to start. There are few legal restrictions (compared with those that come with partnerships and corporations) and few legal papers to complete, with the exception of a business license and a fictitious business license in some states. There are no separate income tax forms to complete; the individual can put the business revenues and losses on Schedule C of his or her 1040. Sole proprietors have relative freedom from government taxes and regulations.

There are many other advantages to starting a geriatric care management business as a solo practitioner. It is easier to maintain control and be flexible because the GCM makes all the decisions and is able to respond quickly to client requests and business needs. Another advantage is financial, in that all the profits go to the owner rather than being split between multiple owners. In addition, solo practitioners can dissolve the business more easily if they decide being a GCM is not for them. As being a GCM is difficult, this may be a distinct advantage.

There are also many disadvantages to being a solo practitioner. There are multiple tasks in running a geriatric care management business, including marketing, bookkeeping, managing human resources, counseling, and being on call. A sole proprietor must either do all of these tasks or outsource some of them, which can be expensive. Many times sole proprietorship leaves a person exhausted, with no salary to boot.

Another negative is that sole proprietors have to be on call by themselves 24 hours a day, 7 days a week, because this is the nature of being a GCM; the only alternative is to outsource some time. If the GCM becomes ill or cannot practice for any reason, there is no one to turn to bear the burden of the cases or run the business. Having an agreement with another GCM to pinch hit is a possibility, but client service will be less consistent.

Sole proprietorship can be tough financially. In this business form, the owner has unlimited liability, so creditors can come after the owner's personal assets. Lenders tend to offer less start-up cash and fewer ongoing business loans to a sole proprietorship. Sole proprietors may have a hard time getting long-term financial capital, which can affect their ability to grow.

Finally, sole proprietors have no one to lean on in times of crisis. Bearing the burden with others means that a GCM gets feedback, support, and respite from the pressure.[4]

People should consult with their attorneys and their accountants about whether to choose this form of business organization. An attorney can help with many issues, including a "right of survivorship" agency agreement in case of the GCM's death or disability. An accountant can explain tax requirements for recording business expenses and profits, Social Security, and employee wage withholdings.[5]

Partnerships

Some GCMs may prefer to have a partner. Legally there are two types of partnerships. First, there are general partnerships, where the business has two or more owners. All individuals are liable if the business defaults, no matter what percentage of the business each individual owns. Each partner must report income or loss in the business. Second, there are limited partnerships, where one partner simply invests in the business but does not make business decisions. In this case, the investing partner is liable for only the amount of the investment. People considering a partnership should see an attorney and an accountant to decide whether a partnership is their best option and which type of partnership to choose.

Partnerships have their advantages. Partners share financial, administrative, and emotional burdens. Compared with corporations, partnerships are relatively easy to set up and are flexible, in that there are only two people to make decisions. Lending sources tend to prefer partnerships to sole proprietorships, although partnerships are still less appealing to lenders than corporations are.

There are also disadvantages. Unlike corporation owners, partners have unlimited liability. Like sole proprietors, partners may still have an unstable business life, with fluctuating incomes and exhausting schedules. If something happens to one partner, the partnership may be dissolved. If a partner decides to leave, it may be hard on the other partner, as buying out a partner can be legally and financially difficult.

Wendy Marks and Carol Westheimer gave a workshop at the 1995 NAPGCM conference entitled "Partnerships: The Good, the Bad, and the Ugly. Why Do They Succeed or Fail? Or Everything You Wanted To Know About Marriage without Sex but Were Afraid To Ask." Partnerships are as delicate as marriage, and people need to think carefully before becoming partners. As Marks points out in her 1996 article about partnerships in the *GCM Journal,* people should first assess whether they are suited to be in a partnership.[6] Some individuals, according to Marks, have problems sharing tasks with other people, whether they are equals, subordinates, or superiors. People with this very domineering personality type are probably not suited for partnerships. Partners are meant to bear a mutual burden and make mutual decisions. Some people have a hard time sharing leadership duties and think of everything in terms of "mine" or "yours," which can also cause problems in a partnership.

Marks also suggests figuring out what relevant skills both people considering a partnership have. This list may include bookkeeping, care management, geriatric assessment, marketing, payroll, hardware and software support, administration, and human resources management. A skill map will show which partner has which skills. Marks points out that areas that are not covered by either partner as well as areas that are covered by both partners are of concern in establishing a partnership.

Another step is to assess how long a commitment each partner can make to the fledgling enterprise. If one partner plans to retire in 5 years and wants to stay in the partnership only for that long, while the other wants to make a 20-year commitment, the mutual venture may need to be reassessed. Does one partner want to have another child in a few years? Does one partner expect to relocate anytime soon? People should assess the present commitment to the partnership, then anticipate what the partnership will look like 2, 5, and 10 years down the line. There may be a period where one partner would be running the business alone, and this may not seem agreeable to both partners.

Next, the partners should list the tasks that their business will require to make it operate well. These tasks may include marketing, being on call on a 24-hour basis, paying bills, doing accounts receivable and accounts payable, and handling human resources. Both partners should decide what level of commitment they have to each task. One partner will have to do each task, or the partners will have to outsource the task. For example, if neither partner understands bookkeeping, the partners will have to hire a bookkeeper.

According to Marks, the ideal partnership has two people who are equally committed. If there is a different level of commitment, then partners may want to explore splitting the profits accordingly (a person who does 40% of the work gets 40% of the profits). This needs to be thought out and explored with an attorney.

What all this leads to is exploring whether the potential partners have a similar vision for the future of the business. In addition to making a business plan, the partners may also want to both write down a 5- or 10-year plan for each partner's involvement in the business, then compare the visions. If the forecasts are similar, great. If they are different, the partners can negotiate and try to agree. Are both partners willing to share the evening and weekend responsibilities in this around-the-clock business? Resentment can build if someone is unfairly shouldering more of the burden.

The best GCM partners make decisions objectively and are comfortable with change. They learn from their mistakes and are not afraid to fail. If one partner cannot stomach failure, that person may blame the other partner rather than see the errors as a way to learn what does and does not work in the business. Together, good GCM partners are prepared for and able to survive a crisis, as crises are an inevitable part of new businesses.

An adjunct to this is the "worst nightmare" scenario: Partners should consider how they would do if the business failed (not an unlikely occurrence). What contingency plans might be set up? How would the partners survive without blaming each other?

Being partners in a business also means spending many hours together working very hard. People considering a partnership need to make sure that they can comfortably spend that much time with another person. Many partners have tested the waters by going off and "playing" with each other (e.g., by taking a trip together). This helps them gauge their compatibility.

Partners should also make sure they have compatible values, Marks says.[6] If one partner believes that earning a profit is immoral and the other partner embraces capitalism, there will be problems. If one partner believes in spending all available funds and the other is fiscally conservative, there will be problems. Partners may complete some kind of values assessment and compare the results. People may also, as Marks suggests, interview friends, family members, and colleagues of a potential partner to see how their potential partner's values mesh with their own. An accountant can help partners assess their beliefs about finances (e.g., should you have credit cards, what should the limits be, what constitutes abuse of those cards), then compare the responses for compatibility. If the responses are not compatible, the partners may try to negotiate or may rethink the partnership.

As Marks points out, partners should also discuss their commitments to their families, especially since geriatric care management is such a time-intensive business. Are the family members on both sides willing to accept the partners' absences? This needs to be assessed before the partnership begins. Can each partner devote the same amount of time to the business? If not, should one partner get more money? If the imbalance cannot be resolved, the partnership should be reconsidered.

Exhibit 3–2 contains a quiz that sums up many of the points discussed above. Potential partners should take the quiz before formalizing the partnership.

Marks sent a survey about partnerships to NAPGCM members in 1996. She found that most GCM partnerships consisted of two people. Most partnerships did not have adequate insurance; usually, they had life insurance but not disability insurance. Only half of the partnerships had formal contracts. However, most partners who felt their business was successful had formal agreements and terms of partnership. Most respondents felt good about being a partner.[6] As these survey results suggest, formal partnership agreements may help partnerships succeed and insurance is important.

Some people may find, in consultation with an attorney, that the "C Corp" or the "S Corp" structure may be right for them.

Exhibit 3–2 Partnership Quiz

___ Do you both have the entrepreneurial qualities to survive the first 5 years of a business?

___ Is either one of you unable to share tasks with anyone else?

___ Can you both commit to this company for the next 7 years?

___ Do you both have all of the following traits?

   ___ Honesty

   ___ Risk-taking ability

   ___ Ability to withstand failure

   ___ Ability to withstand rejection

   ___ Capacity to share

   ___ Ability to argue strongly and courteously lose

   ___ Ability to forgive

   ___ Ability to survive a crisis

___ Do you both look at each other as someone with whom you could spend long periods of time?

___ Can you both say "no" to a plan but "yes" to a person?

___ Do you both have a similar vision of the future?

___ Do you both have the finances to cover expenses until you turn a profit?

___ Can you both survive failure?

Corporations

The third and most complex form of business is the corporation. As with the other forms of business, people should consult an attorney and an accountant before deciding to start a corporation.

Setting up a corporation offers several advantages. Corporations are identified as legal entities within themselves. They exist apart from the stockholders. If a founder or stockholder dies, it does not affect the business' legal status. Liability is limited to the amount of the investment; therefore, personal holdings are not affected if the corporation becomes insolvent. This is an attraction of establishing a corporation when starting a business. Ownership is easily transferred, so if the founder wants to relocate or retire, he or she simply has to sell stock in the company.

Another advantage is that banks or lenders are more open to lending to a corporation that has a good track record or a new corporation that has sufficient equity and promise. The lender may ask for collateral or signatures from stockholders as a precaution. There also can be certain advantages to the corporate form in fringe benefits such as stock plans or pensions.

But choosing the corporation business form also has its drawbacks. First, it is more expensive to start a corporation than it is to start a sole proprietorship or a partnership because of the legal costs. And unlike sole proprietorships and partnerships, corporations are exposed to regulation by state, local, and federal governments and depend heavily on the assistance of attorneys and accountants.

Another limitation is double taxation. Corporate profits are taxed once to the corporation and again as income, when distributed to the stockholders. So the founder pays taxes on his or her salary and any share he or she might have of the distributed profits. A corporation is also required to have bylaws, hold stockholders meetings, and keep records. A corporation may choose to set up as an S corporation. In an S corporation, both income and losses are usually taxed to the individual shareholders, rather than the corporation. As new businesses generally lose money in the first year, this can be a distinct advantage. Any loss can be applied against any other personal income, thus reducing the amount of income tax levied. However, consult an attorney to find out whether you can qualify for an S corporation.[7]

Attorneys help with many essential corporate functions, including

- filing an "articles of incorporation" document in the state where the business is located
- issuing stock
- electing directors and officers
- drawing up bylaws
- helping with procedures for conducting stockholders' meeting, keeping records of these meetings, and creating stock agreements.

Accountants help with corporations' tax requirements and other matters.

CREATING A BUSINESS PLAN

After choosing which form a business will take—sole proprietorship, partnership, or corporation—people need to come up with a business plan. The business plan will clearly organize all of the ideas about the business into a focused description of what the product of the geriatric care management business will be, who will buy that product, who the competition will be, and how the product is similar to and different from that of the competition. Why do this? First, a business plan makes ideas concrete and ordered, turning subjective dreams into objective goals. It also lists the obstacles that a business might face. It explains, step by step, how a person's entrepreneurial dream will become a reality.

The business plan helps people get the money they need to start a business. Bank loan officers and other sources of capital will want to see a business plan. Merrily Orsini, in her workshop entitled "Doing Good Makes Cents: Advanced Business Practices" and presented at the 10th annual NAPGCM Conference in 1994, emphasized the importance of having a business plan at every stage of a geriatric care management business, but especially in the beginning.[8] Orsini, who now helps new businesses, including fledgling geriatric care management businesses, through her company, My Virtual Corp, offers a generic outline of a business plan (Exhibit 3–3). The sections below provide details about how a business plan for a new geriatric care management business should address each of the items listed in Exhibit 3–3.

Business

The first section of a geriatric care management company's business plan describes the business in general terms. It mentions the background of the principals and measurable company goals (e.g., 20 clients and $100,000 in revenue by the end of the first year). It also explains why the plan is being written (e.g., to attract in-

Exhibit 3–3 Outline of a Business Plan

```
     I.   Business
    II.   Products and services
   III.   Industry
    IV.   Location
     V.   Market
    VI.   Competition
   VII.   Marketing
  VIII.   Operations
    IX.   Personnel
     X.   Finances
```

vestors, to show how the operation will work, to show that the business is financially feasible) and the niche that the business will occupy (i.e., what customer needs will be met).

Products and Services

The second section of the business plan discusses the products or services the business will offer to meet these customer needs. Even though the business is selling services, it may be helpful to think of them as products: for instance, geriatric assessment might be one product, placement assistance another product. What is each product? Who delivers the product? What does the product cost?

Industry

The third section of the business plan describes the geriatric care management industry. Helpful information is available from the national NAPGCM office (e.g., what a GCM is, how many GCMs are in the country, how long the profession has been around, the financial performance of the industry, the role of government regulation).

Location

In the fourth section, the plan discusses the place where the company will do business. Is location a factor in getting customers? Is the office going to be in a certain part of town because that is where the customers are? Perhaps the business

will be near a hospital or other building offering services for older people. Geriatric care management businesses are not like clothing stores or other merchandise-based businesses, which need to be located in areas with considerable foot traffic (e.g., malls, busy streets). But locating next to a long–term-care discharge unit might increase business.

Market

The fifth section of a business plan describes the market the business serves. Who is in the target market? Older people? Their families? Developmentally disabled individuals? How big is this market in the area where the business will be located (e.g., how many people over age 85 live in the town, how many trust departments are in the town)? Demographic information may be available from U.S. Census reports, local area agencies on aging, local chambers of commerce, local hospitals, and even members of the local media who have done their own surveys.

The section also mentions the plan writer's own research into the needs of the area. The entrepreneur may have done a needs assessment, including the number of older adults living in the area who need chronic care. Does the local target market need the business? Will older people in the area be able to afford the services?

Competition

The sixth section discusses competition. Are there other geriatric care management businesses in the area? Do home health agencies in the area offer care or case management? Are there physicians' practices offering geriatric care management? Research into these issues can be done using the local phone book or the CMSA or NAPGCM national directories.

Once the competition has been identified, other issues are discussed. What traits does this new business share with the competition? What separates this new business from the competition? How will the new business woo customers away from the competition? By offering lower prices? By offering better or different services?

Marketing

In the seventh section, marketing is discussed. How much will the business's services cost? How will the business go about promoting them, and who is going to do the promoting?

GCMs and people with human services backgrounds are not often familiar with marketing. They may want to get marketing assistance from an outside consultant. No one will fund something that the business cannot sell. Doing research into how other GCMs have marketed is helpful, as is reading marketing articles in care management journals. NAPGCM and CMSA offer tapes discussing marketing (see Appendix A for contact information). Chapter 7 is devoted to the subject of marketing.

Operations

The eighth section discusses operations (e.g., when the office will be open, when GCMs will be on call). It should be a blueprint for the upcoming days, weeks, and months of geriatric care management operations, defining how and when the entrepreneurs will carry out the tasks necessary to run the business and serve the clients. It will give a clear picture of how many people will be needed to run the business. The section should also mention the following:

- all equipment and supplies to be used in running the business (e.g., a computer system, a printer, a telephone, a pager)
- the business's recordkeeping system and how much it will cost to operate (i.e., how client information will be tracked and whether it will be stored in case files, computerized records, or another storage system)
- the business's accounting and billing system (manual? computerized? outsourced?) and how much it will cost to operate
- how stock is divided in the business agreements and its succession in case of the loss of key personnel
- what professionals the business will need to use (e.g., an attorney, an accountant, a cleaning person)

Personnel

In the ninth section, the professional experience of the owner and key employees is described. Each person's daily role in the business is explained. The business's organizational structure (e.g., sole proprietorship, partnership, corporation) is also noted.

Finances

In the last section, finances are discussed. This may include how much money is needed to fund the venture and a history of the owner's finances. It might also mention people who will offer audits of the business's success or failure, such as an accountant.

It is helpful to get expert advice on financial matters. The Small Business Administration (SBA) has small business development centers all over the United States to help small businesses get started. Local chambers of commerce can provide information about where local small business development centers are located. The Service Corps of Retired Executives (SCORE) can also provide assistance. There are also consultants who specialize in helping geriatric care management businesses get started. NAPGCM or CMSA may be able to direct people to these consultants. Appendix A contains contact information for all these organizations.

FINANCING A GERIATRIC CARE MANAGEMENT BUSINESS

According to the SBA, 80% of new entrepreneurs start their businesses without any commercial loan or debt financing.[9] Banks are usually hesitant to make loans under $50,000 because the loan is not cost-effective for the bank.

Since small businesses often need less than $50,000 and frequently have difficulty finding banks to lend them money, they look for other financing. Serious lenders and investors want to finance new businesses with a track record and an excellent business plan. New business owners with some background in geriatric care management, social work, or nursing will probably have an easier time satisfying lenders and investors.

The SBA lists several sources of financing that new care management practices often use:

- personal savings
- personal credit (including credit cards and personal lines of credit)
- loans from friends and family members
- loans from informal investors
- home equity loans (especially in areas where home values have risen considerably)
- financing from credit unions (which tend to be more open to lending to alternative or new borrowers)
- financing through city and county economic or community development programs

The SBA itself is another source to look into. It has loan programs of its own and lists of local economic development offices that may have loan programs for start-ups that respond to local economic development needs. Some of these programs will offer loans and provide information and technical assistance on starting a business.[8]

PROFESSIONAL CONSULTANTS

Professional consultants are a very important asset in setting up a geriatric care management business. Many of these consultants may not require a capital outlay but provide consultation based on the business's future earnings. Even if consultants do charge from the beginning, businesses are usually smart to invest in expert advice because consultants help businesses avoid costly mistakes and make better choices (e.g., an attorney can help a new business avoid lawsuits, an accountant can help people develop figures to help them get funding from the bank, a geriatric care management business consultant can help a business owner come up with excellent geriatric care management services to make the business really grow). This section will discuss the role of different professional consultants in helping to establish a new geriatric care management business.

Attorneys

A new geriatric care management business needs an attorney, and not just any attorney. The attorney should have considerable experience in working with small businesses. The attorney can help set up the legal business entity, help businesses decide how to register or license the business, help businesses meet Internal Revenue Service (IRS) requirements (e.g., whether the business needs an employer identification number), offer advice on whether the business should employ staff or independent contractors, and help businesses with getting a fictitious business name.

Accountants

The business needs an accountant, possibly one that is a certified public accountant. The accountant helps with setting up the business plan by assisting with the financial arrangements. Owners need help determining the funding requirements of the new business, including how much cash is needed to open the business, the terms under which the business will obtain the money, and the type of money desired (loans, personal savings, etc.). Business owners also need to decide with accountants what type of accounting system to use.[9] There are many software packages out there, and many cost under $300, including Quick-Books, Peachtree Accounting, and Mind Your Own Business (see Chapter 6 for more on software). An accountant should also offer advice on what types of business records to keep, including a cash receipts journal, a cash disbursements journal, a sales journal, a purchases journal, a payroll journal, and a general ledger. Unless the geriatric care management business owner is an accountant, has a degree in business, or has owned businesses before, getting help from a professional accountant is important.

Consultants in the Geriatric Care Management Field

Most new geriatric care management businesses will benefit from assistance from a specialist in the industry. A professional consultant can help a business owner gain a thorough understanding of geriatric care management, which can help the business owner develop services. The consultant can help with the business plan and be on call in case a crisis occurs.

Bankers

Bank representatives can help new geriatric care management businesses as well. Even though banks do not operate the way they used to, with one-to-one relationships between bank representatives and customers, some banks (especially small-town banks and credit unions) do have representatives that handle small business loans and can work with the business on an ongoing basis. Ted Turner, now famous for developing CNN, had many secrets to his success, including incredible energy, an ability to fail and pick himself up, and unbelievable vision. But he also had an uncanny ability to work with bankers and borrow money. Owners who find a bank to loan them money should also try to develop a long-term relationship with a representative at that bank, for assistance with both future lines of credit and direct deposit for employees.

Owners who are women should, if possible, try to find a bank that has lent to women-owned businesses in the past. Unfortunately, some banks are still somewhat reluctant to loan money to women. Credit unions are sometimes better alternatives.

Insurance Brokers

Insurance brokers also provide new geriatric care management businesses with an important service. See "Business Insurance" below for more on the contribution of these professionals.

Free Advice

Other sources of advice and assistance are free. One is the IRS. It offers new business owners many free materials and workshops, including information about recordkeeping, tax reporting, and hiring employees and independent contractors. (Business owners should, of course, also work with their attorneys and accountants in determining their tax reporting requirements.)

Another source is the local chamber of commerce, an excellent resource for information on what other help is available in an area to new businesses. Chambers of commerce can point the way to local small business development centers. In addition to helping businesses get started, chambers of commerce can help businesses grow. Many GCMs across the country, like other small business owners, have joined the chamber of commerce to develop relationships to further their business. Some chambers have newsletters that announce new businesses, and chambers usually have mixers where businesspeople can meet each other, talk, offer support to each other, and exchange business cards. Owners might ask local chambers if it would be possible to celebrate the opening of their businesses at one of these mixers.

Professional associations are another helpful resource. NAPGCM and CMSA, as stated previously, have a wealth of resources to help geriatric care management businesses get going. New business owners will seriously want to consider joining one or both industry-specific organizations and purchasing their start-up materials. These associations also put new business owners in contact with (1) more experienced professionals who can either act as mentors or simply offer advice about setting up a business and avoiding pitfalls, and (2) other new business owners, forming an informal support group. These associations also have regional and local chapters, which offer start-up information and information about ongoing areas of interest in the field (e.g., Alzheimer's). Owners should also consider attending the regional and national conferences of NAPGCM and CMSA. They usually have presessions covering issues that owners of fledgling geriatric care management businesses need to understand. Tapes of presessions and regular sessions are also available, as are tapes that cover start-up business issues.

Exhibit 3–4 summarizes this section and lists the individuals as well as groups and agencies that can help a new geriatric care management business get off the ground.

DEVELOPING PROCEDURES

Any geriatric care management business needs procedures to run smoothly, efficiently, and legally. New business owners need to have many procedures in place, from how to do a ge-

Exhibit 3–4 Professional Consultants and Groups To Help a Geriatric Care Management Business Get Started

---

Individuals
Accountants
Attorneys
Bankers
Consultants specializing in geriatric care management
Insurance brokers

Groups and Agencies
Chambers of commerce
The IRS
Professional associations (NAPGCM, CMSA, etc.)
SCORE

---

riatric assessment to how to open, manage, and close cases; store records; open and close the office; and set up and maintain a filing system. The business owner must write out how each procedure will be done. For instance, if the owner is unable to run the business for some time, someone else will need to take over, and unless procedures are written out, inconsistency and other trouble will result.

NAPGCM publishes procedure manuals that can help new business owners get started. These general procedures need to be tailored to each business, and a consultant can provide assistance if necessary. The expense of using a consultant may be worth it in the end. A local chamber of commerce can provide names of consultants who can help.

BUSINESS INSURANCE

Business insurance is taken out to protect people from professional, business, and personal liabilities or risks created by a private practice. Both start-ups and mature geriatric care management practices need business insurance. It protects assets, prevents loss of income, provides expenses in case of illness, provides coverage for errors and omissions, and meets requirements for third-party reimbursement. As in legal and accounting matters, it is best to hire the services of an insurance broker to provide advice about what type of insurance coverage a business needs and help businesses with claims. As geriatric care management is a very new field, business owners should make sure to talk to an insurance broker who understands the needs of businesses in the field.

Beginning geriatric care management businesses need the following types of insurance:

- *Professional malpractice insurance.* This insurance will protect a business and its employees for any (subject to the policy conditions) act, error, or omission that arises out of the performance of professional services to others. Policies may also be extended to cover independent contractors.
- *Business liability insurance.* This insurance covers bodily injury, property damage, product liability, and job completion in the general operation of a business. Personal endeavors are excluded. A business can also decide to insure the building in which it operates as well as improvements or personal property for either replacement value or actual cost. Other options include coverage for loss of business earnings, accounts receivable, and valuable papers and records.
- *Workers' compensation insurance.* This insurance offers disability coverage for work-related illness or disability for employees. All a business's employees must be covered under a workers' compensation policy.
- *Business overhead insurance.* This insurance is designed to cover loss of income due to the disability of a principal in a business. It is based on the monthly expenses of the business, not its earnings.
- *Social Security Disability Insurance and other disability insurance.* Social Security Disability Insurance is paid through payroll taxes and provides a minimal income after a period of 6 months of disability if the disability is expected to last 1 year or more. In various states, short-term disability insurance is available. Long-term disability pro-

vides monthly benefits after the 26-week short-term disability benefits are used up.[5]

SETTING UP AN OFFICE

A geriatric care management business needs an office. Many of the first GCMs started practicing out of their homes. In this era of telecommuting, running a home office may be even more feasible if space is available. Using a home office eliminates the expense of renting office space but may be too distracting. Crying babies, complaining children, and laundry that just has to be done can get in the way of being a GCM.

Whatever the choice of office location, it is helpful to make a timeline listing all tasks that need to be done before the business can open: renting office space or refurbishing a home office; getting insurance; recruiting and hiring staff; ordering a system to handle telephone calls, voicemail, and paging; arranging for a security system and cleaning people; arranging for an answering service or setting up an on-call system; buying office equipment; making arrangements with suppliers of items like office supplies; arranging for credit cards; ordering brochures; and so forth. The new business owner should estimate how long each task will take, put each task on a timeline, and give him- or herself a deadline of opening day. Exhibit 3–5 shows a sample timeline.

If there is no space for a home office or working at home seems too distracting, entrepreneurs need to contact a realtor and look for a small space to rent. They might want to consider renting 400–600 square feet with a small reception area, so clients are not walking right in on conversations with other clients. It is helpful to have the business on a bus line, as many care providers and clients do not drive. The realtor and an attorney will offer advice about how long a lease to take and what terms the lease should have.

Offices should be as professional as possible. Having administrative assistants and other staff members helps. Having an administrative assistant answer the phone is much more professional than using an answering machine. An administrative assistant will also help process paperwork in a professional and timely manner. Good staff can

Exhibit 3–5 Sample Timeline of Tasks To Be Done during the 3 Months Prior To Opening a Geriatric Care Management Business

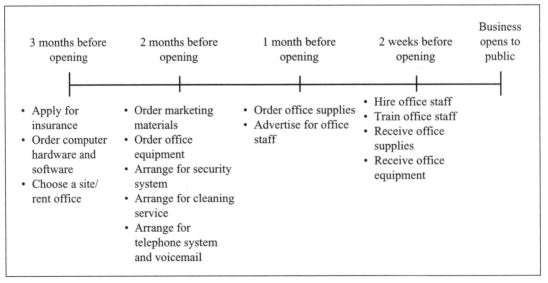

actually help a business make more money. When an owner does everything alone (e.g., answering the phone, seeing clients, doing the billing, responding to emergencies), a business may not make as much money as it would if tasks were handled by others. The business makes money off billed GCM time, and if a GCM spends a lot of time away from clients, less time is being billed.

Also, doing everything alone can send a GCM into a cycle in which too many care managers find themselves. People with human services backgrounds are so accustomed to emergencies that they become "adrenaline junkies." However, when a business is about dealing with clients' emergencies, the business itself should not have daily emergencies of its own. An owner who does everything alone may eventually find him- or herself in this cycle.

HIRING GOOD STAFF MEMBERS

Hiring staff members is an art. Well done, the art will help a business considerably. Poorly done, the art will lead to trouble, making the owner a care manager to staff as well as clients.

Before advertising for employees, an owner should write job descriptions. A sample job description appears in Exhibit 3–6. The description

---

Exhibit 3–6 Sample Job Description

ADMINISTRATIVE ASSISTANT

QUALIFICATIONS:

Minimum	**Desired**
Excellent Communication Skills	AA in Business
Administrative Skills	Case Management Experience
Organizational Skills	Home Health Care Experience
Typing/Filing Skills	Desktop Publishing Skills
Macintosh Computer Experience/Knowledge	
Dependable	
Self Starter	

SUMMARY STATEMENT:
The Administrative Assistant is responsible for general operations of office procedures.
Answers telephones
Opens mail
Prepares and distributes all monthly charting
Prepares and maintains Client Data Books
Prepares and Maintains all Client Charting Books
Prepares and Maintains all Case Site Charting Books
Prepares and Maintains blank charting files
Prepares and Maintains completed charting files
Opens and closes all new intake files
Opens and closes all CMP, PP, CA, and GA cases
Takes minutes at staff meetings
Inputs, copies, and mails all monthly reports
Retrieves messages from answering service twice daily
Takes on-call every third weekend
Creates emergency list
Maintains filing system
Creates and edits Care Staff Newsletter and quarterly Marketing Newsletter

should list the qualifications applicants should have and the responsibilities and tasks of the position. A human resources consultant can offer assistance in writing job descriptions.

Advertising for staff should occur at least 3–4 months before opening your office. An ad should run for at least a full week. It takes another week or two to interview staff. It then may take 2 weeks or a month until someone is on board as a new employee, as he or she may have to give notice somewhere else. You then need to train your staff, which can take up to a month. Again, using the services of a human resources consultant can help you tailor your advertising timeline to your agency's needs.

A business owner might want to put together a professional policy manual, which might include policies and procedures regarding paydays, vacation, and time off as well as all policies required by the Department of Labor (e.g., sexual harassment, nondiscrimination). Sample policy manuals are available in bookstores and through the SBA.

Employers should take care that they are meeting the legal standards for employment. An attorney can help the owner draw up legal contracts to sign with employees. The employer-employee relationship should begin on solid ground, which means making everything clear in a contract.

BILLING

Billing customers is key to keeping a geriatric care management business afloat. A billing system needs to be set up and functioning well before a business opens. A good accountant can help a business set up an appropriate billing system.

Catherine C. Thompson did a survey of GCM members in 1994, and the results were published in an article in the GCM Journal in 1996.[11] She found that GCMs handle billing in many different ways. The frequency of billing seemed to depend upon how much business the GCM did. Thompson suggested that low-volume businesses could probably manage with quarterly billing but that high-volume businesses would do better with more frequent billing. Billing statements used by GCMs ranged from bills handwritten on standard forms purchased at office supply stores or business stationery to bills done on the computer. Timeslips, Quicken, and QuickBooks seemed to be the most popular software to assist with billing, but many GCMs used customized billing programs. Most GCMs billed for their phone calls, often at the same rate as they charged for care management ($20 to $150 per hour). Many GCMs billed more for phone calls with the GCM than for phone calls with a clerical person. Some GCMs did not bill for messages left but billed for long-distance consultation or car phone calls. Some had no differentiation between types of phone calls and billed for all. One-fourth billed for all staff conference time, half did not bill for any conference time, and a quarter billed for some conference time. The GCMs who did bill for staff conferences charged them at their current rate for geriatric care management. The great majority of those surveyed billed for travel time. Some billed at their regular rate, and some billed at half of that rate. Mileage was billed in addition to the travel time by some of the responders. Others responded that they billed for mileage and not for time. The mileage rate varied from $0.22 to $0.50 per mile.

GCMs reported several problems in the survey. Some complained about the need to train staff on handling billing (i.e., installing and using billing software) or learning to do this themselves. Others complained that clients wanted detailed bills and that adding detail to bills was tedious and time-consuming. Some reported that clients did not pay or were slow to pay. GCMs surveyed wondered whether they should charge interest on unpaid bills.

Thompson pointed out that careful contracting is key to successful billing; a good attorney should draw up client contracts for a new business. Contracts should address issues like telephone time, mileage, billing for staff conferences, and different billing rates for different staff members. Another issue to address is whether to get a retainer before rendering services. In addition to a sound contract, Thompson emphasizes how important it is to have clearly stated fees. Everyone should understand how much each service costs and about how many hours it will take to render that service. A business should have not just a client contract but a service description before opening its doors. Thompson recommends looking for templates in the NAPGCM forms manual.

Thompson does not address cash flow in detail but does note that most business professionals are advised to bill as soon as possible and pay bills as late as possible without incurring late fees. Whatever an owner decides to bill for (phone calls, staff conferences, travel time, etc.), he or she needs to remember that their's is a business, not just a community service, and the business is supporting the owner and any staff members. Unbilled time is uncollected revenue, which creates more stress for the owner and any staff members. Many GCMs come into the field from human services, where they have never billed; they may feel guilty about billing.

Designing time cards to capture billable time is important. Getting a good bookkeeper or billing/payroll service to do billing may be helpful. If no one involved in the business can handle the billing, it should be outsourced. Without proper billing, the business and its personnel will not have the money necessary to function.

INTEGRATING A GERIATRIC CARE MANAGEMENT BUSINESS INTO ANOTHER PRACTICE, BUSINESS, OR AGENCY

Throughout the United States, geriatric care management practices are slowly merging with for-profit agencies and private practices (Chapter 15 considers the broad integration that will likely occur in the 21st century), including law practices, trust departments, physician's offices, accountant's offices, and the practices of a myriad of other professionals who deal with the needs of older people. GCMs offer these practices one central and very important skill: the ability to do geriatric assessment. GCMs assess the older client in his or her home and bring back to the trust officer, attorney, accountant, physician, or other professional helpful information about the client's health and psychosocial status as seen through the home setting. Other professionals may see the client in the home but not assess the client's functioning based on the home environment.

Integrating with Physicians

Because older patients represent such a large segment of most physicians' practices, GCMs are naturally helpful to physicians. As the skills of the GCM are increasingly recognized as an important part of solving chronic health problems, physicians' practices may become more open to having GCMs on staff. In 1992 the John Hartford Foundation funded a 5-year initiative to come up with better approaches to caring for the frail elderly.[12] Part of the study looked at how case management became integrated into physicians' practices. In general the study found that integrating a GCM into a physician's practice worked well. The GCM was able to work closely with the family and patients, as the GCM had access to the patient that neither the staff members nor the physician had. The physician's busy office staff found it a relief to "hand off" the older patients when problems involved accessing the continuum of care in the community or dealing with complex family problems. Physicians in the study found the GCMs' home visits very helpful; GCMs could alert the staff to potential patient problems early on, before they became a crisis, so physicians treated patients in half the time, an outcome that impressed the physicians.

The study found that integrating the GCMs into the physicians' practices initially required GCMs to overcome the resistance of the office staff by making a good first impression. Whether the physician accepted the case manager depended on learning and appreciating the value of case management before the GCM was really integrated into the patient's care. GCMs had to build trusting relationships with both the office staff and the physicians before they were fully accepted into the practices.

Integrating with Attorneys

Attorneys have slowly begun to integrate GCMs into their practices. Elder-law attorneys in particular stand to benefit from involving a

GCM in their practice. Both elder-law attorneys and GCMs serve aging clients, have long-term relationships with their clients, and address conservatorships, medical planning, elder abuse, powers of attorney, and geriatric planning. Attorneys understand law as it applies to older people, and GCMs understand psychosocial and health issues as they apply to aging, making these professionals a very good match.

GCM time is not billed at as high a rate as attorney time. GCMs often see clients before attorneys do, reducing the amount of time that clients need to spend with high-cost attorneys.

Very few attorneys employ GCMs at this point, but many may look into employing GCMs because of the benefits of such an arrangement, including one-stop shopping for the client. Benefits to the elder-law attorney are many. If the attorney handles conservatorships, the GCM can assess competency. This can be very helpful when the attorney may suspect that a person petitioning for conservatorships has a questionable agenda in getting the older person conserved; financial abuse is often involved in these cases. GCMs also have valuable knowledge of the continuum of care in the community when cases need to be referred to psychiatrists or medical social workers. GCMs can not only assess the level of confusion but help create care plans to deal with the confusion (either the primary GCM or another GCM can then take on the older person's care).[13] GCMs employed by attorneys have also been helpful in making placement suggestions in cases where the attorney serves as guardian, attorney in fact, or health care agent.

Advance planning for times when the client is unable to make medical or personal care decisions is another area where having a GCM on staff in an attorney's firm can be helpful. GCMs can help clients formulate the questions to which they need answers. Older clients may be confused about the various options available to them. The GCM can have a discussion about the medical planning needs of the client before the client sees the attorney, thereby helping the older client be better prepared to work with the

attorney. The specific needs of the client will determine how the GCM will be of assistance in this area. For example, if the client is fully capable of making decisions and is seeking assistance for the future, the discussion will be about hypothetical situations. If the client is already in poor medical health and needs assistance, the GCM can facilitate communication between the client (and/or family) and the attorney about these often difficult and private matters through precounseling. This reduces the time the attorney needs to spend with the client and raises the quality of medical planning. In a similar way, GCMs can help clients sort through personal feelings about will making and power-of-attorney appointment.

Caregiver education is another general area where the GCM can really benefit an elder-law practice. A GCM on staff can help to educate families, older people, and third parties about Medicare. Medicare benefits are little understood and, unfortunately, the majority of older people and their families still believe that Medicare will cover long-term care. Having a GCM educate clients about what Medicare will and will not cover is very helpful to a law firm because the GCM's time, again, can be billed out less expensively. Clients and their family members quickly come to understand Medicare's limitations and benefits and can do better long-term-care planning, saving themselves money and making smart choices.

GCMs can also educate clients and their families about managed care. As more and more older people are going into managed care plans, this education can be very helpful.

Some law firms have used GCMs as part of the general legal team helping an older client. GCMs can do telephone checks on older clients, make home visits, go with older clients to physician appointments, consult with physicians and other health care consultants about clients, consult with staff and caregivers in a client's facility, or serve as a liaison between the client and family and friends. All these standard geriatric care management tasks enhance the legal firm's services.

Integrating with Accountants

Accountants and GCMs have begun to work together in both formal and informal relationships. Accountants and GCMs both deal with older people, have clients who are in the upper income brackets, have long relationships with clients, have a strong ethical code, and can work with other professionals to meet their clients' goals. Unless accountants specialize in elder-care services, they do not always have extensive knowledge about entitlements such as Medicare and Social Security and can benefit from a GCM's understanding of these entitlements. Accountants understand taxes, long-range financial planning, and resolution of financial problems, while GCMs understand psychosocial issues and the continuum of care, especially managed care systems. All in all, the professions are complementary.

Since long-term care is so costly and considerable financial planning must be done to make it affordable, accountants are a wonderful resource to older people facing long–term-care planning and decision making. Since long–term-care planning hinges on the client's ability to pay for his or her care or have it covered by insurance or third-party payment, accountants and GCMs can complement each other by helping the older client come up with options for long-term care based on the client's finances and the care options available in his or her community. This pairing will benefit the accounting firm and the accounting firm's clients, who will be able to do one-stop shopping.

The accountant and the GCM need to be able to work together, have open lines of communication, and have mutual trust and confidentiality, according to Rona Bartlestone and George Lewis, who have presented workshops on this type of collaboration.[14] The American Institute of Certified Public Accountants (AICPA) has encouraged accountants to move into the elder-care field. AICPA has established an ongoing task force to communicate with AICPA members about elder care. It offers five 8-hour courses (available in self-study or group-study formats) for accountants on elder care and is working on more. In addition, AICPA has published a guide called *Eldercare: A Practitioner's Resource Guide*. Another guide, *Guide to ElderCare Engagements*, is published by Practitioners Publishing Company. The AICPA also has an elder-care marketing kit for accountants. AICPA suggests that accountants create relationships with GCMs as well as other specialists like elder-law attorneys. The accountants can then refer clients to the GCMs and the clients can hire the GCMs independently.

Like physicians and attorneys, few accountants have GCMs on staff. However, accountants are interested in expanding the relationship between the professions and have reached out to NAPGCM to speak at its conferences and begin collaborating.

GCMs AND MANAGED CARE ORGANIZATIONS

Many people believe that managed care plans seek to maximize profits and minimize quality. Improving everyone's perception of the quality of managed care is a challenge that managed care organizations face. In the market-based environment, consumer choice, consumer satisfaction, and client health outcomes will affect the success of managed care organizations. Geriatric care management may help improve older people's perceptions of managed care.

The fee-for-service system that managed care has been replacing did not always, according to Rosalie Kane, give older people fair access.[1] That system was not ideal, although many people today talk about it as if it was. Older people need to fairly compare managed care with the fee-for-service system.

Managed care has tried to contain spiraling costs and ensure greater fiscal responsibility. It has also tried to provide a less fragmented health care system. Reducing fragmentation, which both managed care and case management can do, was critical to curbing the health care cost crisis.[2] In the fee-for-service system, the costly acute care environment (i.e., the hospital) was used more often than it needed to be. Both managed care organizations and GCMs have tried to replace this acute care model with the continuum of care model. The continuum of care model does not simply treat illness but encourages wellness. So managed care, like GCMs, moved away from filling beds to treating clients in an appropriate environment, like the community.[3] Therefore, managed care and geriatric care management have much in common.

Staff GCMs could greatly enhance managed care's present tarnished image, helping the plans increase consumer satisfaction and improve consumer outcomes. Unfortunately, GCMs have only begun to work with managed care.

CONCLUSION

Starting a geriatric care management business is no easy task. There are many decisions to be made, many tasks to be completed, and many systems to put in motion before the business's opening day. Once the business opens, the hard work continues.

In the future, many GCMs may find themselves not running their own businesses but integrated into the businesses of physicians, attorneys, accountants, managed care organizations, and others who can benefit from GCMs' great input.

NOTES

1. Knutson K, Langer S. Geriatric care managers: a survey in long-term/chronic care. *GCM J.* 1998;8:9.

2. Gross EB, Johnson LF. The development of a case management business: the changing paradigms. Presented at the National Association of Professional Geriatric Care Managers Conference; October 22–24, 1998; Chicago.

3. Kraus A. Before you leap: a start-up guide for the beginner. Part I: Do you have the soul of an entrepreneur? *GCM J.* 1993;3:2–10.

4. Brostoff P, Stewart H. *Basic Components of Private Geriatric Care Management, Part II.* Presented at the National Association of Professional Geriatric Care Managers; October 14–17, 1992; Tucson, AZ.

5. Dolen L, Rubin E, Charnow J, Cress M. *The Business of Becoming a Private Geriatric Care Manager.* Tucson, AZ: National Association of Professional Geriatric Care Managers; 1992.

6. Marks W. Partnerships: the good, the bad, and the ugly. Why do they succeed or fail? *GCM J.* 1996;6:6–9.

7. Burstiner I. *The Small Business Handbook: A Comprehensive Guide To Starting and Running Your Own Business.* New York: Prentice Hall Press; 1989.

8. Orsini M. Doing good makes cents: advanced business practices. Presented at the National Association of Professional Geriatric Care Managers Conference; October 19–22, 1994; Paradise Island, Bahamas.

9. US Small Business Administration, San Francisco District, *Women's Small Business Start-Up Information Package.* Denver, CO: SBA Publications.

10. Feller R. Effective record keeping in small businesses. Presented at the National Association of Professional Geriatric Care Managers National Conference; October 31–November 3, 1996; Tucson, AZ.

11. Thompson CC. Billing and invoicing options for geriatric care managers. *GCM J.* 1996;6:15–19.

12. Netting FE, Williams FG. Geriatric case managers: integration into physician practices. *Case Management Journals, Journal of Case Management and The Journal of Long-Term Home Health Care.* 1999;1:3–10.

13. Miller AH, Karasov MA. Elder law and elder care. Presented at the National Association of Professional Geriatric Care Managers; October 21–24, 1999; San Diego, CA.

14. Bartlestone R, Lewis G. CPAs in partnership with care managers. Presented at the National Association of Professional Geriatric Care Managers Conference; October 21–24, 1999; San Diego, CA.

CHAPTER 4

After the Start-up: Issues for Mature Care Management Organizations

B.J. Curry Spitler and Laura Spitler Hansen

INTRODUCTION

As Chapter 3 made clear, the new geriatric care management organization has very particular concerns. It must define itself, decide who it serves, and establish its place in the community. After this flurry of start-up activities, methods of operation have been established and relationships have been initiated. Eventually, the organization comes to a point at which initial premises are reexamined, systems are refined, and directions are adjusted. These are some of the tasks of mature geriatric care management organizations, which often experience periods of reassessment and adjustment.

DEFINING A NICHE

The organization's niche is defined by the services it provides and the population it serves. When contemplating growth, the mature geriatric care management organization may be ready to consider expanding or changing the population it serves and the services it offers. Just as a functional assessment of a new client guides a geriatric care manager (GCM) in planning initial services, and periodic reassessment keeps GCMs responsive to changing client needs, a reassessment of the type of clients served and the services provided can offer guidance in developing a plan for growth and development for the organization.

Organizations finding themselves at this crossroads should answer the following questions:

- What are the geographical location and pattern of the population being served (e.g., within a given city, which neighborhoods have the highest density of older people or older people in certain income brackets?)?
- What is the average income of the clients?
- Are the clients primarily living at home (alone? with spouses or family members?) or in institutions?
- How functionally dependent are the clients?
- Is there a focus on long-term care, short-term care, or a mix?
- Are services primarily consultative?
- Is care coordinated to help the client remain at home, or is the primary focus on helping clients transfer to assisted living or skilled care facilities?
- Are services provided in assisted living or skilled nursing facilities?
- Are conservatorships provided?
- Does the organization provide services in the range of the activities of independent living or in the activities of daily living?
- Which therapies are provided directly and which are coordinated?
- Are fiduciary services provided?

Having answered these questions, the geriatric care management organization can assess its responsiveness to clients and determine if services should be added, dropped, or shared with other providers.

MODELS OF GERIATRIC CARE MANAGEMENT

Geriatric care management has evolved largely as a private professional practice shaped by the unique skills and orientation of the GCM conducting the practice and the identified needs of the clients served. The GCM practicing alone may continue indefinitely or as long as the individual's strength and health allow. Also, single practitioners may practice with other professionals such as elder-law attorneys, certified public accountants, and physicians (as described in Chapter 3).

Practices, large or small, can be divided into two basic models, the brokerage model and the integrated model, on the basis of whether the geriatric care management organization employs and supervises its own caregivers. Some organizations may begin using a brokerage model and, as they mature and grow, adopt the integrated model.

Brokerage Model

In the brokerage model, caregivers are not employed by the geriatric care management organization. The GCM assesses the client's level of functioning and living situation, explores options, develops a plan of care, and either refers the client or arranges client services (e.g., caregiver services, shopping services, transportation services). The GCM monitors and coordinates the care that is provided by one or several independent sources. The question then becomes, What needs does the GCM respond to directly and what relationships must be developed with other service providers in the community? The major concern is when to responsibly and responsively refer clients for required services and when to deliver and coordinate services for clients directly. In general, most of the smaller geriatric care management organizations adopt this model.

Integrated Model

In the integrated model, caregivers are employed by the geriatric care management organization. The GCM assesses the client and the situation, explores options, and develops a plan of care. If caregiver, transportation, shopping, home repair, and other miscellaneous services are required, these resources are furnished by or through the GCM's organization. The GCM employs and monitors the caregivers providing services.

Choosing a Model

Geriatric care management organization owners must decide which model they prefer as they grow. If the organization is to employ its own caregivers, there must be contractual arrangements between the organization and the clients and between the organization and the caregivers. Payroll services, workers' compensation, and tax withholding must be provided. Training and supervision must be established to ensure safety and quality control. These functions are generally beyond the scope of a care management organization operated by a single professional. Larger organizations, however, generally opt for the integrated model.

MAINTAINING THE ORGANIZATION'S IMAGE

A large organization based on the integrated model must focus on maintaining a consistent philosophy and approach. The chief executive officer (CEO) must convey to all new employees—whether they are caregivers, administrative/clerical staff, or professional GCMs—the guiding philosophy and values of the organization. Defining and maintaining the image of the organization is an ongoing task for the CEO of any new or mature organization.

The image of the organization involves everything those outside the organization think and see and hear about the organization:

1. the physical appearance of the people within the organization and the offices or physical building occupied by the organization
2. the observable behaviors of all the employees of the organization
3. the reputation the organization has obtained
4. the collateral material (e.g., logo, letterhead, brochure, print advertising) of the organization
5. the training and experience level of the staff

Reputation depends partly on the professional training and orientation of the organization's leading GCMs. GCMs may have been trained as social workers, nurses, gerontologists, psychologists, health administrators, or educators. Whatever their background, all GCMs should project their competence as seasoned professionals capable of conducting autonomous, independent practices in which the welfare of the client is the highest priority. This image can be projected by having well-organized protocols, an attitude of caring and helpfulness, and respect for the client's need for autonomy and self-determination.

Mature geriatric care management organizations employ several GCMs. Each GCM will have unique skills and strengths, and each will have weaknesses. Regular, consistent, supportive supervision is critical to ensuring high-quality service. At a minimum, GCMs should

- be professionally trained employees who are perceived as being friendly, caring, and cooperative people experienced in serving the client population
- be licensed and/or credentialed by their professional group or the standard-setting bureau of their state
- approach client needs and problems in an organized manner
- be flexible and creative in exploring client options

- assist clients and families in making decisions without imposing opinions or being judgmental
- understand their value as professionals and charge for their time accordingly
- not take on tasks that can be completed by para- or nonprofessionals
- be an integral part of the community
- receive regular, consistent, supportive supervision

Caregivers must understand that the work of the organization is carried out through them and behave accordingly. They are the eyes and ears, heart and hands of the organization. As the mature geriatric care management organization grows, there will be more staff and more caregivers to serve the increasing number of clients. This will increase the need for regular and ongoing training. Orientation to the geriatric care management organization's procedures, protocols, safety precautions, and care guidelines will be required for new employees.

Every member of an organization contributes to the image of that organization, and it is the responsibility of each person to project an image congruent with the mission of the organization. While considerate, professional behavior is the most important factor, it is also important for employees themselves, their cars, and the organization's offices to look clean and neat. When all employees look and behave in a professional manner, the organization's reputation will be enhanced.

MARKETING

In order to thrive and grow, mature care management organizations must refine their marketing approach by examining their marketing philosophy periodically and updating their marketing plan. If the organization has an annual strategic planning meeting, marketing is an appropriate topic for discussion. If the organization is a very small one- or two-person part-time practice, choosing a new marketing strategy may simply mean deciding to develop a new brochure and update marketing materials.

Marketing Philosophy

A dominant thread in the marketing philosophy of the mature geriatric care management organization involves education. Marketing can educate older people, their families, and professionals who serve older people about the spectrum of services geriatric care management provides. A second thread of the marketing philosophy is the building of goodwill. The community's goodwill toward the organization is one of the greatest assets an organization can have. Though it may seem to have little to do with the financial standing of the organization, goodwill is in fact a vitally important element of an organization's equity. The third thread to weave into the fabric of the marketing philosophy is the primacy of relationships. A marketing philosophy focused on relationship building is most consistent with the care management values that drive the organization. It is also most congruent with the way in which services are delivered: through a relationship between the GCM and the client. The clinical and marketing functions of a geriatric care management organization ideally have the same focus: relationship building. Marketing conducted from the perspective of relationship building can demonstrate to potential clients the quality of relationships available to them. Prospective clients choose providers of elder care who they trust, with whom they feel safe, and who they view as competent professionals. It is through a *relationship* that prospective clients develop this trust. The three threads—education, building goodwill, and building relationships—form the fabric of the marketing philosophy.

Marketing Plan

This section discusses marketing plans for mature geriatric care management organizations—organizations that have already had marketing plans in their start-up phase. Seven elements of a marketing plan that a mature organization might look at will be discussed:

1. definition of services and target profiles
2. market research
3. community development
4. advertising
5. public relations
6. inquiries and the intake process
7. tracking and learning

The beginning geriatric care management organization will have become involved in at least some of these seven elements. But most beginning organizations lack the financial and human resources to invest in the development of a full-blown marketing plan. As the organization grows, new challenges and opportunities appear. Additional resources may become available. An annual review of the marketing plan and assessment of the organization's functional capacity are critical to an organization's success.

Definition of Services and Target Profiles

A marketing plan for a mature geriatric care management organization begins with a redefinition of services and a profile of the target markets. For whom do we do what? The organization must clearly redefine the features and scope of its services. Only then is it able to differentiate its services from other services provided in the community. Does the organization provide geriatric care management only? Does it provide caregiving services? Does it contract out for caregivers or employ its own? Are services subsidized or are they paid for privately?

What is the profile of the target market? There are generally three target audiences: the older clients themselves, their families and relatives, and professionals in the community who refer older people to needed services. The question then becomes, Which target market do we wish to reach?

Older people themselves may resist services and be among the last to admit they need assistance. The older person may or may not be making the decisions about purchasing care management services. The decision maker may be a family member, a trust officer, or a conservator. Marketing efforts must be directed to educate older people about geriatric care management as an alternative to institutional care. What is the profile of the specific kind of older person the agency wishes to serve? What is the person's age range, income level, and level of education? What are the person's levels of cognitive and physical functioning?

The adult children or relatives of the older person are frequently the ones to initially reach out for services. Although geriatric care management as a professional service is now almost two decades old, many families do not know it exists, much less what it can provide. Education for this segment of the target audience is a vital function of marketing. Information about the availability of care management services, what specific services a given organization provides, and how these services are differentiated from other services offered to older people in the community are of vital interest to this group. The care management organization must define this target audience. Are its members well-educated, upper-income professionals with busy careers and young families of their own? Do they live out of town or out of state?

The third target market is the professionals who serve older people and their families. These professionals are valuable potential referral sources and frequently participate as members of the support team for the older person. This group includes elder-law attorneys, financial planners, geriatric physicians, psychiatrists, trust officers, private fiduciaries, hospital discharge planners, members of the clergy, and other community organizations that provide services for older people. What is the profile of this population? It will be different depending on the geriatric care management organization and the communities it serves. A geriatric care management company serving an upper-class suburb will target a different kind of professional than a nonprofit agency providing care management services to low-income older people.

Market Research

The second step in updating a marketing plan is to develop a market research strategy. This research strategy will enable the geriatric care management organization to redefine the needs of those residing in its market area. A sense of the character and lifestyle of the older people in the community will guide the practitioner so that services may be tailored to appeal to the community's older residents and their families.

Demographic information can often be obtained from the area agency on aging. Census data can be obtained on the Internet. Chambers of commerce and other local planning bodies may also have valuable information.

When looking at demographic data, geriatric care management organizations should ask a number of questions. How many older people reside in the organization's service area? In what Zip codes are they concentrated? How many of them are between the ages of 70 and 85? How many are over 85? How many live alone? How many need assistance with the activities of daily living? What is their income level? What is their level of education? In addition to research pertaining to older clients, the organization will also want to research area families and professionals, the other two target audiences. The demographic information can inform future marketing decisions such as where and how advertising dollars would be most effectively spent.

Community Development

In this section, the term "community development" refers to developing and nurturing relationships with referral sources in the community. The mature geriatric care management organization will have already identified many people with whom to develop relationships and will have initiated these relationships. Marketing professionals can do relationship development, but experience indicates that GCMs employed by the mature organization are perhaps the best candidates for this role.

Resistance to community development, or marketing, is common among people from a human services background. Administrators may see things one way and GCMs another. GCMs or employees can be encouraged to carry information and small gifts so that it becomes easy to make a gesture to a professional encountered in the process of conducting regular business. For example, an information packet and small gift given to a hospital discharge planner as the GCM is taking a client home from the hospital can result in ongoing referrals. Staff training focusing on how to talk about the services provided by the organization and how to ask for referrals can be very helpful.

Clearly, community development can easily be carried out in the course of daily care management activities. A GCM who accompanies a client to an appointment can educate the physician about geriatric care management in general and the organization's services specifically. The GCM can illustrate the services by talking about how the client's sundowner symptoms have been tracked in a log book that is kept in the client's home or how the GCM is training and supervising the caregiving staff to carry out the physician's instructions. If the GCM works with an elder-law attorney on behalf of a client to arrange estate planning, the GCM can again take the opportunity to inform the attorney about the full range of the organization's geriatric care management services. The attorney will encounter other older clients who need the services of a GCM and will refer them provided he or she understands what geriatric care management is and what services it can involve.

Experience has shown that community relationships take time to evolve. Repeated encounters and first-hand experience with geriatric care management services are often required before other professionals understand the scope of service provided by a comprehensive geriatric care management organization. It takes time for the professional to trust the GCM. In short, relationships are rarely established in one visit. Social workers and many nurses are trained to start any relationship "where the client is." When the desired relationship is with another professional, the principle remains the same. Professionals have a particular point of view: They are trying to accomplish some goal for their client. If geriatric care management organizations can focus on these professionals' goals and learn how to make their work easier for them, the relationships between the care management organizations and other allied professionals will flourish.

While community development can happen in the course of geriatric care management activities, an approach that combines both organized, concerted efforts and spontaneous encounters will yield the best results. The marketing plan must articulate the targets for community development, who is accountable for developing the relationships, and how these contacts will be tracked. Community development activities can be divided by profession (e.g., one GCM is responsible for developing relationships with all the elder-law attorneys in the community). GCMs then attend the association meetings of and network within that one group of professionals. Alternatively, one community development representative can be responsible for a particular neighborhood or geographic area. Within that area, the GCM networks, educates, and develops relationships with physicians, elder-law attorneys, trust officers, hospital discharge planners, assisted living residence administrators, and so forth. How community development tasks are divided is not important. What is important is that they are divided in a manner that clearly defines who is responsible for fostering which relationships. For example, a GCM serving a suburban area encounters a supervising trust officer during a routine call to a trust department. The GCM follows up with a letter and an information packet. He or she alerts the person in charge of marketing, who then follows up with a call to the supervising trust officer in the regional office thereby expanding the company's opportunity to broaden its influence throughout the trust departments in the region.

Advertising

A marketing plan for the mature geriatric care management company must address what advertising will be done. Depending on the local market, different advertising options may be appropriate to achieve the business's marketing objectives. Advertising options for the mature organization include but are not limited to print advertisements, broadcast (television or radio) advertisements, Internet sites and links, billboards, booths at senior health fairs, and sponsorship of community events. Common print advertising options appropriate for geriatric care management organizations include general-interest newspapers (most newspapers have a senior section), senior newspapers, local civic magazines, local business journals, community newsletters, Better Business Bureau consumer guides, elder-care directories, and local professional newsletters. A geriatric care management organization may want to be listed in several categories (i.e., home care, geriatric care management, elder care, senior services) in local directories. The mature organization should have a budget large enough to pay for advertising. Advertising that reaches the most people in the target market at the lowest cost is of course the best choice. For example, is there a radio station that is popular with professionals as they drive to and from work? A timely spot could reach adult children who are professionals as well as professionals serving older people.

Public Relations

The mature geriatric care management organization looking to grow will want to focus on public relations. Major relevant public relations activities can include creating media kits, sending regular press releases, building relationships with media contacts, publishing newsletters, holding open houses, participating in speakers bureaus, attending health fairs, and giving seminars and presentations at conferences. These activities are part of educating the public about the organization's services and building goodwill toward the organization. Some of these activities are discussed in Chapter 7.

The mature geriatric care management organization will want to continue to use media kits to keep the press mindful of the organization's history and aware of information that is in the public interest. Media kits are used to educate media representatives about the organization and to solicit media coverage of the organiza-

tion's services, activities, and events. Media kits can include the following items: company background/fact sheet; company brochure; appropriate press releases; biographies of the executive team, board of directors, advisory board, and GCMs; client testimonials; reprints of articles on or about the geriatric care management agency or about geriatric care management in general; literature on the National Association of Professional Geriatric Care Managers (NAPGCM) or Case Management Society of America (CMSA); photos with captions; a sheet of frequently asked questions and their answers; a sheet with common objections and answers or explanations for the objections; and a narrative of one client's experience with the organization (with the client's name changed for confidentiality).

Press releases can be sent for a variety of reasons: to announce an upcoming event (for inclusion in a newspaper's listing of events), to launch a new service, to announce a new office location, to announce a new contract or affiliation, to announce awards and achievements (awarded to either the company or an employee), or to announce a client's achievements. (A press release about a 100-year-old client who flew cross-country to visit her childhood summer home with her caregiver resulted in a feature article in a metropolitan newspaper.) Press releases should be sent to the following contacts: local press, trade press, business and financial press, investors, and prospective investors. Press releases should be sent on a regular basis by the mature geriatric care management organization because they can build and maintain awareness of the organization. Many organizations providing "home care" are springing up; a good human interest story can highlight the important differences between professional geriatric care management and home care.

Relationships with media contacts begin by sending or delivering the company's media kit. Relationships are fostered by sending regular press releases, monitoring editorial calendars for media opportunities, pursuing appropriate opportunities with the media representatives, inviting editors and advertising representatives to visit the company, and working with media representatives on feature articles and interviews. The more these relationships are nurtured, the more often the organization will be mentioned by the local media.

Company newsletters that educate people about geriatric care management can offer a valuable service to the professional community and serve a significant public relations function simultaneously. A well-written, regularly published newsletter can establish professional credibility and community presence. Holding open houses when an organization opens new offices, moves, or celebrates some anniversary can also serve a public relations function if professional and media contacts are invited.

Inquiries and the Intake Process

Targeted advertising and public relations activities help geriatric care management companies talk to strangers, and companies will always need to make strangers aware of their services. But after an organization does the expensive work of getting people to pay attention, then what? People who have agreed to pay attention want to get to know the organization. They want to know if the organization can help solve their problems. In a marketing (and clinical) model in which relationships are primary, the focus is on educating and creating lasting relationships, not creating instant impressions.

Inquiries are the information-seeking contacts made by family members, older people, or professionals seeking information about the organization's services. The intake process is developed to respond to these calls, from the initial greeting at the reception desk to the information exchange to the point when the caller chooses to work with the organization (as a client, as a relative of a client, or as a source of referrals) or chooses another organization. A critical element of the mature geriatric care management organization's marketing plan is ongoing analysis and improvement of the inquiry and intake processes so that as many inquiries as possible lead to new clients. A monthly summary and analysis of intake calls received, the referral source, and the outcome of

the call is a vital management tool. If the research, community development, advertising, and public relations are working, a steady stream of prospective clients will be calling.

The prospects have varying degrees of information about the organization's services. One caller's friend may have heard an ad on the radio. That caller may know nothing about geriatric care management and not be certain that an older aunt wants or needs assistance. Another caller may have heard about the organization from three different respected sources, have done extensive research on how to best provide care for his or her aging parents, and be seeking information about some of the fine points of the services. How does the organization handle these various calls to maximize conversions from callers to clients?

The mature geriatric care management organization has already designed an inquiry and intake process; however, periodic review and analysis are vital to organizational growth. Several elements are involved in designing and refining the inquiry and intake process. These elements include making sure clear information is provided, checking the information packet, following up on the initial call, referring when appropriate, and refining the intake process itself. Are the first contacts primarily phone calls, e-mail inquiries, written inquiries, or walk-ins? Who fields the first contact? Is it the receptionist? Does he or she convey a good image for the organization? Is he or she warm, inviting, professional, and knowledgeable? This is one of the most important positions in the organization. Does he or she have a script of what to say? Is there an established protocol of how to field inquiries? If not, the organization needs to design a script that includes the initial greeting, the question "How may we help you?" and the assurance that the intake GCM will respond within the hour if he or she is not immediately available. This initial response tells callers how important they are to the geriatric care management organization. The protocol should include early if not immediate recording of the caller's name and phone number (lost calls are costly).

Information Packet. Geriatric care management organizations will need an information packet of materials describing their services. The materials should accurately convey the organization's identity and be of a high quality, to reflect the quality of the services themselves. Remember that relationships are primary and the focus is on educating prospective clients about the organization's services. The material can be as simple as a brochure or as sophisticated as a presentation folder containing multiple pieces (e.g., a brochure, a description of geriatric care management, a sheet of frequently asked questions, a sheet of common objections and answers or explanations for the objections, information about NAPGCM or CMSA, reprints of articles about the organization or about geriatric care management in general, newsletters, and a narrative of a client's experience with the organization).

Intake. The intake process itself is very important. This is where the greatest opportunity exists to educate prospective clients and referral sources about the organization's services. The prospect is giving his or her full attention. The potential to expand the relationship with the prospect is great. It is critical that the intake coordinator keep the prospect's full attention. The best intake coordinators have both strong clinical skills and an understanding of and comfort with sales principles. The intake coordinator will want to use a consistent format to find out as much as possible about the prospect's situation and needs. Questions to be asked include

- Who is the client?
- What is the caller's relationship to the client?
- How did the caller hear about the organization?
- How is the client's overall health and well-being? Where and with whom does the client live? How independent is the client in caring for him- or herself?
- What was the precipitating event that resulted in the phone call?
- What services does the client want?

- What does the caller know about geriatric care management?
- Does the caller understand the geriatric care management model?

It takes time to educate the caller. While seeking answers to these questions, the intake coordinator must spend ample time listening. It is here, in this sharing of information, that the relationship between the prospect and the organization is being formed. Some callers request services immediately, while others require a number of follow-up calls before becoming clients and some are not appropriate for the organization's services at all.

One person must be the designated intake coordinator. Multiple GCMs with widely varying schedules cannot field incoming inquiries in a consistent manner. It is a well-known fact that the organization that responds most promptly to the inquiry is the most likely to be the chosen service provider. It is vitally important that the intake coordinator offer information and referrals to callers who are not appropriate for the organization. The intake coordinator must be familiar with community resources. Disseminating information and appropriate referrals is an important community service and good public relations. It provides valuable education and builds enormous goodwill in the community toward the organization.

Tracking and Learning

The follow-up process is almost as important as the intake process. Intake coordinators at mature geriatric care management organizations can use lulls in the incoming inquiries to follow up on previous calls. Follow-up may be difficult for the beginning geriatric care management organization but should be done as often as possible. A tickler system is used to follow up on prospects who say no or who are not immediately interested in services. There are numerous computer software programs available to assist in reminding to follow-up on prospects. It is important to know that "no" is not always a final answer in this situation; in fact, marketing experts suggest that it usually means "maybe" or "not just yet."[1] Remember, if people have contacted the organization, they are serious prospects. The intake coordinator must pay special attention to nurturing these relationships.

The geriatric care management organization, desiring to build equity, must be a learning organization across the board. According to Peter Senge, spokesperson for the learning organization concept, a learning organization is a new source of competitive advantage.[2] Nowhere is this learning organization approach more important than in marketing efforts. At a learning organization, people are constantly researching the existing business, tracking every dollar spent on marketing, tracking every response, measuring and analyzing the data, and making modifications to the marketing plan based on those data. Learning organizations continually measure, learn from what they measure, and make changes according to what they learn.

Computer software can make tracking manageable. Some of the information to track will be number of intake calls, number of e-mail contacts, number of inquiries converted into active clients, organizations to which callers are referred, and sources of referrals. This and other information will allow the organization to refine its advertising and public relations plans, community development efforts, and intake process. Adequate tracking is part of the vital feedback loop guiding the marketing plan and the organization as a whole.

ORGANIZATIONAL DEVELOPMENT

The information in this section is derived from the direct experience of building one geriatric care management organization and many discussions with colleagues struggling with the same issues. The reader is encouraged to borrow whatever is useful but to ultimately do whatever works best. This discussion of organizational development will address four areas:

1. defining the organization's identity
2. assessing and tending the organization's culture
3. developing leaders and staff members
4. developing systems

Defining the Organization's Identity

In order to thrive and grow, a mature organization must have a clearly articulated identity. Organizations can begin the process of defining themselves by focusing on four elements: mission, purpose, values, and culture. (The first three elements will be discussed in the next three sections. The fourth element, culture, is discussed under "Assessing and Tending the Organization's Culture," which follows those three sections.) Most geriatric care management organizations will develop mission and purpose statements early on. As organizations mature and expand, it is useful to revisit these statements to allow newcomers to participate in their revision.

Mission

A mission statement tells the community what the organization strives to accomplish through its work. The mission statement of Age Concerns, a company in San Diego, California, is "to enhance the quality of life for our clients to the maximum extent possible by fostering the elderly person's health, self-esteem and right to self determination." Ideally, every employee in the organization helps to craft the mission statement. The beginning organization may have only two employees, so it is wise to revisit the mission statement as the organization grows. When employees participate in creating the statement, they are more committed to it than they would be if it were developed by management only.

Once the mission statement is articulated, it becomes a guide for decision making at all levels of the organization. It becomes, in a sense, the organization's true north. Placement of this statement on business cards, brochures, and other informational materials serves to remind the staff of their mission and educate the community.

Purpose

While the mission statement speaks to the organization's community, the purpose statement is an *internal* statement the staff make to *themselves* about *how* and *why* they do their work. According to Collins and Porras, the "core purpose is the organization's reason for being. An effective purpose reflects people's idealistic motivations for doing the company's work. It doesn't just describe the organization's output or target customers; it captures the soul of the organization."[3(p68)] Purpose should not be confused with specific goals or business objectives. The purpose statement answers the question, Why is what we do important to us? The purpose statement of the beginning geriatric care management organization may be suitable for the mature geriatric care management organization, but a periodic review of the statement helps staff to maintain focus. As with the mission statement, staff will feel more committed to the purpose statement when they participate in creating it.

A completed purpose statement reminds staff members about how and why they do their work. It can also guide decisions that impact the culture and work environment. Management can ask "Would implementing this new policy be in keeping with our purpose statement?" The purpose statement of Age Concerns is "By serving our clients, their families, and the community, we seek to enhance the quality and meaning of our lives and the lives of those with whom we work. By growing and prospering as an organization, we make a good income for today's needs and have resources and investments for the future. By working together mindfully, respecting and nurturing our unique strengths and talents, we foster growth, a sense of community, and fun." The purpose statement can help management and staff assess how they are doing. Individuals can ask themselves "Are my unique strengths and talents being nurtured?" "Am I respecting and nurturing the strengths of my fellow workers?"

Values

The third element for the organization to articulate in its process of self-definition is its values. Core values are the essential and enduring tenets of an organization. According to Collins and Porras, "A small set of timeless guiding principles, core values require no external justification; they have intrinsic value and importance to those inside the organization."[3(p66)] They are for what the organization stands. The core

values of the geriatric care management organization may have been defined and articulated at the start and may have remained unchanged; however, the mature organization will do well to revisit these values as part of new employee orientation and renew them as part of a retreat to remind and refocus all staff. The following questions can be posed to staff in order to help them define or review their values:

- What core values do you personally bring to your work? (These should be so fundamental that you would hold them regardless of whether they were rewarded.)
- What would you tell your children (or grandchildren) are the core values that you hold at work and that you hope they will hold when they become working adults?
- If you awoke tomorrow morning with enough money to retire for the rest of your life, would you continue to live by those core values?
- Can you envision those core values being as valid for you 100 years from now as they are today?
- Would you want to continue holding those core values even if at some point one or more of them became a competitive disadvantage?
- If you were to start a new organization tomorrow in a different line of work, what core values would you build into the new organization regardless of its industry?[3(p68)]

For a geriatric care management organization, core values might include the centrality of relationships, the belief that clients are best nurtured by well-nurtured staff, the acceptance of and respect for the uniqueness of every human being, and the acceptance of growth and change as a part of life. Defining values as an organization is beginning is important. To remain effective, the mature geriatric care management organization should revisit values periodically to include new staff in value development, ensure their commitment to the values, and change value statements as the organization evolves.

Many successful organizations publicize their values. For example, three core values of the Nordstrom's retail stores are

1. service to the customer above all else
2. hard work and individual productivity
3. excellence in reputation

Assessing and Tending the Organization's Culture

Work cultures are made up of a variety of elements. These elements, which range from "encouraging innovation" to "maximizing client satisfaction" and "providing secure employment," can be prioritized so that organizations can begin to determine both their current and their ideal cultures. The new organization should assess and define its culture. The mature organization should redefine its culture periodically. The following questions can be helpful in the process:

- What is the overriding strategic intent of the organization? The strategic intent refers to *how* the organization does what it does. The strategic intent answers such questions as
  1. What do customers want?
  2. How does the organization deliver it?
  3. How is the organization different from other organizations?
- How is the organization structured (e.g., hierarchical, flat)?
- How is work organized (i.e., teams versus individual contributors)? How do teams and individuals interface?
- How are decisions made?
- What behaviors are encouraged? What behaviors are discouraged or prohibited?
- What kind of people work for the organization?
- How do they think?
- How do they act (e.g., in a task-oriented way)?
- How much power do they have?
- How much risk are they allowed—and do they wish—to take?
- How are they selected and developed?
- How are they rewarded?
- How is pay viewed? Is it seen as an investment or merely a cost of doing business?

Once an organization has clearly articulated its mission, purpose, and values and assessed its culture, it can more effectively continue the process of *developing*. At any point that the current reality does not match the desired state, efforts can be made to improve the situation. Development is not a one-time event but a continuous process—improvement is always possible. With a clear picture of the current reality, the organization can begin to define *how* it would like to develop as an organization. The organization's culture must be tended if the organization is going to remain robust and dynamic. Cultures differ from organization to organization. There is no one right answer. Whatever *works* is what is "right" for that organization.[4] However, the centrality of relationships appears to be one tenet that is essential to the cultures of geriatric care management organizations.

In the delivery of geriatric care management services, it is the quality of the relationship between the GCM and the client (and the family) that makes this service unique and is a key criterion for success. It is, in part, the absence of human relationships in the nation's bureaucracies, medical system, and elsewhere that creates the need for geriatric care management.

If relationships are the lifeblood of the organization, what is the organization doing to foster them? This element of the culture must be focused on, nurtured, and developed in order for the organization to continue to mature. It is often said that a child learns what he or she lives. In a sense, we all learn what we live. If management wants the GCM to develop mastery in his or her relationships with clients, then managers must develop mastery in *their* relationships with the GCMs (and other staff members). If the organization wants GCMs to nurture their clients, then the *organization* must nurture the GCMs. If the organization wants to support the autonomy and self-determination of older clients, it must also support the autonomy and self-determination of its employees. Organizational practices that foster staff autonomy and self-determination include participative management and self-managed teams.[5]

Developing Leaders and Staff Members

Geriatric care management organizations focused on growth must attend to leadership and staff development. Fostering professional development improves individual and team performance, strengthens an organization's effectiveness, creates a more cohesive culture, and encourages staff loyalty. An organization's plan for professional development should be based on an assessment of the organization's needs. Leadership and staff development based on an assessment can include training in building teams, conducting meetings, resolving conflicts, supervising, balancing work and life, managing time, making presentations, and handling countertransference. (Countertransference is the totality of feelings experienced by the practitioner toward the client, whether conscious or unconscious, and whether prompted by the client or events in the practitioner's own life. The countertransference process is an appropriate, natural, emotional response of positive value; important therapeutic tool; and the basis for empathy and deeper understanding of both the client's and the practitioner's processes.) Table 4–1 lists different kinds of staff training and their impact on business, leadership, and clinical skills.

The leader of a mature geriatric care management organization must begin to delegate tasks to staff. Leaders who are accustomed to being solo operators experience difficulty in delegating and supervising. A clear job description, well thought out in advance of hiring a new worker, helps the leader to clarify what is expected from the employee. Delegation must confer on the worker the authority to carry out the assigned responsibility. This is a basic tenet, often overlooked as geriatric care management organizations grow. Regular supportive supervision (a set day and time each week) is a way to ensure that the new employee will have opportunities to ask questions and provide feedback. As the numbers of staff increase, it is vital to divide the work into professional/clinical functions and business/support functions, thereby always en-suring that every worker has a supervisor. Adequate delegation frees the GCM for leadership roles. Remember, it is not possible to play all the instruments when one is conducting the orchestra. Delegated tasks create opportunities for staff development.

Caregiver Training Development

As geriatric care management organizations grow, many of them begin to employ their own caregivers. Geriatric care management organizations that employ their own caregivers should develop training to educate the caregivers in the mission, purpose, and culture of the organization. This training should focus on how to work as a team to foster the client's well-being. It should address these issues and more:

- the caregiver's role and responsibilities
- the organization's guidelines
- communication skills

Basic caregiving duties must be addressed (e.g., nutrition, hygiene, grooming, exercise, medications). Universal safety training is important in order to prevent caregiver or client injury. Safety training may include body mechanics (positioning, transfers, lifting), environmental safety (slips, trips, falls), disaster preparedness (earthquake, fire, utility outage), universal precautions (infection control), crime prevention (home security, weapons, theft, loss), and what to do in case of an injury to a client or caregiver. Training that addresses problems of caring for clients suffering from dementia, depression, diabetes, arthritis, Parkinson's, and other conditions helps caregivers to provide excellent care.

Developing Systems

Procedures, policies, processes, and systems must be documented as organizations mature so that institutional wisdom is preserved and so that processes and procedures become reproducible and transferable.

This documentation can begin with creating a personnel manual articulating the organization's policies regarding holidays, vacations, sick

Table 4–1 Impact of Staff Training on the Development of Business, Leadership, and Clinical Skills

Type of Training	Business Skills	Leadership Skills	Clinical Skills
Team building	Teaches process skills that enable staff to work together to achieve business objectives.	Teaches leadership skills within the team context. Shared leadership is experienced.	Teaches people to work with family "teams" and caregiver teams.
Conduct of meetings	Teaches business leadership.	Teaches how to get results in teams.	Teaches people to handle family meetings and caregiver team meetings.
Conflict resolution and mediation		Teaches this core leadership competency.	Teaches how conflict resolution skills improve clinical effectiveness with clients, families, caregiving staff, and allied professionals.
Supervisory skills	Teaches communication and relationship skills. Teaches legal responsibilities and laws affecting supervision.		
Annual company retreat		Encourages personal and professional renewal.	
Renewal	Anchors individuals in personal values and a sense of purpose. Results in increased motivation and professional commitment.	Encourages personal and professional renewal.	Results in work/life balance and an increased connection to one's sense of purpose.
Time management	Improves overall business effectiveness.	Increases the awareness of what is important.	Assists with prioritizing competing client demands. Assists with work/life balance.
Presentation skills	Improves business presentations and professional image and credibility.	Improves communication and leadership skills.	
Countertransference			Increases clinician's awareness of his or her own issues. Teaches strategies for skillful interventions.
Continuing education. Allows staff to customize learning according to personal goals.			

leave, health insurance, and so forth. The organization must also develop a policies and procedures manual that specifies the tasks of each job function. Manuals may also be developed for the various types of training the organization provides for its staff. Growing organizations are not static; therefore, it is vitally important to periodically renew and update the policies and procedures manual. An annual review of the personnel policies should be a part of the human resources function. If there is a human resources manager, this should be part of his or her job description. If human resources is not a separate department, the review and update can be outsourced to a consulting firm. However updating is done, it is imperative that personnel policy manuals reflect current legal requirements. In the mature geriatric care management organization, timely revision of the procedures manual is generally the responsibility of each department head and the overall concern of whoever is in charge of operations.

ESTABLISHING WORKING RELATIONSHIPS WITH KEY ORGANIZATIONS IN THE COMMUNITY

When one is a company's CEO, it is extremely important to be known in many circles in the community and be perceived as a leader. In the mature geriatric care management organization with numerous employees, the CEO should make the development of these kinds of relationships a priority. If the leader of the organization lives and works in a major city, one cannot realistically aspire to be known as a leader citywide, but one can seek to spread one's sphere of influence.

Some wise person once observed that the best way to obtain one's goals was to help others obtain their goals. This may or may not be universally true, but one who is perceived as helpful can generally build a referral network of allied professionals. Relationships, as previously stated, grow only with time and nurturing. Thank-you notes for referrals and other assistance will help maintain and nurture good relationships.

The CEO of the mature geriatric care management organization may want to consider the following avenues in order to expand the organization's presence in the community:

- *Memberships in service clubs* (e.g., Rotary, Kiwanis, Lions). The businesspeople in these groups may not have a clue about care management but they probably have aging parents. Membership gives one an opportunity to educate and spread the word. From these diverse contacts may come invitations to speak and other opportunities to educate. Referrals of clients usually follow.
- *A seat on the board of directors of advisory committees and community organizations* (e.g., the Better Business Bureau, Community Chest or United Charities, or the YMCA/YWCA). Participation by the CEO on community boards can widen the organization's involvement in the community and enhance the organization's image. Participating in advisory committees for the planning of neighborhood, city, or county services is also an excellent way to extend one's involvement.
- *Active involvement in the religious community.* Active involvement in the religious community can provide the CEO with opportunities to educate volunteers and clergy working with older people. Every church or place of worship in every community in the United States is grappling with the problems of serving a rapidly aging population. Older people tend to look to their churches for support. By building a role in the ecumenical conference of churches, synagogues, and other places of worship, one can often educate those who are attempting to guide the efforts of volunteers. By supporting or training volunteers who serve older people, one can contribute to the well-being of many older people. Religious leaders can be a valuable source of referrals of clients who need more services than volunteers can provide.

CEOs may also want to take the following steps:

- *Attend attorneys' community meetings.* A significant group of professionals serving older people are attorneys specializing in wills and probates, estate planning, or other elder-law issues. Elder-law attorneys are becoming aware of the invaluable services GCMs can provide. Educating attorneys by attending their community meetings, providing information on health or psychosocial issues affecting older people, and making referrals to them when appropriate can foster relationships with this group of professionals who can become valuable supporters of a growing care management organization.
- *Call regularly on trust officers, departments, and accounting firms.* These professionals are seeing the number of older people in their practices increase rapidly. Many of them become trusted counselors to their clients, but frequently there comes a time when the client's ability to make safe and sensible personal decisions diminishes or he or she becomes physically dependent and requires more personal care from others. These professionals are not trained in assessment of need, provision, or supervision of home care. The mature care management organization's reputation for cooperation and service can be built by making personal calls, speaking at group meetings, and providing educational information regarding the role of geriatric care management.
- *Call regularly on senior centers and when possible give small presentations.* In almost every community, senior centers provide education, recreation, and socialization programs vital to the well-being of active older people. The activity directors of these centers are often the first people to see signs of deterioration or disease. Day care centers providing support and activities for special groups such as people with Alzheimer's or muscular dystrophy serve a very vulnerable group of older people who can often benefit from care management services. Ongoing contact, occasional talks to groups, and sponsorship of special events build awareness and trust of the geriatric care management organization.
- *Maintain contacts with support organizations.* In larger cities there are organizations providing counseling, specialized information, and referrals for older people and their families. These may be regional caregiver resource centers, Alzheimer's associations, or associations organized for the education of people with other diseases and their families. The area agencies on aging provide information and referrals exclusively focused on the needs and issues of older people. Keeping these people regularly supplied with printed material describing the care management organization can be an important way to increase awareness of the care management organization. Occasional talks at in-service training sessions are also helpful to keep new staff updated about the organization's services.
- *Attend coordinating councils.* In most areas there are associations of professionals who come together to share information, give mutual support, and network. These are often known as councils on aging or coalitions of elder services. Attendance and participation can foster good relationships with people in a wide circle of related service organizations.

There seems to be no limit to opportunities for networking with allied professionals. Tracking of referral sources will yield clues to which activities result in direct referrals. Goodwill is harder to measure. Building community awareness and good relationships is, for the mature care management organization, not only building the business but also building the value of the organization.

JOINING ORGANIZATIONS AND NETWORKING NATIONALLY

From the acorn grows the mighty oak. That is the manner in which many of the national organizations dealing with the concerns of aging have grown. Many professionals who are still active in the field participated in the formation of these associations. Gerontology is a new field of study, less than 50 years old. Geriatric care management, as reported by NAPGCM, has yet to celebrate its 20th birthday and is still unknown to many. Media coverage of aging issues in general and care management specifically has increased markedly in the past 2 years as a growing awareness that the baby boomers are aging is creating new interest among businesspeople, health care providers, and politicians. The age wave is upon us.

Continued participation and networking in national organizations can inform the growing care management organization of legislative trends in health care, the results of scientific studies, and developments in clinical practices. In a new profession such as geriatric care management, everyone is traveling in uncharted territory. The interaction with colleagues is enriching. Mutual support and open dialogue can be invaluable. The mature organization has the opportunity to present material to educate and mentor newer colleagues. Opportunities to participate in the development of professional organizations inform efforts to develop a geriatric care management organization. The mature geriatric care management organization can join as many national groups as it has time or staff to become involved.

- *NAPGCM* and *CMSA.* Long-term NAPGCM and CMSA membership by the mature geriatric care management organization will allow the leader to get involved in the organization's activities and perhaps run for office. This level of participation allows the leader to develop a broader understanding of national trends in aging policy, the policy development necessary to ensure supportive care for older people, and the opportunities for the national organization and its members to strengthen and expand the services that will be needed.
- *The National Council on Aging (NCOA).* NCOA, one of the older associations addressing issues relating to aging, also fo-

cuses on the issues and concerns of service providers, but its scope is much broader than that of organizations focused on provider issues. The needs and concerns of many different groups serving older people, such as home care providers, senior centers, activity programs, or housing projects, to name a few, are addressed. NCOA also provides a legislative advocacy function.
- *The American Association of Retired Persons (AARP).* AARP is the largest of all the geriatric associations. Its financial base is insurance and other business ventures. It exerts a strong legislative advocacy presence and ensures the participation of older people through volunteer groups at the local, state, and national levels. It publishes *Modern Maturity,* a magazine that addresses a wide range of geriatric issues and targets older readers.
- *The National Gerontological Society of America (GSA).* GSA deals primarily with research and the interests of academia. There are four primary sections: biological, psychological, behavioral, and policy. Emphasis at the annual meetings is on the presentation of research findings.
- *The American Society on Aging (ASA).* ASA was originally named the Western Gerontological Society. The emphasis was on training at the undergraduate level and sharing information regarding advances in the field. From this beginning, ASA has developed a strong program of seminars, often clustered around annual or regional meetings as preconference educational opportunities. The focus is on a wide array of services provided to older people, including care management. From a small regional association based in academia, it has grown to a broad international organization.
- *The National Association of Elder Law Attorneys (NAELA).* NAELA is open for membership to attorneys only. There appears to be growing interest within this group to share information with members of NAPGCM. Opportunities to participate

on panels and to promote cooperation between the professions can work to the benefit of both organizations.

Contact information for these seven organizations appears in Appendix A.

There are other care management organizations focused on insurance coverage services or hospital/health maintenance organization concerns that may interest growing care management organizations.

The mature geriatric care management organization can benefit from participation in the conferences and activities of numerous national organizations. Choices are clearly necessary. Membership in national organizations can be costly in terms of money, time, and energy. Establishing priorities for national participation and sampling conferences can help determine the extent to which the mature care management organization involves itself in networking at the national level.

CONCLUSION

As the geriatric care management organization matures, it will revisit many of the steps it undertook in its infancy and take new steps on new pathways. These steps begin with redefining the organization's niche, confirming or changing the model of practice, and strengthening or adjusting its image in the community. The mature organization will need to rethink its marketing program and its strategy for organizational development. Finally, the organization will need to solidify its working relationships with key organizations in the community and reassess its involvement with national professional organizations.

NOTES

1. Taylor W. Permission marketing. *Fast Company.* 1998;April–May:198–212.
2. Senge P. *The Fifth Discipline: The Art and Practice of the Learning Organization.* New York: Doubleday; 1990.
3. Collins J, Porras J. Building your company's vision. *Harvard Bus Rev.* 1996;74:65–77.
4. Wheatley M, Kellner-Rogers M. *A Simpler Way.* San Francisco, CA: Berrett-Koehler Publishers; 1996.
5. Anderson B. *Pathways to Partnership.* Whitehouse, OH: Soulworks; 1998.

CHAPTER 5

Fee-for-Service Care Management in Not-for-Profit Settings

Monika White, Robyn L. Golden, and Cathy Cress

INTRODUCTION

The senior services industry has become big business and has enormous potential for profit. With increased length of life comes an array of needs, ranging from services such as health care, housing, home care, and nursing facilities to opportunities for recreation, leisure time activities, and education. While most people manage their aging fairly well, older adults may face health, cognitive, financial, legal, and housing problems with little or no idea of where to get help. Many families also struggle with these problems when caring for older relatives.

One of the important components of the aging business is helping older individuals and families through care management services. Many families are willing—and able—to pay for assistance with older relatives. The growth of the for-profit care management business has demonstrated the need to provide the service on a fee basis and the fact that there are customers to purchase those services. The presence of the not-for-profit (NFP) agency in the fee-for-service (FFS) care management business has been slowly but steadily growing.

Probable reasons for the slow growth lie in both philosophical and operational issues. As NFPs have considered adding FFS services, NFPs' leaders have found themselves in debates about their organizations' missions. Many large NFPs have taken the position that if there is no profit margin, they cannot continue their primary mission of serving people in need. Others resist the new emphasis on the market. The debate is not a simple one nor has it been resolved.

Contrary to the past, today NFPs and government agencies are no longer the only trusted providers of services for older people. Quality services are now found in the for-profit sector as well. As public funds shrink, NFPs are at risk of being left to serve only the poor and to operate at a deficit. Thus, to expand the client base and to offset the expenses of serving those that cannot pay, many NFPs are competing with private for-profit entities for clients who can afford to pay for service.

Initial interest in establishing FFS case management programs within NFP agencies was twofold: to develop the capacity to meet the needs of multiple income groups and to generate revenue. FFS case management evolved very slowly within NFP agencies during the mid- to late 1980s, then picked up during the 1990s. Knutson and Langer, in a survey of geriatric care management practice, found that by 1997, NFPs made up 16% of the membership of the National Association of Professional Geriatric Care Managers, an organization formerly accepting only for-profit practices as members.[1]

This chapter focuses on the development of FFS case management programs. It draws on the experiences of two agencies that have successfully implemented such programs: the Council of Jewish Elderly (CJE) in Chicago, Illinois, and Huntington Hospital Senior Care Network (SCN) in Pasadena, California. CJE, a large NFP agency, has always provided some form of case management services. FFS care management was started in 1995 to address the need for producing revenue from services to offset budget deficits. By the late 1990s, FFS care management was a part of CJE's continuum and a self-supporting service. SCN developed FFS case management in response to a clear need; namely, people with higher incomes had no access to case management services even though they experienced the same problems as people with lower incomes. Another objective was to generate revenue. Over the next 10 years, the program grew from one to six care managers and incorporated a variety of care management services, including long-term care insurance underwriting and claims assessments, elder care services for employed caregivers, and other fee-based contract services.

TERMINOLOGY

The term "case management" has long been considered undesirable; calling people "cases" and thinking that their lives are something that can be "managed" has come to seem both negative and paternalistic. Despite numerous contenders (e.g., "care coordination," "service management," "service coordination"), "case management" continues to be the most commonly used term. Slowly, the name "care management" is gaining popularity, especially with private practitioners and FFS professionals. But, as pointed out by Bodie Gross and Holt, while professionals continue to carry on debates about language usage, "from a consumer's perspective, there is no difference between a care and case manager. The sole standard of judgement is one of satisfaction with the services being delivered."[2(p23)]

For the purposes of this chapter, "care management" is most frequently used, especially when referring to fee-based services. However, "case management" may be utilized when referring to a particular program or where that is the common terminology.

Just as no one name or title is used for case management, no single agreed-upon definition of case management exists. However, there is

consensus on the key tasks performed by the case manager: assessment, care planning, coordination, follow-up (including monitoring of client status and service delivery), reassessment, and termination or case closure. While the focus here is on care management for older people and their families, it is important to note that care management is utilized in a wide range of settings for a variety of populations.[3]

BRIEF HISTORY OF CASE MANAGEMENT

It is difficult to definitively trace the beginnings of case management, since most disciplines lay claim to inventing at least some element of it.[4] Its principles can be found as early as the turn of the century in the settlement movement, but public nursing, mental health, disability, and other fields can all point to historical beginnings of case management within their own discipline. Clearly, identifying and solving problems by assessing needs, linking people to needed resources, and coordinating the delivery of services are central themes of case management throughout the history of human services.

Case management programs for older people have been offered by NFP agencies for the past 25 years, primarily for frail, low-income populations at risk of institutionalization. Case management grew more popular because of the increasing costs of long-term care and continued fragmentation, duplication, and gaps in services. The case management programs of the 1970s and early 1980s were largely financed by public sector dollars—specifically Medicaid—for the purpose of decreasing the utilization and expense of nursing home care by keeping individuals at home. Through these and other national demonstration projects, case management became an important part of long-term care programs.[5] Many of these projects were implemented in NFP agencies as part of a continuum of services provided for older people. They all utilized case management, which rapidly became a popular approach to linking clients with needed resources.

By the mid-1990s, individuals practicing some form of case management could be found in virtually every service setting, including private practice. In fact, the private practice business was enjoying enough success that professionals and paraprofessionals from a wide range of educational and disciplinary backgrounds were opening care management businesses catering to families of means. This trend continued through the late 1990s and is expected to grow.

PRIVATE PRACTICE CARE MANAGEMENT VERSUS PUBLIC AND NFP CARE MANAGEMENT

With the proliferation of case management programs focused on low-income populations, the development of private FFS care management was not surprising. Higher-income families ineligible for income-based case management programs provided the ideal market for the for-profit care management business.

The need for assistance in accessing information, locating services, and solving problems associated with aging is not linked to income. Parker delineates the reasons why families hire care managers:

> The need for a professional assessment;
> The need for an objective opinion regarding service options;
> Help with the feeling of being overwhelmed;
> The inability to resolve family conflicts;
> Help in transitioning a relative to a nursing home;
> Long-distance caregiving issues;
> The need for respite care; and,
> Help with filling out forms.[6(pp4–5)]

Families at all income levels share the same sense of helplessness when crises occur, and all lack knowledge of available resources.

There are many similarities in geriatric care management services offered in an NFP and a for-profit setting. Both perform the same tasks, including assessment, care planning, service coordination, referral, and monitoring. Both need after-hours access to staff. Both need professionals with good skills and a strong background in working with older people. Because geriatric care management cases tend to be complicated, it is important to hire staff who have the professional background to deal with the complexities of difficult situations and to build in mechanisms to ensure that client needs are met. Both limit caseload numbers to enhance the quality of service delivery. Forms, procedures, and billing may be similar in both types of agencies; however, the NFPs are likely to have federal, state, or local regulations; external funding requirements; or internal policies and guidelines that may affect their practice and procedures.

Overall, the private FFS practice has the major advantage of enabling an intensive and personal relationship that is important to clients looking for a surrogate family member. Parker explains how private practice is different from public and NFP geriatric care management in this way:

> *Eligibility*. While there are strict eligibility requirements to participate in a publicly funded program, the ability to pay a fee is usually the only criteria for becoming an FFS client.
>
> *Availability*. Private practitioners will typically be on call or actually available 24 hours a day and weekends.
>
> *Staff Turnover*. Unlike the public agency with high caseloads and more frequent staff turnovers, the private care manager is more likely to be able to offer a more stable, long-term relationship.
>
> *Conflicts*. There appear to be fewer conflicts about providing direct services in addition to care management including home aides and companions.[6(pp4–5)]

The FFS geriatric care management program within an NFP offers other kinds of advantages. Many NFPs provide services other than care management, giving clients served by the agency more choices. NFPs often employ professionals from multiple disciplines. This is beneficial because it enables cross-training and collaboration with the geriatric care managers (GCMs) that may result in a better-quality product for the client. A well-established NFP can offer greater fiscal security to a fledgling program. Unlike many of the small for-profit companies, a well-funded NFP is more financially secure and able to support the care manager in times of slower business.

Another advantage of the NFP is its standing in the community. Through its established community relationships and reputation, it can help the GCM program be accepted and grow. In such a setting GCMs have an entire agency behind them and great support in the beginning of the program when many crises are to be faced and much is still to be learned.

Because the NFP programs serve a mix of income groups, there is a risk of losing the private-pay clients to NFP if available options are not clearly presented at intake. All available options should be presented at intake including fee-for-service geriatric care management and fee-for-service home care, if offered.

Vocker discusses both positives and negatives of integrating FFS geriatric care management into an NFP agency.[7] Many NFPs receive case management funding through the Older Americans Act (OAA). In order to be a recipient of OAA-funded case management services, a client must be at least 60 years old and live in the geographic area served by the agency. OAA also requires that the agency be open 8 hours each weekday and never closed for 4 or more consecutive days. When the agency is closed, alternative assistance must be offered. This could include access to staff pager numbers or arrangements with police and fire departments. In addition, the agency must meet the needs of non-English-speaking and physically challenged clients. Other types of requirements cover case assignments, care plans, and supervision.

Since geriatric care management is an around-the-clock business, it can be hard to get staff to participate in this service. Also, because of its time-intensive nature, FFS geriatric care management typically means smaller caseloads; thus, keeping track of client caseloads is especially important. Typically, FFS clients are not the only clients served by any one care manager in the NFP agency, so it is important to monitor the GCM's ability to respond to the needs of FFS clients.

Friction may arise between staff who serve the FFS clients and staff outside this program. Since geriatric care management is so labor-intensive, staff not delivering FFS care management may resent the disproportionate amount of time spent with the paying clients.

NFPs' FFS PROGRAM DEVELOPMENT CHALLENGES

In making the decision to implement FFS care management, NFP boards and staff address many questions. How will the commitment to serve those most in need be maintained? Will revenue-seeking activities compromise other social service involvement? If building the business means selling services, how can client interests come first? Are we being driven by profit motives? Should services be different if people are paying? What would it mean to have a two-tiered system? How can we work with demanding customers when we went into this to help the needy and vulnerable? Will we be asked and have to do things that seem unprofessional, such as escorting someone to the opera?

NFPs continue to struggle with these fundamental questions as they develop FFS programs and must consider and resolve them if programs are to succeed. Among the biggest hurdles is overcoming the reluctance to charge fees. Other major challenges include developing a customer orientation and marketing FFS care management services.

Overcoming the Reluctance To Charge Fees

Charging fees in exchange for services remains one of the most difficult challenges in developing FFS care management in an NFP setting. Generally, charging for services has been considered inappropriate for the NFP sector. The reluctance to charge for services most likely stems from traditional attitudes that the NFP sector's mission is to provide access to those who are unable to pay or to meet other criteria such as need, status, condition, location, race, ethnicity, or religion. In many cases, services are given to clients who are not eligible for public sector case management or prefer not to use it. But decreasing opportunities to acquire public dollars and private donations for direct care have led more NFPs to generate revenues through fees.

While there are clinical as well as fiscal and operational reasons to collect fees, there has been significant resistance within NFPs to implementing FFS programs. This resistance has come from all groups: staff, volunteers, administrators, and clients who have been receiving free services for many years.

Many human service professionals who have worked in publicly funded social services and the NFP sector appear to suffer from a type of "fee phobia." For example, when SCN first developed its FFS program in 1985, it was difficult to find professionals who were comfortable with charging for care management. These professionals felt that social services should be free to clients and that clients would not pay or would refuse help if they were charged. The professionals were inexperienced in setting rates and did not feel confident about negotiating fees. Many of them objected to the idea of "selling" services, stating that they did not choose to become a social worker (or nurse or other human services professional) to work as a "salesperson."

CJE struggled with many of these same issues. CJE began its FFS private geriatric care management service with a few interested staff members who took on cases. The intake worker who responded to initial inquiries played a significant role in engaging callers to view the service as viable. An after-hour call system was developed, and only supervisory staff responded, to protect staff time. As the number of cases grew, the staff became excited, particularly by the positive feedback they received from clients. CJE staff members were soon sold on the idea and requested beepers so they could respond to their own after-hours calls. The few specialists'

enthusiasm was infectious, and other staff members became interested in providing care management services.

Most practitioners who provide care management in NFPs have backgrounds in helping professions in which revenue is not discussed. Many of these practitioners believe that older adults have no disposable income and should be taken care of because they are needy and frail. It is difficult for these practitioners to see their services as products and think that older people should pay a fee for those services.

Early in SCN's FFS program, staff noticed that clients also created barriers to "selling" care management as a service. Many clients said that they should not have to and could not afford to pay for this kind of service. Others thought that since they had already donated to the organization, they were entitled to get free services. Still others believed that if they did pay for both case management and a service provider, they would spend more money than necessary.

In his study of nontraditional in-home services, Hereford reports that older people did not see case management as a distinct product worthy of a fee.[8] Prior to implementing its FFS care management program, the CJE conducted market research that reinforced this perspective. CJE found that fees of $50 to $100 per hour were considered too high; a few older adults would pay $20 per hour, but most wanted to pay nothing. Family members, on the other hand, supported the concept of paying fees for this service.

Many of today's older adults still have what is known as "Depression era" thinking—the desire to preserve every penny to save for a "rainy day." Many services to seniors have been based on entitlement, and consequently, many seniors expect services to be provided for them. Older adults also find it distasteful to pay for something they could previously do for themselves. Others resist outside involvement by a professional because they fear a greater loss of control than they already experience due to aging.

A reorientation of practice philosophy is necessary to shift staff members' thinking about charging fees for these services. An NFP needs to help staff see the need for revenue to offset deficits and survive in a time of more limited resources. Full-paying clients are needed so the agency can continue to serve those who cannot afford to pay.

Sales training sessions, sessions to increase understanding of NFP funding mechanisms, and sessions teaching about marketing and appreciating the value of care management as a professional service were all held for FFS staff at SCN. Letting staff members articulate their objections and do role-playing helped them be comfortable with charging fees. SCN care management program managers focused on establishing a business mentality, paying attention to changing attitudes as well as language. Figure 5–1 shows an example of training materials used to help achieve this shift.

In response to similar issues, CJE spent considerable time defining care management so that staff could comfortably articulate the benefits of the service. Then staff could better help older adults and families understand the value and necessity of care management when it was indicated. Staff worked on increasing their comfort with fees through outlining and challenging staff biases and paternalistic views about what older people could understand and afford. Discussions were held with private practice GCMs about their views, which helped staff members realize the value of their services in the marketplace. Role-playing was utilized to increase everyone's comfort level.

This type of a practitioner paradigm shift takes time. The reality is that some care managers have an easier time with charging fees than other care managers do. To integrate a private care management philosophy into NFP structures, an organization needs to allow for some anxiety and sadness about the change. It is important, wherever possible, to create mechanisms for staff input into the development of the service. One way to begin is to identify staff who are comfortable with fees and create specialist positions. They can then act as champions as the program develops. The organization's leaders should think about similar changes from the organization's past and what helped ensure staff commitment as those changes were taking place.

Developing a Customer Orientation

Care management, for a fee, provides many of the case management services traditionally offered by senior and social services agencies at no cost to clients. When an NFP decides to develop an FFS care management model, it must also develop a customer orientation rather than the traditional client orientation. Customers expect to have choices and to be treated in a special way, with privacy, flexibility, control, quality, and a personal touch. The balance of power between clients and case managers is different, with the case managers making most of the decisions for the client.

In traditional case management, the case manager identifies what he or she thinks the client needs, then tries to ration services to meet those needs, where possible still relying on the support of family members, neighbors, and other people in the client's life. This is very different from the "surrogate child" or "substitute family member" model associated with private geriatric care management. Private GCMs are available weekends and evenings to provide the personalized

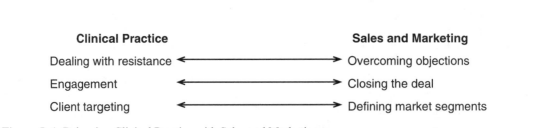

Figure 5–1 Balancing Clinical Practice with Sales and Marketing.

touch that accommodates requests above and beyond just client need.

At CJE every effort was made to develop an FFS geriatric care management business that reflected an integrated practice model. This model balances customer wishes with assessed needs and priorities in order to maximize independence, reduce risk, and strengthen family support. For both paying and nonpaying older people, the values and goals were similar.

A major goal at SCN was to develop a true care management continuum with a full range of opportunities for older people to receive services regardless of income or condition. Centered on a triage model with professional telephone screening, consultation, information, and referral, SCN established case management programs with several public and private funding sources. The addition of FFS care management made the service available to virtually anyone. It also created a customer service approach that eventually permeated the other programs.

Marketing

A critical factor in creating an FFS geriatric care management business in an NFP is the image of the organization. A marketing plan needs to be developed that communicates that the agency is broadening its program. To seek services from an organization viewed as serving lower-income clients, FFS customers must realize that FFS services are being offered and trust the organization to provide high-quality services. Conversely, residents of the community may well be drawn to the NFP's care management program because they view the NFP as having no profit motive. Outreach and marketing staff must be prepared to deal with both perspectives. In either case, the reputation and credibility of the NFP organization are the most important factors in the success of the new program.

Marketing of FFS care management is rarely focused directly on the person who will receive the service. Rather, it is aimed at adult children and other individuals (e.g., attorneys, physicians, financial planners) who help older people make decisions. Different marketing strategies are needed to reach these different audiences. An NFP can look to the for-profit business sector to learn about successful marketing and, at the same time, build on the NFP's history and tradition of service to set itself apart from the for-profit business sector.

Before developing FFS care management, an NFP's leaders must consider whether there are enough potential customers in the community. The leaders should also consider whether the community already has enough organizations providing these services.

The success of the services will depend on a network of trusted, caring service providers committed to quality and open to suggestions for improvement. A trusted provider network is an important part of what is being sold.

COSTS, RATES, AND BILLING

One of the first questions typically asked by potential clients is "How much will it cost?" Setting rates takes a good understanding of direct and indirect agency expenses. Profits can be built in but must be reasonable, keeping prices competitive with those of similar service providers in the community. Many NFPs are able to keep their prices somewhat lower than those of for-profit businesses because of their size and funding from other programs. However, FFS care management fees are billed by the task or hour; thus, staff productivity becomes an important element in the program.

Productivity in an FFS program most commonly means the number of hours each care manager can bill. This is a strange concept to those unaccustomed to billing and requires training and experience to become second nature. As noted by Bellucci and her colleagues, productivity can be raised through methods such as objective feedback.[9] A study in an NFP's FFS case management program serving human immunodeficiency virus/acquired immune deficiency syndrome clients showed a 13.4% increase in billable hours after an expected number of billable hours and weekly reports were provided to each team of case managers. These findings show the importance of good supervision, target setting, and ongoing staff development.

CONCLUSION

Many decisions must be made prior to implementing an FFS care management program in an NFP setting. Choices must be made about the program's purpose, staffing, structure, rates, relationship to other programs, and marketing strategies. In the years to come there will probably be more questions than answers as NFPs further develop for-profit enterprises. These debates will help ensure that the mission and values of NFPs can be maintained while paying customers are accommodated. Moving into the FFS world will enable NFPs to survive and serve more people.

NOTES

1. Knutson K, Langer S. Geriatric care managers: a survey in long-term/chronic care. *GCM J.* 1998;8:9.

2. Bodie Gross E, Holt E. Care and case management summit—the white paper. *GCM J.* 1998;8:22–24.

3. White M. Case management. In: Maddox GL, ed. *The Encyclopedia of Aging*, 3rd ed. New York: Springer Publishing Company; in press.

4. White M, Gundrum G. Case management. In: Evashwick C, ed. *The Continuum of Long-Term Care: An Integrated Systems Approach*, 2nd ed. Albany, NY: Delmar Publishers; 2000.

5. Austin CD, McClelland RW, eds. *Perspectives on Case Management Practice*. Milwaukee, WI: Families International;1996.

6. Parker M. Positioning care management for future health care trends. *GCM J.* 1998;8:4–8.

7. Vocker M. Care management from the perspective of a not-for-profit agency. *GCM J.* 1996;6:11–15.

8. Hereford RW. Private-pay case management: let the seller beware. *Caring.* 1990;9:8–12.

9. Bellucci M, Tonges MC, Kopelman R. Doing well by doing good: the case for objective feedback in case management. *J Case Manage.* 1998;7:161–166.

CHAPTER 6

Improving Care and Profitability through Integrated Information

Rick Zawadski and Michael Zawadski

INTRODUCTION

Effective use of information and information technology is essential for the efficient operation and management of any business today. Geriatric care management practices that have grown beyond the "one-person shop" are businesses with distinct and demanding information systems needs. At one time, all an organization needed to succeed was an organized office, caring staff, and good common sense, but today's organizations need more.

Several factors have contributed to the need for the integrated information system (IIS) within the contemporary geriatric care management agency. First, as the number of persons served by geriatric care management agencies increases and the cases become more intricate, there is heightened pressure for more effective and consistent care monitoring, service coordination, and planning. The complexity of operating a geriatric care management practice increases not only with the addition of new clients, but also with the addition of new case managers. Second, many geriatric care management practices today have multiple sources of funding. While new reimbursement sources are a reason to celebrate, each new funding source unfortunately comes with new reporting requirements. Third, there is an increasing interest in outcome measures; funders, potential funders, clinical staff, and consumers want to know the benefits of geriatric care management services. Specifi-cally, funders want benefits described in objective, rather than anecdotal, terms. Geriatric care management companies must, therefore, become efficient at capturing and disseminating information to ensure that new reimbursement sources create more cash flow and do not just add to administrative costs.

This chapter focuses on the role of information and the IIS in the development and operation of geriatric care management practices. It briefly reviews some operations that have implications for information management. The chapter then presents a model IIS for the modern geriatric care management practice and practical issues associated with the development and implementation of such an IIS. The chapter ends with a discussion of the value of the IIS, issues involved with data sharing, the role of the Internet in building national databases, and the ability of this medium to help bring new clients to a geriatric care management practice.

INFORMATION AND GERIATRIC CARE MANAGEMENT ORGANIZATIONS

Why do geriatric care management organizations need information? Every successful business needs to know who its customers are, what services and benefits it provides, and what it costs to do business. Geriatric care management organizations have the typical information needs of a business plus the additional information needs and information management problems of a new and growing service. At the macro level, information can help geriatric care management organizations create new funding sources by demonstrating their services' value. At the micro level, information can help individual practices use data to increase the quality of care provided and to cut clerical costs.

Growing Role in Long-Term Care

Geriatric care management will play an increasingly important role in the nation's health care system as the population ages and its need for long-term care grows. Geriatric care management organizations serve persons needing support with a range of medical problems, cognitive impairments, and other personal assistance needs. They fill a variety of liaison and organizational roles that traditionally have been filled by older family and friends. Although families usually have the best understanding of a client's needs, good geriatric care managers (GCMs) are often better advocates for the client. There are several reasons for this. Not only do GCMs have a superior knowledge of care providers and options, but they also are able to use established assessment tools to carry out an objective review of a client's needs. In addition, as an objective third party and experienced professional, they bring a higher level of credibility to meetings with providers.

According to the U.S. Census Bureau, the number of persons aged 65 and older has increased by a factor of 11 during the 20th century. Fifty percent of those 85 years and older need assistance with activities of daily living (ADLs).[1] Many of these individuals are candidates for the services of a GCM, but only a few are now served by GCMs. Although the exact number of GCMs currently in practice is not known, the National Association of Professional Geriatric Care Managers (established in 1986) has directory listings for more than 1,000 GCMs.[2] It is almost certain that the geriatric care management field will continue to grow as the population ages and families' need for assistance with their older members' care increases.

Information Management Needs

At present, information management systems within the geriatric care management field vary widely and there are no industrywide standards, for several reasons:

1. Geriatric care management is a fledgling field.
2. GCMs perform many different functions.
3. There are many varieties of geriatric care management agencies.

There are, however, certain types of functions that most geriatric care management organizations perform and thus certain information management needs that they share. GCMs are professionals who specialize in assisting older adults and their families in understanding their options for long-term care and making arrangements for such care. They may have training in gerontology, social work, nursing, or counseling. The term "GCM" covers providers who offer a wide variety of services, including screening clients; arranging and monitoring in-home assistance services; reviewing financial, legal, and medical issues; offering referrals; providing crisis intervention; acting as a liaison among the client, family, and professional service provider; providing consumer education and advocacy; and offering counseling and support. Some GCMs also provide family or individual therapy, money management, and conservatorship or guardianship assistance.

Although most GCMs have similar duties, they are part of many different types of organizations. Some GCMs are stand-alone, single-person providers. Others may be part of an agency that has multiple providers that may offer additional services, such as home care. Still other GCMs may work as part of an affiliated group of regional or national providers. This can be as a part of an alliance or through a traditional franchise model.

While each organizational type will, of course, have different needs and methods for managing information, the data they need to collect to assess needs, make referrals, schedule care services, and manage and bill for services are remarkably similar. At the same time, the diversity of the industry and the need for individual geriatric care management practices to stand out in the marketplace present barriers to the creation of a single information system that can meet the needs of a large number of providers. Looking to the future, it is likely that GCMs will opt for the benefits from working together to create common standards that allow for the creation of industrywide tools. At least this has been the endpoint in most mature industries. Common standards would not only make high-quality information tools available to providers at a lower cost but also create a large store of comparable data.

The absence of any national industry standard means that funders and consumers are not able to compare providers' effectiveness or know, in other than anecdotal terms, about the effectiveness of the services GCMs provide. Such information is becoming increasingly important, particularly given the growing trend for funders such as Medicare and health maintenance organizations (HMOs) to operate at a multistate level. Although not currently funders of GCMs, health care funders are increasingly willing to consider funding community services for clients with significant health needs where the level of care can be defined and the benefits demonstrated. Unfortunately, within the geriatric care management industry there is no ongoing collection of cross-site, cross-state data that can address outcomes. Individual providers do typically spend significant time collecting data for assessment, funding requirements, or licensing, but this work is seldom entered into a database within an agency to help people benchmark for outcomes and rethink care decisions. Furthermore, this information is almost never shared with other agencies.

In contrast, home health agencies, rehabilitation centers, and adult day services providers have established common, cross-state definitions of their role, clients, and services, making it easier for them to establish funding relationships with national funders such as Medicare,

private insurers, and HMOs. The investment in industry-specific software for this purpose is now the norm for these other community provider types. Access to these increasingly sophisticated information systems and networks will help GCMs demonstrate outcomes, gain national funding, and win a larger share of the long-term care dollar.

It has been demonstrated that investment in information tools yields dividends in the long run. Many organizations, however, are tempted to forgo these long-term returns because of the required initial investment. It is the challenge of software makers to lower this barrier sufficiently to attract enough geriatric care management organizations to create a viable market. Similarly, geriatric care management organizations face the challenge of selecting the best product available today, with an eye toward tomorrow. Unless geriatric care management organizations are able to work with good software makers to create a viable product for their industry, the organizations will never be able to share data efficiently or benefit from the economies of scale that an industrywide standard product can provide. The development of low-cost, consumer-friendly information systems and tools for tiny markets such as geriatric care management is possible only when both players—in this case, software makers and geriatric care management organizations—recognize that a symbiotic relationship must exist between them. By helping geriatric care management organizations to share and compare data across agencies and across states, such systems and tools will prove to be critical in establishing geriatric care management organizations as key players in the future landscape of long-term care.

INFORMATION SYSTEM BASICS

What Is Information?

Information consists of facts, figures, and other data put together in a meaningful way. Data exist in various forms, including simple observations (e.g., Mr. Jones became a client today; he was born on April 10, 1907; or he answered three out of seven questions correctly on a mental status test). These facts and figures are data. A lot of unanalyzed data can be overwhelming. To make data more useful, they are often summarized in some meaningful way. For example, the data about Mr. Jones and other clients might be summarized as follows: "Geriatric care management agency X has an average active client load of 56; they range in age from 64 to 94; and more than half (68%) are cognitively impaired." An information system organizes raw data and transforms them into useful information. One page of aggregated information is often worth more than 1,000 pages of unprocessed data.

What Is an Integrated Information System (IIS)?

An IIS is basically a black box: people put in the information they have and extract the information they need. Most service providers and managers do not care how the IIS works as long as they can get the information they need, when they need it, with accuracy and minimum use of resources. This is not as simple as it sounds.

An IIS offers significant advantages to the organization and its clients. Single data files are capable of holding and manipulating one information set, such as a list of clients and their addresses. Multiple data files take data processing capability one step further by linking different information sets together (e.g., linking the list of clients to the services they received, then to the center's accounting records). Different members of the service agency can collect these information sets at different points in time to meet different needs. An IIS is a more efficient way of organizing information because data used throughout the system only need to be entered once. The IIS eliminates the need for repetition of data collection by providing a framework for holding and accessing multiple data files in an organized and user-friendly fashion.

Geriatric care management organizations have much to gain from investing in the new and expanded use of information offered by an IIS. In order to deliver a single service, a geriatric care management organization must identify information on the patient or client, assess service need, track and describe services provided, and bill multiple funders (the client, family members, long-term care insurance, employers). Often, even within a single agency, multiple users collect their own overlapping information. Multiple sets of overlapping information are inefficient, and with each duplicated data entry the chance for human error doubles. Isolated data sets also limit the usefulness of the information gathered. An IIS offers geriatric care management organizations a well-defined plan that will link the various information sets collected by different units in an agency and make them available to meet the needs of multiple users in the most efficient and effective manner. By making more information available to all users, an IIS helps to improve service quality and increase efficiency.

Does an Information System Require a Computer?

Computers process data very quickly and accurately, which makes computers an ideal tool for implementing an information system. However, the computer is just a tool; what is important is creating an information system that identifies appropriate items of information and organizes those items in a meaningful way. In and of itself, a computer cannot accomplish these ends. Creating a good information system is like writing a book: the typewriter or word processor can help put the words on paper, but it is the quality of the content and the thought that went into it that make a book worth reading. So too with an information system, it is the quality and usefulness of the information that matters. Just as no smart author would ask a typist to write his or her book, no knowledgeable GCM should expect a programmer to create a useful information system on his or her own. GCMs may get involved either directly or by proxy. In an ideal world, an IIS would be developed by a team of GCMs, researchers, and software designers. Such a team could accurately identify important data elements, archive them properly, and provide an easy and reliable way to interface with the data.

It is important to understand that while computers may be the most visible component of an IIS, they are far from the most valuable or costly. In a typical IIS, the least expensive component will usually be the computer. This, of course, makes sense, as it is the most mass-produced component. With every computer sold each year, hardware development costs are shared by more people, making each computer less expensive.

If computers are the least valuable and costly part of the system, what is the most valuable and costly part? To start using a system, a GCM will need training. This can be self-directed time spent learning the system or time with a professional trainer. Next, someone will need to enter all the data into the system. Obviously, these tasks take time and money. Between the low cost of the computers and the high cost of data collection and training, the middle area of the IIS cost spectrum is the GCM's IIS software.

DIFFERENT MODELS FOR HOW ORGANIZATIONS USE INFORMATION

Information systems technology, including the hardware, software, and techniques for using information, has advanced dramatically over the last 20 years. In the geriatric care management field, information management has also been evolving from paper systems toward Internet-based networks. Today, a number of information system models coexist, varying according to the reason for collecting information and the tools or technology used. Each information system model has its strengths and weaknesses. Most agencies will use more than one of the following information user systems. (The scoring sheet in Exhibit 6–1 will help a geriatric care management organization assess its "information systems quotient" [ISQ].)

The Paper System

The first information systems were built with paper. Client intake sheets, indispensable "black books" listing service providers used in the past, schedule books filled with appointments, post-it notes with updated information, folders filled with progress notes, invoices with summary lists to record payments—these are all too familiar examples of paper systems. Probably every GCM uses some paper systems and many GCM organizations rely on paper for meeting their day-to-day information needs.

Efficiently producing accurate invoices for clients is often the driving motivation for creating an information system. When paying for services, the primary concern is usually accountability: Did this service get delivered? Often, citing when the service was delivered (October 15 at 10:30 AM), where it was delivered (client's home), and what the service was (interview of home care worker) is sufficient information for the payer of an invoice. If a geriatric care management organization has more than one payer, however, different billing formats may be required for each one. This can lead to overlapping billing reports with high administrative costs and limited management or clinical benefit.

Paper-based systems may seem straightforward to create, but in reality they are time-consuming to develop, maintain, access, and analyze. As a result, they are underutilized and often are eventually abandoned. Moreover, while paper forms can be as helpful as an electronic system in reminding users what to collect, they are unable to do anything with the data collected without time-consuming hand sorting and manual calculations—both of which are prone to human error.

Electronic Systems

Information technology—computers and software—can be used to automate the information management function for GCMs. Good computerized systems address the same basic needs of the paper systems but ideally simplify the data collection process, improve access to the information, and use the same collected information in many additional ways.

Building an IIS and using technology to link data sets and make data collection easier can

Exhibit 6–1 Assessing a Geriatric Care Management Agency's Information Systems Quotient (ISQ)

Information Use

7   The agency runs on information, continually monitoring its performance against goals.

6   Information is being used by service staff to guide and track client services.

5   Service and billing staff use the same information files.

4   Funder reports are produced by computer and/ or service billing is done electronically.

3   Lists are produced for appointments using a word processor.

2   Information is collected on paper for funders or others.

1   Agency collects no information, does not know how, and does not want to do so.

Staff Skills

7   Agency staff develop customized software and provide assistance to other agencies.

6   All staff are skilled users of all applications and use the Internet to get information they need.

5   All key office and service staff have basic computer skills and use the technology.

4   Key staff are skilled users of geriatric care management software packages.

3   Some staff are skilled users of office, word processing, and spreadsheet software.

2   Staff are interested in technology and ready to learn.

1   No one on staff has ever touched a computer.

Tools (Hardware)

7   The agency has a networked computer system that is linked with geriatric care managers on-line though an intranet.

6   Modems link the agency's computers with computers in a second location.

5   Multiple computers in the agency are linked together as part of a network.

4   Multiple computers are sharing the same printers, but there is no network for data sharing.

3   There are one or two personal computers in the agency, and they are not linked.

2   There is a data entry terminal only.

1   The agency uses nothing more automated than a mechanical pencil.

Tools (Software)

7   Software electronically links the agency information to outside databases for regional, state, and national comparisons.

6   There is a single integrated software package meeting all information needs of the agency.

5   There is specialized software for specific tasks (e.g., billing, funding reports).

4   Database systems are used.

3   Spreadsheets are used.

2   Basic word processing software is used.

1   Information and forms are stored in folders in a file cabinet.

---

produce better information for both payers and providers. In addition to using billing data to create bills, an electronic system can use billing data to provide GCM efficiency reports. It can provide quick answers to questions such as the following: Which GCM is billing the most hours in the agency? Who is doing the most assessments? How long do a given GCM's clients remain with the agency? With each question answered, it becomes even more clear that an IIS is more valuable than a paper system.

Common PC Tools

The revolution in personal computers (PCs) during the mid-1980s and the growth of user-

friendly tools brought significant changes to the field of information management. Such tools have begun to make their way into geriatric care management organizations, but the process has been slow. This slow rate of growth can be explained by two factors: (1) GCMs are trained as caregiving professionals and as such are focused on interacting with people, not on establishing management systems, and (2) there are few software products designed specifically for geriatric care management organizations.

As was typical in other community long-term care organizations, at geriatric care management organizations the first PCs sat idle for a while before anyone could find a use for them. At first, geriatric care management organizations began to use generic software tools to meet specific needs. Word-processing programs were used to produce mailing lists and attendance schedules, and even to prepare service bills. Spreadsheets were being used to summarize client characteristics and services, prepare fiscal reports, and sometimes even do payroll. Over time, many geriatric care management organizations found that they did not lack an information system; rather, they had too many! There was one for client contacts, one for providers, another for client case notes, and so on. When each new issue arose, a new system would be created to address it.

Evolution toward Integrated Systems

These general-purpose tools and homemade solutions did improve the quality and usefulness of information, and they reduced the time needed to produce and update it. Word-processed documents and spreadsheets, however, are not ideally suited for many of these information functions. They seldom link information across different lists and reports (leading to duplication of effort and data inconsistency), and they are usually confined to a specific organization—that is, they are not shared or standardized across different geriatric care management organizations. Intuitively, what GCMs who used these generic software tools were doing was creating parts of what could be a whole IIS. Unfortunately, these components, not designed to be linked, are incapable of being directly connected into a single system. In order to be linked, the elements would have to be stored in a database table and accessed properly through the use of database code.

Function-Specific Applications

Specialized software packages—for example, accounting systems—have been developed to do specific tasks. Yet a customized accounting package for a single organization can cost well over $100,000. When an application is developed and sold to a large group of users, the cost for each user can be kept very low, just as with hardware. In the 1980s, standard accounting packages could be bought for $10,000 to

$25,000, with the development costs, in effect, being shared by the 10,000 companies that purchased the product. Today, a PC-based accounting package like Peachtree Accounting or QuickBooks, with more capabilities and features than a $100,000 customized system, can be purchased for less than $200. Competition and a large market (500,000+ users) keep the cost for each user low.

These specialized packages, if they meet a geriatric care management organization's needs, can be a great value, since functions like payroll and accounting are the same for most organizations. Programs for billing case management and nutritional assessment can also be useful. On the downside, some specialized packages may not fully meet the geriatric care management organization's needs, creating more work to change or accommodate the differences. In addition, using different packages for many different functions can lead to errors and wasted time duplicating data entry.

Customized Geriatric Care Management Information Systems

Computerized information systems specific to community long-term care have been around for almost 30 years. In large businesses, including large health providers such as hospitals, mainframe computers and minicomputers developed in the 1960s were being put to use in the 1970s for operational needs such as billing and accounting, but computers were generally too expensive at the time for community service programs. This began to change with the development of minicomputers in the mid 1970s. For example, On Lok Senior Health Services used a minicomputer to develop an information system for its first Adult Day Center, later adapting this to an on-line minicomputer to meet the clinical and management needs of its expanded community long-term care system.[3]

When they were introduced, customized multiuser systems were useful tools in meeting the specific information needs of some of the larger and more innovative community long-term care agencies. Unfortunately, these custom systems were too expensive for most community organizations. Not only was the hardware still costly at that time, but developing such systems required programmers, technical staff, and, most important, managers with information systems skills to design, develop, and manage these information tools—staff members these organizations generally did not have.

Multifunction Integrated Geriatric Care Management Packages

The PC and powerful database programs have made it possible to develop an affordable IIS that is tailored to geriatric care management organizations. When a system meets the needs of a number of similar programs, the cost of development, which can range from $30,000 to over $500,000, can be spread across many geriatric care management organizations. The larger the market, the lower the cost per organization. While the number of geriatric care management organizations is small compared to the number of organizations in most industries, some multifunction IIS packages have been developed just for geriatric care management organizations.

Multifunction integrated systems are a good solution to many geriatric care management organizations' information systems needs. The best of these packages can, for a very low cost, meet the information needs of program managers, GCMs, and payers. Not only can an information system provide greater access to more information; if it is a good system and has been properly implemented, it should more than pay for itself in reduced staff time within the first year. Properly implemented, an IIS is a significant strategic advantage for any business. It cuts clerical costs and increases the amount of information managers have so that resources may be more intelligently distributed.

Even the best off-the-shelf geriatric care management packages will not meet all the needs of all geriatric care management organizations. The variation in geriatric care management information needs across program type, service mix, and funding source makes it important for geriatric care management organizations to choose the right system and, if possible, adapt the system to meet their needs. Groups of similar geriatric care management organizations can work together with system developers to build new packages or adapt one of the existing packages to meet their particular needs. Even the perfect system will not provide any benefits if the geriatric care management organization does not invest the time and resources to use it effectively. Effective use of the system includes an ongoing investment in staff training and upgrades to the IIS as a geriatric care management organization's needs change.

THE ROLE OF INFORMATION IN SPECIFIC CARE MANAGEMENT FUNCTIONS

Information can be useful in a number of different arenas within the field of geriatric care management. Computerized referrals and billing procedures speed up program operations and support the efficient provision of services. Information can be used to produce general management reports on costs, demographic profiles of the client population served, the caseload of each GCM, and so on. Program managers can also benefit from access to cross-site comparison information collected from other GCMs, including the success rate of different placements, the effectiveness of outreach by type, and other operational outcomes. This information can assist GCMs in completing a self-assessment of their strengths and weaknesses and guide their future management efforts. To demonstrate the value of such a system, a thumbnail sketch of a model system's major components is provided below: managing outreach, assessing clients, creating a service plan, matching clients and services, monitoring service delivery and quality, and billing for services.

Managing Outreach

An information system should start helping with clients from the time of their first contact with an agency. Switching from pen and paper to an IIS for recording inquiries has several advantages. Once the client's name and address are typed in, the client is in the system. This means mailing labels can be quickly produced to follow up on the call. Notes can be recorded that will allow the agency staff member who does the follow-up to personalize the next contact. By recording what prompted the call and how the caller heard about the agency, the organization can evaluate its marketing efforts. For example, the ad in the *Gazette* may generate the most inquiries, but referrals from Dr. Brown may actually yield the most clients. When the length of time between inquiry and enrollment is reviewed, it will become apparent when follow-up contact is needed and when it is no longer cost-effective.

Assessing Client Needs

Determining what level of care a client needs is arguably the most important function of a GCM. Standardized tools are commonly used to improve the accuracy of the assessment of a client's acuity and the level of care needed to meet his or her needs. These standardized tools can be incorporated into an IIS and administered at multiple points in time. Assessment data can then be compared item by item at these different points to assess changes in client health and functional status that may indicate a need to alter the care plan. The IIS can also help GCMs to track and compare outcomes for clients with similar problems who have received different packages of services and rate the effectiveness (or ineffectiveness) of a plan.

Creating a Service Plan

Armed with an information system that contains client assessment data, GCMs can create information-driven service plans. An IIS can isolate how clients with specific traits or a particular general level of acuity fared with different provider and service types. By implementing this system of continuous quality improvement (CQI) to client assessment and placement data, geriatric care management organizations can

make placements that not only meet clients' obvious needs but also have had the highest level of success with similarly assessed clients. Outcome data not only allow improvements in service quality but also furnish the data necessary to demonstrate the value of a geriatric care management service.

Matching Clients and Services

A core function of most geriatric care management practices is finding clients the best provider to meet their needs. In any given metropolitan area scores of providers will be able to meet the basic needs of a given client. The value of a GCM is his or her ability to make referrals that can fulfill the client's care needs, to provide services that are within the client's price range, and provide care in such a way that the client is satisfied with the placement.

The experienced GCM today is likely to have a "little black book" of providers. Names and notes are recorded in this book. To make referrals, a GCM flips to the pages listing providers that the GCM believes will be good matches. To make the referral, the GCM provides the client with notes on the provider; less commonly, notes on the client are prepared for the provider.

This paper method may, at first glance, appear to be efficient. However, the GCM may have failed the client by overlooking potential providers. Because people are, well, people, they may subconsciously overselect certain providers. Referrals often used in the recent past may be overselected "out of habit," whether or not those providers are the most appropriate for a particular client. The organizational structure of a hard-copy list will also tend toward overselection of certain providers simply because of their location on the list (e.g., AAA Home Care). Lastly, GCMs' anecdotal experiences with providers tend to skew their opinions.

Another shortcoming of a hard-copy system is that once appropriate referrals are selected, the client and provider data cannot be readily shared. Sharing this information in an organized, professional manner means retyping the selected list of providers for the client. A quick but still unsatisfactory alternative in a hard-copy system is an impersonalized collection of photocopied provider sheets or a collection of brochures with a note.

In an electronic system, this matching process is different. Instead of providers being selected by intuition and a scanning of provider notes, the client's assessment data are compared to the services of available providers. If an insufficient number of providers is returned in a search, desired characteristics of a placement can be added or dropped until a sufficient number of providers is returned. In evaluating which providers to keep on the list, a GCM has the opportunity to review who he or she has sent to the provider in the past and the outcome of that placement. Once the list contains a selection of providers whom the GCM is comfortable matching with a client, a click on "print" produces a referral list of all the selected providers, along with the search criteria they meet and do not meet for the client. At the same time, the GCM can print out a client characteristic sheet, omitting identifying data, to distribute to providers to see if they will accept the client. On either list, a brief personal note can be added. Each referral made is then recorded in the database.

The electronic referral reduces the clerical effort needed to create a referral. It also helps the GCM to avoid the tendency to unintentionally over- and underselect certain providers. It accomplishes this by searching for objectively defined criteria and comparing these criteria to the information in the provider database. This data set continues to increase in value over time as operational experiences are added to it. For example, when Mr. Jones returns for another Home Care Agency referral, it is already known to whom he was referred previously and who he selected. An agency may decide to omit certain providers from referral lists if it is found that clients rarely select those providers or are often dissatisfied with their service.

Another advantage to the electronic "little black book" is the ability to quickly update provider information. If a provider's address or phone number changes, one quick editing session will update the provider's information throughout the entire system.

Monitoring Service Delivery and Quality

After the referral is made, can an IIS continue to provide value? Yes. Once a client has selected a provider from the referral list, all that has to be done to track the client's enrollment on an ongoing basis is to update his or her status from that referral list. This allows one to view all of the client's active and past enrollments. Additionally, it is easy to create a list of all the clients that are actively enrolled with any one provider. For providers, this list will be concrete proof of the value of the agency's referrals. And any time GCMs are speaking with specific providers, the GCMs can easily look up with which clients the providers are working and ask for a progress report on those clients. Lastly, electronic progress notes can be created. These notes can later be linked to other important information: the client for whom the note was written, the provider mentioned in the note, the date of the note, and the care manager who wrote the note.

Billing for Services

Since the IIS has been used to input information on each client throughout the delivery of services, it is possible to use the system to create bills. The IIS simply reviews the system for all of the services provided to the client during the specified period, then creates a bill that lists the service dates and it is ready to be mailed out.

A MODEL INFORMATION SYSTEM PLAN FOR GERIATRIC CARE MANAGEMENT ORGANIZATIONS

Often deemed cumbersome and costly, when used correctly and consistently, an IIS is a feasible and worthwhile investment for geriatric care management organizations today. Below is a basic breakdown of what is needed to set up a cost-effective IIS in a geriatric care management organization.

Hardware

This chapter will not make specific hardware recommendations. Instead it will put hardware in perspective and will provide an overview of key hardware specifications. The most important thing to remember about hardware is that it is just part of an information system's budget and should not account for more than a third of this budget. Hardware includes not just the computer and monitor, but also the printer, modem, and network.

When purchasing hardware, people should remember the "$n - 1$" rule. In this equation, n represents the newest technology and 1 stands for one generation. Therefore, $n - 1$ means that it is best not to buy the newest version but the next to newest version. For instance, if an Intel Pentium III 500-megahertz chip is the best on the market, one should purchase the chip that came out before this chip. This rule is helpful because it helps highlight two truisms about hardware: (1) everything becomes outdated quickly, and (2) by not chasing the cutting edge one will lose little performance and save significant amounts of money. (See Appendix 6–A for a detailed explanation of specific hardware components.)

To Network or Not To Network

Agencies that own more than one computer have another question to address: Should the agency computers be networked? The likely answer is yes. Networking refers to the connecting of multiple individual computers together to allow the sharing of data and resources (e.g., printers). If more than one person will need to work on the same files or the agency decides to invest in an IIS, a networked system will be a necessity. The cost of networking a few machines in an office is quite minimal. All that is needed are network cards for each computer, cable between the machines, and a hub. All told, the cost of a simple local area network is less than $100/machine.

Laptops in the Field

Increasingly, GCMs want to take laptops into the field with them. This allows the rapid record-ing of notes and can eliminate the need for paper recording. Since the goal of taking a laptop into the field is to enter client data into the agencywide IIS, it is important that procedures be developed to ensure data integrity. The potential pitfall in collecting data that will later be transferred to the central database is that one can end up with two different pieces of information for one item in the database. For example, GCM A is in the field meeting with Mrs. Jones. During the visit, it is decided that Mrs. Jones will move into an assisted living facility tomorrow. GCM A promptly changes the address for Mrs. Jones in the IIS on her laptop. Later that day, Mrs. Jones' son calls to report that his mother has changed her mind and will instead begin living with him the next day. The receptionist at the agency promptly enters the new address for Mrs. Jones in the IIS. The next morning GCM A returns to the office and dutifully uploads all of her changes to the central IIS, thereby erasing the correct address for Mrs. Jones that was entered in the afternoon.

There are ways to avoid these problems. In theory the best way is to set up each laptop with a modem so that it makes all system changes directly on the main database at all times. This solution is, however, expensive to set up and maintain, and the speed at which the database may function over phone lines can be frustratingly slow. Another solution is to not allow anyone to make changes to Mrs. Jones' record while a GCM has her file on the laptop. In the scenario above, the receptionist would have notified GCM A upon her return that a client file she had "checked out" had a possible change. GCM A would then be responsible for reconciling which address was correct before she uploaded her changes to the main database. The complications involved in having people enter data into a holding database and later share it with the main database require vigilant adherence to well-defined processes. If the data in the database are not accurate, the point of having an integrated database is defeated. Once it is unclear if the data in the central database are accurate, one is forced to pick between two unpleasant options: erase all of the information, or reconcile it item by item.

Software

There are two types of software a geriatric care management practice will need to purchase for its information system: general applications and operations software. Software should account for about 30% to 40% of the total information systems budget, with the remaining portion of the budget reserved for training, support, and other implementation costs.

General applications, such as word processing and spreadsheet programs, are an essential resource in any office. They can be purchased as part of a software suite, or collection of software titles (e.g., Microsoft Office, which contains a word-processing program, a spreadsheet program, a presentation maker, and, in some versions, Web site design software and a simple database language for making small databases). A basic software suite should be considered an essential purchase for a geriatric care management practice.

The operations software (or IIS) will be the most expensive portion of a geriatric care management organization's software budget. Operational software is designed for a specific service (e.g., payroll, intake assessment, client referral). Some geriatric care management organizations may choose a custom-designed system. Those opting for a custom-designed system should expect to pay at least 300% more than those using or adapting an existing software product. The most cost-effective and efficient system is a market-tested, readily available, affordable system (with technical support) that will enable the collection and processing of the data an agency wants.

Just as people building houses follow an architectural plan, the geriatric care management organization building an information system should start with an overall IIS plan. Whether one develops a custom system, buys a ready-made system, or chooses to use paper, it is useful to understand the different types of information that can be collected and how information elements fit together. Figure 6–1 presents a general information system plan for a typical geriatric care management organization. Rectangles in the figure identify different sets of information

or files that GCMs need in order to manage and deliver high-quality, cost-effective services. Lines show some of the ways different files should be linked to each other.

The following sections discuss the major data components of a model geriatric care management information system. The sections give examples of items that should be included in each of the two major areas of information (patient and fiscal) and a recommended frequency of data collection.

Client Information

Identification and Description Information. Identification and description information is basic information that identifies and describes the client. This information is collected at the time of application or enrollment and is used by everyone within the system. The master client record should include the following:

1. identifying information: name, address, phone, family contact, and Medicare, Medicaid, and insurance numbers
2. demographic information: gender, ethnicity, date of birth, marital status, and living arrangement
3. program status information: membership status, application date, referral source, reason for referral, enrollment, and closing date

Information will be recorded at enrollment and updated as changes (e.g., change of address or change in program status) occur.

Assessment Information. Before a GCM can determine a client's service needs, the client's health and functional status must be assessed. Assessment information can then be used to define major health conditions, classify clients by condition or level of care needed, and help in service decision making. Change in assessed health and functional status is a useful outcome measure derived from the comparison of time 1 and time 2 assessments. The client assessment record would include the following:

1. health status information: major medical conditions, active medications, review of

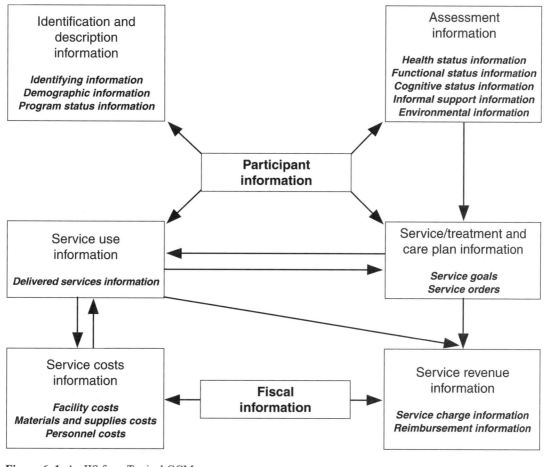

Figure 6–1 An IIS for a Typical GCM.

major health systems, and general health status

2. functional status information: level of assistance needed to support activities of daily living and instrumental activities
3. cognitive status information: short- and long-term memory, reasoning skills, and the ability to make decisions affecting personal well-being
4. informal support information: assessment of the informal support available to the client and the assistance this network (which can include family, friends, and neighbors) provides or could provide
5. environmental information: assessment of living environment to identify barriers to

maintaining independence and safety (e.g., stairs, bathroom facilities)

Assessment information changes over time and needs to be reassessed at regular intervals (e.g., quarterly, semiannually). Multiple assessments across these fixed time intervals should be stored and used to measure change.

Service/Treatment and Care Plan Information. A service or treatment plan is developed by the GCM based on assessment information and information received from the client and/or family. This plan is integrated and cuts across all service areas. The service/treatment plan record would include the following:

1. problem list: list of prioritized consumer problems identified from the assessment
2. service goals: measurable goals developed by the client and GCM for each problem
3. service orders: specification of the type and amount of services ordered for the client to meet service goals (e.g., the number of home health visits, scheduled medical procedures, active medications)

This information changes constantly as client needs change. An initial plan, developed at the time of assessment, would be stored with the assessment record as a snapshot of the client's service plan at a fixed point in time. The service plan record would then be continually updated to reflect progress achieved and changes made in the service plan. Information from this updated plan will be used for service scheduling.

Service Use Information. The service use record tracks all of the health and human services provided to a client through the GCM. This information is collected and organized by service type and amount and is summarized for a given time period. Service patterns can then be compared across clients and geriatric care management agencies and tracked over time. Service use can also be compared to the service plan to assess compliance, which is one measure of service quality. The client's service record would include the following:

1. delivered services information: date, type, and amount of health and health-related services provided through the GCM for the client

This information will be collected on an ongoing basis for each individual client. Individual service records will be summarized and reported for specified time periods (e.g., monthly, quarterly) as a measure of geriatric care management service benefits.

Fiscal Information

Service Revenue Information. Geriatric care management services are reimbursed in a number of different ways: fixed annual program payments; monthly, daily, or hourly service fees; and fees for specific services such as assessments, crisis intervention, and care plan development. Many geriatric care management organizations will have multiple funding sources, and each may use a different payment mechanism. Geriatric care management organizations could evaluate their reimbursement systems to identify those that best reflect cost or provide the best return. The comparison of amounts billed and received from clients for services is a measure of profitability, also useful data. The service revenue record would include the following:

1. service charge information: the date and amount charged for each health and health-related service provided to participants
2. reimbursement information: the amount of payment received for each service from each funding source

This information can be collected on an ongoing basis from the geriatric care management organization's billing system. Service use records may be used to automatically compute bills for each participant. Total service charge information by client can be computed on a monthly basis. Revenues for all geriatric care management services could be tracked separately for each funding source.

Service Costs Information. Charges do not necessarily reflect costs. Where possible, an attempt should be made to capture the cost of services. This information can be ascertained through the agency's fiscal system or independently gathered from cost estimates of time, facilities, and materials needed to provide the service. A chart of accounts would be established for the geriatric care management organization, and expense information would be collected. An expense reporting system would integrate different types of expenses and group them by service area. The program cost record would include the following:

1. facility costs: cost of facilities, equipment, and general overhead involved in the delivery of the geriatric care management organization's services

2. materials and supplies costs: cost of materials and supplies used in the delivery of the geriatric care management organization's services (accounts payable)
3. personnel costs: salaries and benefits for staff involved in the delivery of the geriatric care management organization's services (payroll data)

Cost information would ideally be derived from the agency's general ledger system and reported on a monthly basis. Alternatively, cost information could be estimated on a periodic basis from multiple sources (e.g., through time analysis or prorating of facility use). Cost per unit of service can be measured by comparing total expenditures by cost centers to service counts for the same time period. Cost information can be compared to revenue received by service and overall by client.

INFORMATION SHARING AND THE VALUE OF AN IIS

Sharing information and combining or integrating a data set with other data sets can increase the value and usefulness of information. Integration can occur at a number of levels within a program, among multiple services in a multiservice program, or across programs of the same kind. An IIS provides benefits at each of these levels.

Within Geriatric Care Management Organizations

The geriatric care management model system described above is predicated on the principles of integration within a geriatric care management agency. Integrating information within an agency provides many benefits. For example, an IIS can allow GCMs to share referral sources within an agency, members of the staff can readily take over for a fellow GCM who has a crisis, and all members of an agency can compare their outcomes to peers' outcomes to further hone their skills. Different service plans can be compared to assess what service plans help

clients remain in the community longest. Changes in assessment scores over time can be used to evaluate the effectiveness of the services and, in turn, refine service planning. The integration of fiscal and client information would allow for the measurement and tracking of service cost and enable the assessment of cost-effectiveness and cost-benefit analysis.

Across Service Programs

Geriatric care management clients can have multiple problems and needs and receive services from multiple providers. Increasingly, GCMs may find themselves part of a multiservice program either through their parent agencies or as part of a community service network. In a multiservice agency, vertical information integration (the sharing of information across different services) offers additional coordination benefits. Integrating information across the provider network can provide a more comprehensive picture of each client, his or her health needs and conditions, the services he or she receives, his or her treatment outcomes, and the total cost of his or her care. Sharing client information within a coordinated service network can also relieve the burden on consumers of repeated data collection. By linking information across different services, an IIS would support care management decisions that improve the quality and limit the total cost of care. This issue is especially appropriate as GCMs become partners in managed care. The sharing of information across programs serving similar populations would also yield valuable research data and support the development of cross-site performance indicators.

Across Geriatric Care Management Organizations

As part of a relatively new profession, geriatric care management organizations can also benefit from sharing information across agencies at the local, state, and national level. Horizontal information integration (the sharing of information across geriatric care management organizations) would provide advances in practice and performance management, would facilitate the standardization of information, and would enhance national funding for this service.

For the individual geriatric care management organization, the creation of a multiagency database would provide a reference point for comparison. Geriatric care management agencies could access standard management reports that would provide useful feedback comparing their performance to normative data for similar agencies. This form of monitoring would help geriatric care management organizations identify their strengths and weaknesses and guide the allocation of agency management resources. The database could also help further strengthen programs by identifying optimal service plans and standards for cost and care outcomes.

In time, horizontal integration would lead to the creation of a national database on geriatric care management programs and clients. This would support the development of common standards, definitions, and terminology and provide a valuable tool for clinical, program, and policy research and development. A multiagency database would make it possible to conduct ongoing cross-site research. An IIS would provide a framework for understanding differences among geriatric care management organizations. Agencies could be compared by state, type, and funding source. Researchers would be able to address a range of questions, including whether providers with an ancillary service like home care serve participants with higher levels of impairment; whether geriatric care management costs vary by licensing category; and whether geriatric care management organizations in different states are comparable. Key performance indicators and changes brought about by service innovations could be routinely monitored.

BARRIERS AND BENEFITS OF AN IIS

If the benefits of information are so clear, why haven't more organizations developed these systems? The development of an IIS is not easy; it often involves many changes in an organization.

Moreover, many new information systems have created more problems than benefits, especially during the initial development period. This section first reviews some of the factors that have been identified as concerns or impediments to information system development and then reviews some of the benefits of an IIS for different audiences. Appendix 6–B presents a guide to what a geriatric care management agency needs to get started in developing an IIS.

Barriers

Management Commitment

Many senior executives give "lip service" to the benefits of information but are not willing to make it a priority. An effective IIS cannot be built without a substantial commitment of time and resources. Information systems are not appliances that can be simply plugged in to work. They need to be selected and developed with input from key staff, they require ongoing support and training, and they often require changes in the way the organization does business. Halfhearted commitment and noninvolvement lead to system failure. The key ingredient of a successful system is the commitment of senior management to make it happen.

Shared Objectives

The development of an IIS requires agreement on objectives from all the parties concerned. The clinician wants timely and complete participant information, the manager wants summary information on all areas, and the fiscal manager wants to track and control costs. An IIS can meet the information needs of many audiences; however, these different objectives must be clearly stated, agreed on by all parties, and built into the system.

Willingness To Change

Change is difficult even when an alternative is clearly better. Most people would prefer the familiar; change takes time and effort. A new IIS will cause problems, and the organization should be prepared for them. The best way to minimize resistance to change within an organization is to involve those affected by the change in the development process.

Resources (People, Time, and Dollars)

The development of a good IIS will take considerable time, money, and organizational energy. Lack of resources is a common reason people give for not developing an IIS. This argument indicates a lack of commitment; if something is important, time and funding can be found. Geriatric care management organizations must realize there are costs associated with not integrating and using information. Duplicate records, missing information, and lost reimbursement cost the organization. While difficult to measure precisely, the cost-benefit of an IIS can be estimated. This task should be done before implementation.

Technology

Technology has also been cited as a barrier. Some managers believe there are technical problems preventing full integration. These excuses are simply not valid today. The available technology now exceeds almost all needs. Fast and powerful computers, low-cost memory, mass storage, flexible networks, communication options, and a wide variety of data entry options, from data sensors and bar code readers to scanners and pen-based notebooks, are available today. The tools and technology are available to overcome almost any technical barrier. Others cite fear of technology as a barrier. Yet even the fear of technology is diminishing as computers using graphical user interface make the technology increasingly user-friendly and new staff entering the field come with basic computer skills.

Confidentiality

Confidentiality concerns are raised by integration. Sharing of data across multiple services and providers will increase the threat to confidentiality. Protections (e.g., password-controlled access and confidentiality agreements) can be built into the IIS to safeguard confidentiality. However, the threat remains—increased

access means greater potential abuse. Increased vigilance will be required, and clients may be asked to sign releases of information. The benefits of an IIS for the client should outweigh the costs and justify these risks.

Interagency Cooperation

Perhaps the biggest barrier to integrating information in a geriatric care management agency will be the cooperation between competing agencies. Most service organizations are unaccustomed to sharing information; information can make them look bad. Changing the way they do business to meet an external request is difficult. It is relatively easy for a single organization to move once management has made a commitment. A collaborative effort is more complicated and requires the commitment of many. Cooperating agencies will have to see clear benefits if they are expected to extend the effort required. Geriatric care management organizations will also have to get comfortable sharing information, both good and bad, with each other.

Benefits

While not easy to implement, having an IIS is worthwhile. An IIS is an important tool in service delivery that potentially benefits all the players in the system. In general terms, an effective IIS would

1. reduce recording time by eliminating duplication of information
2. enhance service planning by expanding the amount of available information
3. support service delivery by using service plan information to automate scheduling
4. improve care outcomes by studying the cost and effectiveness of different clinical practices over time and across individuals

A geriatric care management organization has a number of different audiences or consumers of information that will each draw specific benefits from an IIS.

Managers

Managers can use the IIS to actively manage, rather than administer, their practice. The IIS can produce timely reports on the number and characteristics of participants served, the type and number of services provided, the cost of care, and GCM productivity ratings. Managers could set cost and service use goals and use the IIS to monitor performance. A good IIS would reduce administrative costs by eliminating duplicated data entry and by automating internal and external reports. Finally, the IIS would provide information to help the manager track costs and outcomes, across individuals and over time, to continually evaluate and refine the service program.

External Funders

External funders impose many reporting requirements. An IIS can help organizations meet those requirements in an efficient way. By coding services and revenues according to their funding source, the same IIS could be used to produce separate reports for each funding agency. In addition to cost data across time and place, demographic and assessment information could be provided for funders with increasing evaluation data requirements. An effective IIS could help with monitoring program development and implementation and meeting the needs of any external evaluation.

Program Developers and Researchers

An IIS is an ideal tool for the program developer and researcher and makes a geriatric care management agency a service development laboratory where program changes can be studied and improved upon on an ongoing basis. For example, services and costs can be tracked over time to study changes in care management and financing. Clients could be studied overall or grouped by condition. Assessment data from one time period to another could be compared to assess changes in health and functional status. These scores or outcome measures could be correlated with service use to evaluate service effectiveness and refine care plans.

Policy Makers and Shapers

Facts speak louder than words. Policy makers and shapers want to know about the impact of service delivery and financing models. An IIS can provide this information. Which geriatric care management services reduce the use of hospital days? Which ones enhance independence? By tracking costs and revenue information by funding source, organizations can determine the financial participation of different public funders. The proposed IIS could be used to assess the impact of different funding methods on client characteristics, services, and costs. Simply tracking costs across geriatric care management organizations will provide important but rarely captured information.

Clients

Most important, the client can benefit from an IIS. As noted above, an integrated system would reduce the need to provide data to each different provider. More easily accessed information can improve the quality of service plans. Changes in health and functional status could be used to measure outcomes and monitor quality. Finally, improvements in the system because of IIS-enabled research, development, and evaluation would enhance the effectiveness of the service plan and increase the quality of care, improving the outcomes for clients.

Growing a Business

While an IIS provides information advantages for many different audiences, the best reason for purchasing an IIS is that it makes good business sense. Any IIS package that cannot pay for itself within a year in reduced clerical staff time and improved payment processing should not be purchased. Throughout the business world, the efficiency of enterprise software has increased productivity and profits. Businesses have embraced information tools because they save businesses money. For financially challenged geriatric care management organizations, effective information tools can make the difference between a marginal business and a thriving enterprise capable of competing in a world increasingly dominated by managed care.

COMMUNICATIONS AND COMPUTING: THE INTERNET AND THE WORLD WIDE WEB

The Internet is a powerful new tool that is opening up many new possibilities for data sharing, knowledge building, and information exchange. It provides an excellent communications link for GCMs, researchers, policy makers, and consumers. The Internet is a perfect example of the benefits of combining computing and communication technology, enabling a new dimension of information sharing and data integration.

To access the Internet, one needs a piece of software called a browser. Currently, Microsoft Explorer and Netscape are the most popular options. Most state-of-the-art computers come with one or both of these browsers already installed. Once the browser is installed, it is necessary to set up an account with an Internet service provider (ISP). Some popular ISPs today are AOL, Juno, Mindspring, Altavista, and Yahoo.

Marketing a Geriatric Care Management Practice on the Internet

Marketing is one of the most obvious uses of the Internet for geriatric care management organizations. Consumers and their family members can learn about the benefits of geriatric care management and find an appropriate provider in any community on-line. A Web site provides a geriatric care management organization with a new outreach tool, enabling it to make information about its location, hours, services, and fees more available to its consumers and their advocates.

There are two basic ways in which a GCM or geriatric care management organization can market a practice on-line: (1) on-line directory listings, and (2) agency Web sites.

On-Line Directory Listings

The option requiring the least cost, and probably the least work, is entering a listing in an on-line directory. These listings can include just the name, address, and phone number or offer more expanded information, such as the number of clients the practice serves, accreditations, and services offered. Costs of such listings will depend on the directory and the amount of detail the listing contains. Many professional associations offer on-line directory listings to their members. For example, the Web site for the National Association of Professional Geriatric Care Managers (www.caremanager.org) contains a national directory listing of GCMs that consumers can search, containing basic name and address information for each listing.

Other on-line directories available, however, are geared more broadly toward long-term care services in general rather than one specific service type. An example of such an on-line directory is www.GetCare.com, a comprehensive long-term care directory that contains over 60,000 provider listings, including hundreds of GCM listings. Listing in these "broader" directories creates a marketing advantage in that consumers searching these directories may not be looking for one specific service type. These consumers will, therefore, be unlikely to search for services through specific professional association sites. As these listings are free, however, GCMs can list their services in multiple directories.

There are many advantages to listing a geriatric care management practice in an on-line directory. One advantage is that it requires no knowledge of Web design. The GCM or geriatric care management organization simply submits his or her information on-line and is then given instructions on how to update the listing when needed. Another advantage is cost. A basic listing is often free. Even using a more expanded listing, which often requires a fee, will cost less than setting up a Web site, or even a Web page (the GCM or geriatric care management organization is essentially just renting space on an already existing Web site). Setting up a Web page or Web site requires many start-up costs, including the costs of registering a domain name, purchasing or renting server space, and publicizing the site.

Listing a service in an on-line directory, however, does not necessarily preclude having a

Web site or page of one's own. Often, on-line directories will provide a way to link a listing to an individual Web site or page. This mechanism can actually increase the chances that consumers will find a particular geriatric care management site, in that large on-line directories are more likely to be found by search engines and more likely to be known by consumers and referring providers than individual geriatric care management Web sites or Web pages.

Agency Web Sites

Some GCMs and geriatric care management organizations will want to create a Web page or a Web site describing their practice. A Web page will contain just one "page" of information, while a Web site will contain multiple pages, internally linking to one another. Just like directory listings, Web pages and sites can vary greatly in their level of detail and complexity. Some sites contain many links to external sites, some have elaborate graphics, and some have only basic contact information. What a GCM or geriatric care management organization decides to put on a site depends partly on how much money can be spent and how much knowledge of Web programming staff members have (hiring an outside consultant is more expensive).

To set up any new site or page, one must register for a domain name. For example, if Joe Smith wants to create a Web site for his geriatric care management practice, he may want the address to be www.JoeSmithGCM.com. If the domain name "JoeSmithGCM" is available, he can register under that name. A recommended source for information on registering domain names and other aspects of setting up a Web page or Web site is www.networksolutions.com.

Some Web sites and pages are created by a GCM or a member of a geriatric care management organization's staff. Many books explain how to use Hypertext Markup Language, the code necessary for displaying information on the Web. Choosing this option can help build one's skills set but may result in a very simple Web page. The advantages of this option are that it is low cost (one is only paying for the cost of the domain name and the server) and easily maintained (because the page has been created inter-

nally, there is no need to rely on outside sources to update information).

Another relatively low-cost option for creating a Web page or site is to use a "template" Web page. Some Internet-based companies provide a service allowing customers to customize a template Web page to meet their organizational or personal needs. One option for this is www.GeoCities.com, which is a site that allows one to create a free home page. In order to provide free services, GeoCities reserves the right to place advertisements on its customers' Web pages. Other companies who offer this service may require a fee. The advantages for this option include low cost and ease of maintenance. If GCMs or other staff members have limited Web programming skills, they may be able to create a slightly more elaborate site than if they created the Web page themselves from scratch.

Another option, which is more costly, is to hire a consultant to create a Web site. Depending on the experience of the consultant and how complex a site is desired, the cost can range from a few hundred dollars to tens of thousands of dollars or more. The advantage of choosing this option is that the Web site or page may be very extravagant and high-tech. However, there are several disadvantages to this option. First, this option is the most costly. Also, because the site has been created by an outside organization, maintenance of the information on the site, over time, could become very difficult or even impossible. This could result in paying the consultant for each update or having to create a new site from scratch. Additionally, Web consultants often will know a great deal about Web programming and very little about the subject of the Web site or Web page. It is important for the GCM or geriatric care management organization to monitor the page or site content and the general message the site or page is sending.

It can be helpful to look at other geriatric care management sites, or even sites on other subjects, to get ideas for creating a new Web site or Web page. It is important to keep in mind that a Web page or site is not worth much if it is out of date. If it contains date-sensitive materials and those do not get updated, this can send a message that the business is not on the ball. And if a site is too flashy and expensive for an organization or GCM to maintain, the site may have to be shut down, which will send a negative message to site visitors about the business's stability.

E-Mail and the Internet

E-mail is a useful tool that comes free with almost all ISP accounts. This method of sending notes, electronic files, and even pictures is a great way to communicate, especially for making referrals. E-mail is usually less formal than a traditional note, so response times are usually faster. Plus, there is no postage to pay. Clients or their families may prefer to communicate through this medium. This mode of communication can be more private than talking on a phone in a crowded office, and clients or their families can respond at their leisure. E-mail should be checked regularly, typically at least once each business day.

In addition to the account received from the ISP, it may be helpful to set up a Web e-mail account. Several sites offer this service for free (e.g., www.hotmail.com). These services allow easy Internet access to e-mail anytime, no matter how or where the user is logged on. This can be a lifesaver when one is away from home.

Learning On-Line

The Internet has a wealth of information available, from new referral sources for clients to medical research. To search for sites efficiently, people should visit a Web portal site like www.yahoo.com. The last three letters of a Web site's address will identify its type. Three of the most common designations are ".com" (commercial), ".org" (nonprofit organization), and ".gov" (government). Keep in mind that not all information found on-line is verified. Caveat emptor is the rule when on-line.

Consumer Access to Services and On-Line Directories

The Internet provides an ideal vehicle for the creation of a dynamic on-line GCM directory. While helpful and sought after, printed directo-

ries become outdated quickly. One example of the magnitude of this problem was the California Adult Day Care directory that was published in 1994. A review of a sample of listings 2 years later illustrated that 30% of the information in the directory was out of date by 1996.[4] In comparison, Internet-based directories with on-line user updating are able to remain accurate and up-to-date. New Web sites are being developed to list community services, including those of GCMs. As discussed above in the section on marketing geriatric care management on the Web, hundreds of GCMs and 60,000 community long-term care services are listed on-line at www.GetCare.com, a Web site devoted to long-term care. Families from next door or across the country can search this site for GCMs and other community services by center name, city, Zip code, or area code. Hot links and electronic buttons connect basic directory information about a GCM to more detailed information from the GCM's individual Web site. User-friendly indexing or search systems, such as point and click maps, can quickly help users locate up-to-date information about GCMs anywhere in the country. Additional information on GCMs can be collected and used to classify GCM providers based on the types of services they provide or the client populations they serve. Once developed, GCM classifications could be added for ease of reference to this directory. As the Internet grows and develops, consumers will have the information to select the most appropriate center and services for their needs.

Communicating Information across GCMs

The Internet is also an excellent vehicle for disseminating geriatric care management program and policy information. A search of www.google.com, using the term "geriatric care manager", produced over 8,000 links, including GCM directories, individual GCM Web sites and news articles.[5] Web pages linked by keywords provide GCMs with a good medium for collecting, organizing, and disseminating information across services and across agencies. Membership organizations like the American Society on Aging (www.AmericanAging.org) and state associations are developing their own Web sites to connect their members and share information. The California Association for Adult Day Services, for example, has developed a Web site (www.caads.org) to disseminate information on new developments in the field and to provide technical assistance to its members through member-only Web pages and message boards. The association will be testing Internet data sharing. The Web site for the National Association of Professional Geriatric Care Mangement, www.caremanager.org, also provides resources and news/event updates to those in the field.

The Future of the Internet and Potential Concerns

The popularity of the Internet offers new promise and creates new concerns. On-line directories and geriatric care management news services can provide consumers and providers with easy access to the latest information. The Internet can be used to share client information across providers, reducing the need for duplicate assessment, and can make on-line national databases for clinical and policy research possible. However, easier data sharing also presents new threats to confidentiality. In time, confidentiality problems will be overcome and the growth of the Internet will encourage greater information sharing and cooperation among clinicians, managers, researchers, policy makers, and consumers and lead to better community-based services.

The new Health Insurance Portability and Accountability Act[6] recognizes the need for data exchange and is creating a number of new requirements surrounding the sharing of client health information. While good in principle, these requirements will pose new challenges to providers, funders, and researchers.

CONCLUSION

There is a wealth of information available for GCMs and geriatric care management organizations. Most GCMs and geriatric care management organizations are using only a fraction of the information tools available to them. The best GCMs will change that in the years ahead. They will use information systems to simplify their work, improve their effectiveness, and build national databases to strengthen their service.

With health care at the forefront of public concern and scrutiny, accurate records and cost containment are more important than ever. Competition among health care providers and the rise of managed care now necessitate not only that GCMs provide a satisfactory service and are financially viable, but that they also cooperate as partners in a continuum of care ranging from senior centers to hospitals. Information sharing will be integral to those partnerships.

Geriatric care management organizations, like many other types of organizations in the health and human services sector, are finally realizing the importance of the IIS in improving the quality and controlling the cost of care. Leading businesses are using information as the cornerstone to their efforts at improving service quality. Techniques such as CQI involve setting goals and using information to monitor progress continually. Service dollars are limited, and service need is growing. The effective service program needs to monitor cost as well as quality and use information to make the most of limited dollars.

GCMs need to overcome their ambivalence about collecting information on clients and services and their fear of establishing new reporting requirements. They need to recognize that their service infrastructure, their knowledge base, and their investment in computing and communications technology have not kept pace with other long-term care service providers. Investing time and resources in an IIS will be a significant step for any individual GCM. GCMs must be willing and able to make this step if they want to be players in the future.

Funders are moving rapidly toward electronic billing. New government regulations are expected to require computerized records from health care facilities within the next few years.

GCMs are currently behind in the IIS effort. Other industries have been more aggressive in the development and use of information systems. With standardized information on clients, services, and costs; with population-based data on GCM benefits and outcomes; with data systems linked to service partners and funders; and with viable business models, GCMs can become leading players in the integrated long-term care service systems of tomorrow.

NOTES

1. U.S. Census Bureau. "Sixty-Five Plus in the United States." http://www.census.gov/socdemo/www/age brief.htm (8 February 1999). Accessed 17 August 2000.

2. National Association of Professional Geriatric Care Managers. "Benefits of Membership." http://www. caremanager.org/gcm/BenefitsofMembership. htm. Accessed 17 August 2000.

3. Zawadski RT, Gee S. A practical guide to integrated computerized information management. In: Schwartz MD, ed. *Using Computers in Clinical Practice.* New York: Haworth; 1984.

4. California Association of Adult Day Services (CAADS) Directory, 1996.

5. Search, http://www.google.com/. Accessed 18 August 2000.

6. Health Insurance Portability and Accountability Act (HIPAA), Department of Health and Human Services, Health Care Financing Administration, 1996.

SUGGESTED READING

Alter S. *Information Systems: A Management Perspective.* 2nd ed. Menlo Park, CA: Addison Wesley Longman; 1996.

Barnett O. Computers in medicine. *JAMA;* 1990;263:2631–2633.

Gallo J, Fulmer T, Paveza GJ, Reichel W. *Handbook of Geriatric Assessment.* 3rd ed. Gaithersburg, MD: Aspen Publishers; 2000.

Goldberg IV. Electronic medical records and patient privacy. *Health Care Manag.* 2000;18:63–69.

Kane RA, Kane RL. *Assessing the Elderly: A Practical Guide to Measurement.* Lexington, MA: Lexington Books; 1981.

Laudon KC, Laudon JP. *Essentials of Management Information Systems.* 3rd ed. Upper Saddle River, NJ: Prentice-Hall; 1998.

Lutes M. Privacy and security compliance in the E-healthcare marketplace. *Healthc Financ Manage.* 2000;54:48–50.

Hardware Fact Sheet

The first step in setting up your integrated information system involves knowing what equipment to buy in order to make the system work best for you. Below is a fairly comprehensive list designed to help arm you with the knowledge needed to make good hardware purchasing decisions. Where possible, background information has been provided that is not time-sensitive; for this reason, specific product names and brand names have been omitted. With the speed of change in computer hardware, some information may become dated quite rapidly. Regardless, this list contains the basic information you need to get started.

THE MAJOR COMPONENTS

CPU—The CPU (central processing unit) is the part of the computer that actually computes. The faster the processor, the better. Processors should be judged by two factors: (1) their speed (measured in megahertz), and (2) the model number (e.g., 486, Pentium III). Please note that a 486 100-megahertz machine will be slower than a Pentium 100-megahertz machine. The higher the number for both classifications, the better. Remember the rule of "$n - 1$" when selecting a processor (choose not the latest model but the next-to-latest model).

Hard Drive—The hard drive is where your computer stores information. In most computer ads you will see hard drive capacity measured in "gigabytes" (1,000 megabytes = 1 gigabyte). Unless you plan on storing a lot of pictures or are

using the hard drive as a file server for your office network, any hard drive with 5 gigabytes should serve you well for a few years.

RAM—Random access memory (RAM) is like a hot file for your computer. Information held in these easily accessed files can quickly be sent to the CPU. RAM is measured in megabytes ("megs"). RAM is one component of your system on which you do not want to skimp. Although it is possible to add RAM later, starting at 64 megs is best, and in no case is it recommended to start with less than 32 megs of RAM.

KEY PERIPHERALS

Compact Disk Drive—A compact disk (CD) drive is included with most computers sold today. The speed at which CDs transfer data will be noted by a number followed by an X (e.g., 24X is an average read rate for CD drives today). A CD drive with a read rate above 24X will be of little value for most users.

Variations on this option include writable CD drives and digital video disk (DVD) drives. You should consider paying extra for a read/write CD drive. If your machine has one, you can back up your files to CDs. This avoids the necessity of purchasing an Iomega Zip drive or tape drive backup system. A CD drive may also be able to read DVDs. Whether or not this feature is valuable is a personal preference.

Modem—To get on-line you'll need a way to send and receive information to and from your computer. Unless you have a nonstandard phone line, a DSL (direct service line), ADSL, ISDN, or a T1 or T3, a standard modem will work just fine. For such users, a 56.6 kbps (kilobytes per second) modem speed is the best choice. Modems with this speed have been around for a few years so the price is low, and 56.6 kbps is the fastest speed at which standard phone lines can transfer information. Any slower modems should be avoided.

Monitor—Whether it is a laptop or desktop machine, a monitor is, of course, a necessity. Since monitors are typically compatible with a new machine and tend to change less over time, some people keep the costs of upgrading hardware down by keeping their old monitors. If this is your plan, you want to splurge a bit on your monitor. For a desktop machine a 17-inch monitor will work well. Going below a 15-inch monitor is not recommended.

When reviewing monitors, be aware of the following terms: (1) *pixel size* (a number of 0.25 or lower is advisable), (2) *refresh rate* (a quick refresh rate will lessen eye strain, a good refresh rate being 80 per second or higher), (3) *viewable image* (monitor marketing materials will give you two monitor size figures; the number in the big print will be in whole inches [e.g., 15"], but the other number, viewable image, is actually more important). When comparing prices, be sure to compare viewable image sizes.

Laptops, and now some desktop machines, have LCDs (liquid crystal displays), also known as flat-panel displays. These monitors should be rated on one additional criterion: active matrix versus passive matrix. The only type of passive matrix commonly sold today is dual scan. While dual scan screens are a lot cheaper, there is a good reason for the price difference. Active matrix screens are definitely superior.

Printers—The two major classifications of printers are laser printers and inkjets. Laser printers offer a crisper image for printed documents. Although the ratings for an inkjet and a laser printer may be identical, the process that transfers ink to the paper will result in a different quality product. The laser printer fuses ink to

paper, whereas the inkjet spray paints the paper.

The standard for rating printers is dots per square inch, or dpi. The higher the number, the better. A current benchmark of quality is 600 dpi for both laser printers and inkjets. An office network can be efficiently served with one quality laser printer coupled with easily accessible inkjets for drafts of documents. Color inkjets are not much more expensive than one-color inkjet printers and are probably worth considering. Color laser printers are currently prohibitively expensive.

3.5-inch drive—A 3.5-inch drive is a standard feature on all machines except the Apple iMac.

NETWORKING

Hub—If you are connecting more than two machines, a hub will be a useful piece of equipment to purchase. A hub takes information from one source and sends it to all of the recipients it can find. For this reason it is easy to set up: you simply plug the 100 base T wires into the hub. If you have selected 100 base T as suggested, it is important that your hub and all network cards be using this speed line. If you have an older machine using a 10 base T line, you can purchase a switchback cable to synchronize this machine with the rest of your network. As the number of linked machines in your network grows, a hub will become a less efficient solution.

Network Card—To network your machines you will need a network card in each machine. A network card is a modem that sends data only to other machines in your network. A network card purchased today should be "100 base T" or better. This new standard, replacing 10 base T, allows the transfer of data at 100 megabytes per second. A 100 base T cable will plug into the back of the network card just like a phone line into a phone.

Router—A router is a smart hub. Whereas a hub sends all the information to all the recipients it can find, a router sends things on the fastest available route and only to the desired recipient.

What Does My Agency Need To Get Started?

Getting started can seem like an impossible task, if your care management agency has never used information systematically or used computers to manage its information needs. Standing back from everyday demands and taking the time to plan for a change in the way you manage information and for the introduction of computers into your organization is a good first step. Once you have done this, everything else will be easier.

There are five basic components to consider:

1. *Equipment.* The first rule in buying any computer equipment is not to invest in more hardware than your agency is likely to need and use over the next 2 to 3 years. Salespeople will be happy to talk you into buying the latest and greatest gizmos, but remember, if you do not need it, or do not have the resources to use it effectively, then you should not make the investment. If you do, your computer equipment is likely to become obsolete before you get to the stage of using it to its full capacity. Hardware costs today are becoming the smallest part of the investment. In 1999, a capable PC could be purchased for as little as $600. For a small additional cost, two or more computers could be linked together in a network, which is very useful if staff plan to share information.

2. *Software.* Appropriate software enables a geriatric care management agency to keep pace with the always changing, increasingly complex world of health care. The success of a geriatric care management agency today is largely dependent on its ability to handle larger caseloads, keep track of multiple sources of client funding, and provide funders and potential funders with data-driven proof of benefits. In business today, a state-of-the-art IIS is not just a tool but a strategic advantage. Much can be done with word processors and spreadsheets, but an integrated database system is the best way to coordinate data collection across staff and programs. There are software packages developed specifically for GCMs. One option is to work through your state association to develop or adapt an existing software package to address common needs of GCMs in your state.

3. *Training.* Never underestimate the importance of training. A car has little value if you do not know how to drive. A software package will be useful only if you learn how to use it. Without training, your staff members are not likely to use software tools to their full potential. If you are buying a software package, make sure that it comes with a good manual and that technical assistance is readily available. Organized training programs are often the quickest and best way to become familiar with a new software application. Allow staff time to learn new software and en-

courage staff members to help each other. If data entry staff have a high rate of turnover, training is all the more important.

4. *Support.* Consider investing in technical assistance and support when designing and developing your integrated information system. There are many user-friendly tools, but the new technology is constantly changing and the options can be confusing. If you are not comfortable with the technology, making a small investment in support will often save time, build confidence, and help you make the right decisions along the way. It is a waste of time and money to "rediscover the wheel." Take advantage of the experience and knowledge of others. Ask similar organizations for recommendations and talk to several people before deciding with whom to work. Make sure you find someone who can speak your language and who will help you find your way around all the computer jargon. Don't, however, let the *programmer program your program*, that is, define your services for you. The good support provider *helps you implement your vision.*

5. *Commitment.* Commitment is the most important element in developing and implementing an IIS. Change is never easy and the commitment of everyone involved will be a key factor in your success. Commitment of senior management is needed to shape a system appropriate for the organization, find and make the resources available, and inspire staff support for the change.

PART III

Growing and Managing the Business of Geriatric Care Management

CHAPTER 7

Marketing Geriatric Care Management

Cathy Cress

Without customers, geriatric care managers (GCMs) do not have a business, whether they are part of a for-profit or nonprofit structure. Marketing is the way to attract and retain customers.

Why market? Customers have choices. They can choose one GCM instead of another, or they can choose not to use geriatric care management at all. Most communities have more than one GCM. In addition, communities have practitioners in other professions who can do part of what GCMs do (e.g., medical social workers, medical case managers, physicians, and case managers in home health agencies and hospices). Competition is stiff.[1] Marketing tells customers how geriatric care management will help them and why they should choose one GCM instead of another.

BEING A CARE MANAGER AS WELL AS A SALESPERSON

Many GCMs today are not just care managers but business owners, and therefore salespeople. GCMs used to wearing the care manager hat frequently have a hard time with the new role. As care managers, GCMs are always giving to clients, offering advice, direction, and professional expertise. As salespeople, GCMs ask rather than give. This role reversal, with the GCM in need of the client instead of the client in need of the GCM, can be unsettling. A salesperson is not in control in the same way that a GCM is.

Not everyone can make the leap from care manager to salesperson. Women in particular may have difficulty, and most GCMs are women. In a recent survey of members of the National Association of Professional Geriatric Care Managers (NAPGCM), 89–90% were women.[2] In our culture, a traditional woman's role involves constantly giving—to partners, to children, to clients, to friends. A giver is praised for supporting, loving, and compromising in the interest of the group. This is essentially a very passive role. In the role of a salesperson, a GCM must be assertive. This is a difficult transition for many women. Before they make it, women should ask themselves some questions: Can I ask someone for his or her business? Can I close a sale? Can I be aggressive rather than passive?

Many GCMs come from fields in which little formal marketing is done. Nurses and social workers do not do a lot of marketing, and many GCMs come from these professions. Someone who once owned a hamburger stand and is now buying a pizza parlor is also making a transition but has already had some experience with marketing and running a highly competitive business. Human services professionals do not often advertise their skills and rely instead on referrals. Most human services professionals have worked for nonprofits that serve a need rather than sell a need. The customers were at the door because of their need, so attracting customers was not a problem. The problem was finding funding to support the clients, and the funding did not usually come from sales. Furthermore, nonprofits do not outwardly seek to make a profit.

Many human services professionals also have traditionally considered marketing their services to be unsavory, unprofessional, and demeaning. They view their profession as providing ethical caring and needed services and perceive sales as sordid because it reeks of manipulation—getting someone to buy something. Salespeople have been seen as cajoling, maneuvering, and just plain tricking other people to make a sale. GCMs will need to eliminate this bias if they are trying to start a geriatric care management business.

But people from human services backgrounds have one distinct advantage when it comes to marketing: They know how to establish relationships. Marketing is about not just sales and advertising but relationships. A client is buying not just a GCM's expertise but a relationship with the GCM.[3] In doing sales, GCMs can tap into what they already know: how to establish and nurture a relationship with a client. For example, an adult daughter living far from her older parent is purchasing both the GCM's expertise and a relationship with the GCM. She wants the GCM to be solicitous, offer a shoulder to lean on, counsel her when she is suffering, and allow her to call day or night in times of trouble with her parent. A trust officer wants to be able to rely on the GCM for help with older clients' problems.

In deciding whether they can make the transition from care manager to salesperson, GCMs should take several steps. As mentioned above, they should consider whether they can be assertive enough to sell their services and whether they can eliminate their bias against sales and marketing. Getting workshop tapes on marketing and sales from NAPGCM and Case Management Society of America (CMSA) conferences is an easy first step. Second, GCMs can attend regional meetings of NAPGCM and CMSA and speak to other GCMs or medical case managers about what it takes to market their services. If they are not able to attend a regional meeting, people can get the telephone numbers, e-mail addresses, or Web site URLs of association members and see if they will discuss their experiences in marketing. People can also attend the marketing workshops at the CMSA and NAPGCM conferences. In general, people should read all they can about marketing and sales.

SEEING THE CLIENT AS A CUSTOMER

To make the leap from being a GCM to being a GCM who markets his or her business, people have to learn to see their clients as customers. This change in outlook is critical to the success of a geriatric care management business.

Who are customers? Customers are people who need a product and shop around until they get what they want. Everyone is a customer at least some of the time. Customers are the people on whom a business depends. Therefore, every employee of a geriatric care management organization should treat customers as well as possible.

Human services professionals are used to seeing the people with whom they work as clients or patients with needs. But the world of geriatric care management is about more than needs; it is about preferences. Many providers can help clients, so clients are customers with many choices. They are likely to give their business to a GCM who sounds professional and solicitous over the phone, has a bright and attractive office, has a logo that is pleasing to the eye, returns phone calls right away, and takes a lot of time to discuss their concerns.

Human services professionals are used to providing people with high-quality services. GCM entrepreneurs need to learn to extend that quality beyond care management to these many other matters that affect consumers' purchasing choices (e.g., letterhead, phone manner).

WHAT IS MARKETING?

This chapter uses a very simple definition of marketing and discusses two aspects of marketing: public relations and advertising. Exhibit 7–1 gives definitions for marketing, public relations, and advertising.

Figure 7–1 shows the many groups of people that may be part of a geriatric care management agency's target market. The first major step in developing a marketing strategy is defining the target market. Any group that will buy the geriatric care management product or refer someone else to the product is part of the target market. Not every geriatric care management service will have the same groups in its target market.

Exhibit 7–1 What Is Marketing?

Marketing
Recognizing, defining, and understanding a target market and then directing a message to that target market to achieve desired goals

Public Relations
Low- or no-cost methods of reaching and influencing the public and ultimately a target market

Advertising
Utilizing paid media or other channels (e.g., direct mail, flyers) to disseminate a message

Each group in the target market has different needs and different reasons to hire a GCM or refer someone to a GCM. Trust officers, for instance, need someone who will get up in the middle of the night to take care of a very important client's needs and save the trust officers from having to get out of bed themselves. Trust officers need an agency who will handle all the things they are not always paid to do, like finding suitable home care attendants, making sure their client gets to the physician, arranging for medical equipment in the home, or arranging for a friendly visitor or Meals on Wheels. Knowing that trust officers have these needs, geriatric care management organizations can send a message tailored to trust officers: "We do X, Y, and Z for your clients, making your job a lot easier."

Public relations include many no- or low-cost marketing efforts, such as seminars and copromotion. Public relations may be less expensive than paid advertising, but it can be very time-consuming. Beginning geriatric care management businesses owners may want to invest more of their marketing effort in public relations, as they often have less cash. But new business owners are often overwhelmed with tasks

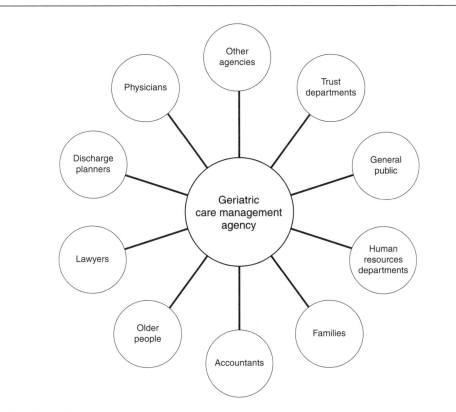

Figure 7–1 Target Market.

already and should consider how much time may be lost to public relations. Public relations is discussed in greater detail below.

Unlike public relations, advertising can be expensive. Some advertising for the beginning GCM businessperson is essential. Placing an ad in the Yellow Pages and putting together a good brochure are important for a beginning geriatric care management business. However, placing ads in magazines and newspapers may not bring immediate results and may be too expensive for a new business.

DEVELOPING AN IMAGE

Even businesses without active marketing strategies are presenting an image to the public, which is a form of marketing. Marketing involves everything that contributes to a business's image (e.g., the company's name, location, and business cards; how every employee treats clients; how community members talk about the business to others). So whether they like it or not, all businesses are doing marketing every day.[4]

Everyone in a company is responsible for marketing. Everything each employee does or does not do for a customer is marketing. More than half of all Japanese companies do not have marketing departments because they believe that everyone in the company has marketing as a job.[3] This means that every point of contact between a customer or potential customer and an employee contributes to that customer's image of the business: the way the phone is answered, the extra steps a GCM takes to solve a client's problem quickly, a staff member's call to an adult child assuring him or her that everything is all right with his or her dad, a GCM's attendance at an older client's birthday party.

Many human services professionals have not thought much about image. Their goal has been to serve clients, and they have thought little about the place where they served clients or the materials they handed clients. But when human services professionals decide to start a for-profit business, they must learn one of the cardinal rules of business: Image is everything. For in-

stance, people do not usually patronize restaurants with waiters in messy uniforms and confusing menus; there are better restaurants at which to spend their money. Geriatric care management businesses are no different from restaurants when it comes to image building. Customers are paying a lot for the service, and they can always go to another geriatric care management business if they are not pleased with the first.

An important component of image is the office. Is it in a neighborhood to which the target market will come? A GCM business has few walk-in customers, but customers will come to the office. Older people, family members, attorneys, trust officers, and others will expect an upscale office in a welcoming location.

Although start-up businesses are usually operated on a shoestring, having a receptionist or administrative assistant to greet clients and answer the phone adds a lot to a business's image. When a client's family member walks in and a GCM is frantically answering the phone and typing reports at the same time, the GCM does not seem like someone who has the time to help other people with their problems. A business's image is tarnished when new clients who need immediate attention encounter an answering machine or when clients are trying to call but are repeatedly put on hold. A fragmented office and answering machine do not portray an image of great service. Hiring someone to serve as a receptionist or administrative assistant can be a great investment.

Another part of image is client services. Geriatric care management services should be thought of as products. GCMs have many different products to offer customers, including assessment, placement, and home care aide monitoring. Describing services in terms of products helps customers understand the GCMs' offerings, which may otherwise seem abstract; everyone understands how to buy products.

GCMs should make sure to offer products that customers are really going to buy. How do GCMs make these predictions? Some do needs surveys in their community. A GCM could survey all the other agencies that offer geriatric care management, find out what services are missing in the community, and offer them. For instance, if no one is offering placement assistance, GCMs might make that one of their services.

Having chosen the services to sell, GCMs need to figure out how to package those products attractively. How would they do this? First, they should write an understandable, user-friendly description of each product. Second, they should put those product descriptions clearly on their Web site, their brochure, the tabletop display they take to senior fairs, and other advertising materials. All of these marketing materials will need to be designed carefully to make sure that the words and images complement each other and present the GCM's services in the best light. Unless they are professional designers or copywriters themselves, GCMs may seek help from copywriters, graphic artists, or marketing consultants. Their services are a good investment. GCMs may also want to collect what they consider to be good brochures and other marketing materials (from NAPGCM and CMSA conferences and other places) to serve as models.

Another part of image involves word of mouth about the GCM and the company. How present or past customers talk about the GCM and the company to other potential customers can really affect business. It is what an agency network says about a business to clients or referral sources. Word of mouth either encourages people to call or stops them from calling a GCM business. A good percentage of referrals comes from word of mouth. A business cannot control what others say but can control the quality of services and relationships and its image in general so that word of mouth is usually positive.

An additional part of image is staff. Just having staff members sends the message to customers that they will get good service. Everyone who comes into contact with staff members should walk away with a positive image of the business. Having good staff members starts with hiring people who are team players, will represent the business well, and will follow the GCM's direction. Once hired, these team players should get to know the company's mission statement. If, for instance, the mission is "to give customers good service," everyone on the staff should know that mission and keep it in mind as they work each day.

The first contact is the most important contact, so every staff member should try to give customers that great first image. Lots of factors affect that first image: how staff members dress, how they answer the phone, how they greet someone who enters the agency, and even what they say to their friends after hours about the GCM and the business. Each aspect of employees' behavior has to be positive to enhance and build the business's image.

Staff can be trained in how to present the best possible face to clients. GCMs may want to consult with human resources consultants about staff training and customer service. GCMs may also want to do a lot of reading on the subject and map out a plan for how to encourage everyone in the office individually and as a group.

Exhibit 7–2 shows a mini image checklist to test a geriatric care management agency's image. It will help show where an agency is doing well and where an agency might improve.

POSITIONING THE AGENCY

Positioning is critical to any marketing effort. But what is positioning? Positioning is discovering what makes a geriatric care management agency different from its competitors. It shows the customer what makes one agency a better choice than another. Writing a positioning statement will help an agency position itself in the market.

A positioning statement should begin with an outline of what the geriatric care management agency offers the customer, listing all the agency's services. People writing a positioning statement should then consider the strengths and weaknesses of each service. One agency might be the only one offering placement services in a community; that would be a strength. The agency's weakness might be that it is undercapitalized and cannot afford to market those services effectively to all target markets.

Next, the needs of each target market should be listed. Trust officers may want to work with someone experienced in social services to help

Exhibit 7–2 A Mini Image Checklist

Give your agency a 5 if your image is high with that group and a 1 if it is low. Give yourself a 0 if most people in that group have little or no knowledge of the agency at all. In each cell, you will be measuring the group's opinion of one aspect of your agency's image.

Image Element	Clients/ Families	Potential Clients	General Public	Professionals (Attorneys, Accountants, etc.)
Knowledge of geriatric care management				
Ability of services to meet community needs				
Quality of services				
Quality of marketing materials				
Professionalism and customer service skills of staff				
Appearance of office				
Location of office				
Agency reputation				

160 points = superb image
120–159 points = great image
80–119 points = good image that needs improvement
40–79 points = mediocre image that needs a lot of improvement
Under 40 points = poor image

them make decisions they are not professionally prepared to make. Attorneys may want help for older clients with bill paying, Medicare, Social Security assistance, and difficult family situations; they may want to use geriatric care management services because they have neither the time nor the expertise to render these services themselves.

The positioning statement should also list how the agency can benefit each target market. What needs can the agency help with now? Which needs might the agency be able to help with later, when new services are offered? For example, if attorneys are looking for private conservators and an agency does not now handle conservatorship, might it plan on adding the service later?

Next, the position statement should discuss the agency's competitors. Who are each of the competitors? What services does each offer? What are the fees? What communities are covered? To do this competitor survey, people will have to call other local geriatric care management agencies and other types of agencies that also offer geriatric care management (a sample competition survey appears in Exhibit 7–3). Agencies should ask competitors to send literature discussing their services and costs.

This information on competitors will help a new geriatric care management agency position itself within the local market. For instance, a new agency that is the only one to offer a written geriatric assessment by a registered nurse and a

Exhibit 7–3 Competition Survey

Agency Name/Phone: _____

Contact Person: _____

I'm trying to get some information. My mom has Alzheimer's and my dad just died. My dad was her primary caregiver. She wants to move in with us, but I don't know whether we should do that, get care at her home, or what to do. Someone told us we need a geriatric care manager to help us. Is this something your agency can help us with?

1. Do you employ a geriatric care manager? _____

2. How much do you charge per hour for geriatric care management? _____

3. Will you come to our home to look at the problem? _____

4. Will you give us a written report? _____

5. What is the background of the geriatric care manager? _____

6. Does your agency belong to any associations like the National Association of Professional Geriatric Care Managers? _____

7. Do I have to pay for mileage? _____

8. Does your geriatric care manager have any credentials? _____

9. Are your care providers bonded? _____

10. Do you accept insurance/are you a Medicare agency? _____

11. Do you employ care providers too? What do they do? _____

    Personal care? _____ Light housekeeping? _____

    Laundry? _____ Meals? _____

    Medication? _____ Pet care? _____

    Driving? _____

12. What if something happens in the middle of the night? _____

    _____

13. What if the regular person doesn't show up? _____

14. Will my mom always have the same person? _____

15. If they have to drive mom somewhere, they can use our second car, but how do you know if that person is a safe driver? _____

16. My mom can be very irritable—are your people trained to deal with this? _____

17. What kind of training do you have for your people? Do you train your people in Alzheimer's behavior? _____

18. What are your rates? _____

    Hourly for companion/aide? _____

    Hourly for Certified Nurses Aide (CNA)? _____

continues

Exhibit 7–3 continued

Sleepover? _____

How many hours are sleepovers? _____

Live-in? _____

Number of hours for a care provider (2 hours, 4 hours, etc.)? _____

Do you have a minimum? _____

19. I need to discuss this with my husband. How much notice do I need to give you? _____

Notes: _____

_____

_____

_____

_____

Rate the following on a scale of 1 to 5 (1 = great, 5 = awful):

Customer service	1	2	3	4	5
Hold time	1	2	3	4	5
Attitude	1	2	3	4	5
Helpfulness	1	2	3	4	5
Knowledge	1	2	3	4	5

Staff member name: _____

Date of call: _____

social worker should let customers know of this unique service. The agency will stand out from its competitors, and customers will have a good reason to choose the agency instead of another.

The positioning statement should end with a discussion of the trends in geriatric care management and the economy generally. How will the agency anticipate and respond to these trends? If more corporations in the agency's area are starting to offer elder-care benefits because their employees are missing time from work to care for their parents, are the agency's services responding to that trend? If the trend is for more attorneys to specialize in estate planning and conservatorship, is the agency handling conservatorships? People can learn about these trends from professional journals as well as general publications such as the *Wall Street Journal* and weekly news magazines. An agency must know what the present market is like and what the future might bring to know whether its services are and will continue to be useful.

Positioning takes into account the real benefits an agency offers to its target markets. Benefits are ways that someone else's life is improved by an agency's service. Do the services give target audience members the benefits they really want? Many trust departments want someone who will solve clients' personal problems on a 24-hour basis without bothering the trust officer frequently; is the agency really providing what trust officers want? Many attorneys want GCMs to solve the lesser problems of older clients and reduce the number of calls the attorney receives; is the agency really reducing the number of calls? Agencies need to analyze their list of benefits and make sure they are all honest-to-goodness benefits.

Are the benefits the agency offers better than those offered by competitors? Is the agency the only one in town where an attorney can get a client's messy stack of unpaid bills paid and cleaned up and have a client's Medicare and Social Security problems taken care of? If other agencies provide the same service, is this agency less expensive or does it get the job done more quickly?

Exhibit 7–4 summarizes some of these points about positioning.

REVAMPING AN AGENCY'S IMAGE

An agency can use the mini image revamp chart in Exhibit 7–5 to begin to improve its image.

First, agencies should reconsider their list of target markets. Agencies need to make sure that they offer as many services as possible that re-

Exhibit 7–4 Positioning

Positioning is
  • what makes you different from your competitors
  • why you should be chosen
Customers have choices:
  1. choose you
  2. choose your competitors
  3. do it themselves
  4. do nothing
What makes your agency different from your competitors? _____

_____

_____

What advantages do you have over your competitors? _____

_____

_____

Exhibit 7–5 Mini Image Revamp

  1. Target market:
  2. Desired image outcome:
  3. Current image:
  4. Desired image:
  5. Major motivation of target market:
  6. Message to be sent:
  7. Media to be used to send message:

spond to all their target markets' needs. The desired outcome would be that all members of their target markets know about those services. If local attorneys want GCMs who will help with conservatorships, the message that needs to be sent to these attorneys is that the agency's written geriatric assessments can help with conservatorships. How will the agency send attorneys this message? One way might be to speak to the bar association, if the agency can get an invitation, about the geriatric assessment services. Another way might be to put together some good prevention folders describing the agency's services, including geriatric assessment, and make appointments with all local attorneys handling conservatorships to review the agency's services. Another way might be to put an ad in the *Journal of the American Bar Association*.

WRITING A MINI MARKETING PLAN

A marketing plan is critical to the success of a geriatric care management business. There are many ways to develop a marketing plan. Consulting with professionals (e.g., marketing experts or people from the Small Business Administration and the Service Corps of Retired Executives—see Appendix A for contact information) is always a very good idea. The positioning statement should be the basis for the plan because it lists the strengths and weaknesses of the agency's services, the needs of each group in the agency's target market, details about competitors, trends in geriatric care management, and other important details that affect a marketing plan.

Exhibit 7–6 shows a mini marketing plan, a simple tool for taking the information from a positioning statement and using it to develop a plan for marketing a geriatric care management business.

A mini marketing plan will help an agency define what marketing strategies have already been used, how well they have worked, and what marketing strategies might be used in the future. For example, an agency seeking to reach attorneys who do estate planning and conservatorships has already tried the following marketing methods: speaking to the bar association, putting an ad in the local bar association's journal, and calling the attorneys and trying to make appointments to meet with them and tell them about the agency's services. Speaking to the bar association was successful because agency representatives met several attorneys who later referred clients to the agency. Putting an ad in the local bar association journal yielded little: Not one attorney who referred a client mentioned having seen the ad. Making appointments with individual attorneys was successful but proceeded very slowly. All in all, speaking to the bar association produced the best results at the lowest cost. A new marketing method might be getting a list of every local attorney who belongs to the National Association of Elder Law Attorneys (NAELA;

see Appendix A for contact information) and calling each one to ask to make a one-on-one presentation. Since NAELA already has a relationship with NAPGCM (the organizations have had several joint conferences, and both work with older clients), its members might be receptive to talking to GCMs.

Complete marketing plans usually start with a description of the industry, both its history and what it is expected to look like in 5–10 years. Next, there will be a marketing analysis discussing the characteristics of the target market (e.g., size, critical needs, how the agency is meeting those needs). Competition will then be considered. What is the agency's market share? Where does the business fit in to the local market? The marketing plan will also probably include a marketing strategy (e.g., which products are meant to attract which target markets, the difference between the agency's products and its competitors' products, the sales staff and how they are supported, the cost of a budget for advertising).

DOING PUBLIC RELATIONS

Public relations is the no- or low-cost method of marketing an agency. Public relations may not cost a lot, but it does take a substantial amount of time. It involves arranging special events, something that few professional social workers or nurses have ever done. But people new to public relations should not be daunted. With some good preparation and organization, these special events are not so hard to pull off. Events such as seminars, speakers bureaus, and health and senior fairs can help publicize an agency and attract new clients. Either owners or "star" care managers usually represent the agency at these events.

Speakers Bureaus

By organizing a speakers bureau, an agency promotes its representatives as experts in geriatric care management. To begin, agencies should choose up to four subjects of real interest to the general public and organize a speakers bureau around them. For instance, "The Sandwich Gen-

Exhibit 7–6 Mini Marketing Plan

1. Which marketing method is best for communicating with each of your primary target markets?
   • Target market 1:
   • Target market 2:
   • Target market 3:
2. Which marketing methods have you used in the past with success?
3. With which marketing methods have you tried but had little success?
4. Which marketing methods got the best results for the least amount of money?
5. Which marketing methods will you try next?

eration: How To Help Your Aging Parents and Survive Yourself" might really attract the target market of adult children of aging parents. Through the speakers bureau, the agency informs people that its GCMs are experts at helping address some difficulties associated with aging. Every listener is either a potential client or referral source.

Speakers bureaus may generate articles in local newspapers, another form of good free publicity.

Choosing Topics and Writing Speeches

People should choose up to four "hot topics" (e.g., "How To Help Your Parent Adjust to Living in a Nursing Home") to launch a speakers bureau. Once they have a topic, they should write an outline of the speech. To grab the audience's attention, speakers should start with something interactive. If they are doing a speech about aging, they could hand out a brief quiz about getting old and ask the audience to take it. The questions should be brief, and speakers should review the answers with the audience. Next, the middle of the speech should cover four to six stand-out facts about the subject, providing some brief detail about each fact. Group participation should be used with every point, framing each point as a question. For example, a speaker could say, "Why are people living so darn long?"

Speakers should end with a list of solutions that the audience members can implement themselves. If the subject is the sandwich generation, for example, a speaker could suggest "Take time for yourself" and "Involve your siblings and other family members." Audience members should walk away feeling like the speaker handed them something.

Booking Engagements

Next, agencies should select community groups that might be interested in the speakers bureau (e.g., women's clubs, men's clubs, corporations with employee assistance programs). An interactive marketing database is very helpful here. It can be used to make a list of groups to contact, create template letters, and send the letters out to the group. If there is no interactive

marketing database, individual letters should be written to each contact. Sending a photocopied form letter is too impersonal.

Where does one find a listing of community clubs? A chamber of commerce or local library will probably maintain a list. One local club (e.g., Kiwanis) may keep a list of all local clubs. Agencies should choose 20 clubs likely to be interested in aging (e.g., the Junior League, not the Bach Society).

Once the list of 20 is complete, agencies should call each club and ask for the club member who arranges for speakers at meetings. This may be the president or another member, and this is the person to whom to send the introductory letter.

The letter should have a brief, catchy introduction, should list the selection of topics, and should have a brief ending summarizing how the presentation will benefit the club and club members. A fax reply form should be included with the letter so recipients have an easy, instant way to respond. The letter should also list an e-mail and Web site address, if applicable. Exhibit 7–7 includes a sample letter, and Exhibit 7–8 includes a sample fax reply form.

No more than 7 days after sending the letter, agencies should follow up with a telephone call to the club representative to whom the letter was written, unless they have already received another response from the representative. After more than 7 days, the letter may have been forgotten. The caller should ask if the club is interested in having a speaker. Callers should smile when speaking; that will come across in their voice.

Clubs tend to book months in advance. The important thing is to get onto the club's schedule.

Making Presentations

Most club presentations are followed by a not-very-tasty lunch. Agency representatives can liven up these "rubber chicken circuit" events by delivering interesting presentations.

Agencies should be sure to prepare the group for the speaker, helping to promote the event. Along with a letter confirming the speaking engagement, agencies should send copies of their

Exhibit 7–7 Sample Letter

December 10, 2000

Cathy Snyder
230 Palm Avenue
Pacific Grove, CA 93950

Dear Cathy:

The pressures of quality child care are a major issue for American families. Unfortunately, the new problem of elder care creates equally as much difficulty. A U.S. House of Representatives study recently indicated that the average American woman spends 17 years caring for her children and 18 years caring for her elderly parents.

Cresscare, Case Management for Elders, has been providing care management services for almost 20 years in Monterey and Santa Clara Counties. We are nationally known for our innovative services to families. One of our missions is to serve the needs of the sandwich generation and long-distance care providers of older people.

Cresscare is presently scheduling for its 2000 free speakers bureau. If this would be of interest to your organization, we would be happy to make a presentation at one of your meetings. Some of the topics you can choose from are:

The Sandwich Generation: Caught between the needs of your elderly parents and your kids? Solutions to relieve a major stress for family members of the 1990s.

When Your Parent Must Be in a Nursing Home—Making the Adjustment: How to help your parent make the best of nursing home life and also get support for yourself.

When Siblings Aren't Doing Their Share: The loneliness of the primary caregiver. Making a new alliance with siblings. Communicating your needs and getting assistance.

Travelers in Time—Understanding the Aging Process: The fastest growing segment of our population is 85 years old or older. What is in store for these older people?

I will be calling you in a few days to discuss speaking to your group. I look forward to talking with you. For more information about Cresscare, visit our Web site: www.cresscare.com.

Sincerely,

Donna Albert, MA, CMC
Geriatric Social Worker

brochures, newsletters, press releases, personal invitations to the office—anything that will encourage attendance at the presentation. The agency should also include a brief biography of the speaker so that the moderator knows how to introduce the speaker.

Speakers should ask the person in charge of the luncheon meeting if they can speak before lunch. Before-lunch speeches should be relatively brief. People are hungry, and having to wait too long to eat may make them think less of the speaker and the agency. Speaking during or

Exhibit 7–8 Sample Fax Reply Form

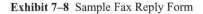

FAX REPLY

Send to: Cresscare
230 Palm Ave.
Pacific Grove, CA 93950

Fax: (408) 372-0392

From: Name _____

Club _____

Telephone _____

Best time to reach me: Day(s) _____ Time _____

_____ I would like more information about speaking to a group

Possible date _____ Time _____

_____ Please send more brochures for distribution to our members.

---

after lunch is not a great alternative; clanging dishes and full stomachs can distract audiences.

Speakers should distribute handouts before speaking so the audience has something to look at before the speech. Handouts can include agency brochures, press releases, and brochures from national associations to which the agency belongs and that lend the organization credibility (e.g., CMSA, NAPGCM). After the speech, speakers should hand out business cards and ask the audience members to put their names on a sign-up sheet if they want more information about the agency. It is important to remember that this is a sales event as much as an opportunity to educate people.

After the event, speakers should follow up with a thank-you note to the club president and add everyone from the sign-up sheet to the agency's mailing list. All those people should receive future press releases, newsletters, and information about the agency's services. Their interest in the agency was captured during the presentation. It is important to keep the agency's name in these people's minds by keeping information about the agency flowing to them.

Senior Fairs/Health Fairs

If an agency wants to promote its services, health fairs and senior fairs are good places to get exposure to a broad group of potential customers. Some fairs are attended by thousands, so each fair should generate at least some business for the agency. Fairs are also an excellent opportunity to network with similar agencies and get a sense of what competitors are selling. During these fairs, agency representatives should take the time to talk to other agencies' representatives about the services their agencies offer.

To pull these fairs off well, agencies need some basic items, including a professional-looking display, printed materials, and items to give away. First, a tabletop booth display should be set up and decorated. It is best to decorate with photos that really convey what the agency is about—photos from the agency's printed materials, for instance. The photos should be blown up and laminated on half-inch cardboard with Velcro on the back so they can be attached to the tabletop display. Brief messages about the agency should be placed under the photos. The text of the messages should be at least 6 inches high and easy to read. The text could include the agency's mission statement, list the agency's services, and mention the benefits of using the agency. The messages should be printed and mounted in the same way as the photos. The agency's logo could also appear on the display. Local copy shops can help with some of the details of making these displays.

There should be printed materials for staff to hand out to booth visitors. Possible materials include brochures, copies of articles about the agency or its owners or staff, press releases, and brochures from national associations (e.g., NAPGCM, CMSA). There should be a sign-up sheet for people who want more information about the agency's services.

Next, there should be some items to give away. Pens, mugs, and other items with the agency's name on them are good candidates. Offering food and beverages (e.g., coffee and gourmet cookies) also attracts passersby. People love to walk away from a booth with something.

Last but not least, excellent staff members must be posted at the booth. They should be friendly, outgoing, energetic people who like to talk, are knowledgeable about the agency's services, and have a background in sales. They should be attractively dressed. Most of all, they should be focused on getting new customers.

How can an agency find health fairs or senior fairs? A chamber of commerce will be able to help. Agencies should ask the chamber of commerce for the 25 largest corporations in their community and then call human resources representatives at those corporations and ask them if they have health fairs. If those corporations do have health fairs, agencies should ask if they could have booths at those fairs. Local area agencies on aging will be able to provide information about local senior fairs.

Seminars

Seminars are a great method of getting new customers by showcasing an agency's knowledge of the geriatric care management field. To begin preparing for a seminar, agencies should (1) select a "hot topic," something that has recently been discussed in the general media and is of concern to the general public, and (2) consider whether to have a cosponsor. Agencies might want to ask a local area agency on aging or trust department to be a cosponsor. Why have a cosponsor? There are several reasons.

1. Cosponsors share costs and organizing duties.
2. Having a cosponsor with an excellent reputation in the community can enhance an agency's image (agencies are known by the company they keep).
3. Cosponsoring an event helps establish a bond between organizations, and this bond can prove fruitful down the road.

Seminars, like speakers bureaus, must be planned in advance. Having picked a date and time for a seminar, agencies should create a timeline showing when different tasks will be done in preparation for the seminar. A room that is easily accessible and known to the target market should be chosen as the seminar's location. For instance, if an agency is targeting seniors, it should consider an upscale senior housing facility, perhaps even having that facility as a cosponsor. Next, agencies should pick the audiovisual materials they are going to use, keeping in mind that the seminar should be both informative and entertaining. Useful materials include overheads, a slide show, or a very brief video. Audiences are accustomed to television and expect slickness and fast-moving images. Unless audiovisual materials are used, seminars may seem boring. All speakers should be given a time limit.

Speakers should include yourself as the GCM, as well as someone from your co-sponsorship group, i.e., the head of the trust department if you are co-sponsoring with a trust department. Utilize outside speakers who are experts in your topic. For instance, if your topic is long-term care insurance, select a speaker who is an insurance agent who specializes in long-term care insurance. Also consider if the speaker makes a good presentation and speaks well. Many times someone will know the content but be a very poor speaker, marring the quality of the seminar. Find speakers in your network of aging providers and in the target markets you serve. Remember, building and maintaining relationships is a major part of marketing.

Handouts should include promotional materials like those used at speakers bureau presentations as well as materials about the seminar topic. A cosponsor should also provide materials. Agencies should prepare an evaluation to hand out at the end of the seminar to ask how the seminar could be improved next time.

Presenting at and Attending Conferences

Presenting at conferences related to aging is an indirect method of getting clients. Colleagues who hear a presentation by an agency representative may refer clients to that agency. If the conferences are local, the likelihood of referrals increases. As colleagues gather and network, helpful tips will be shared, business cards exchanged, and information about competitors collected. Information about conferences that are taking place may be obtained through various local groups focused on aging, clubs, or service organizations (e.g., the Rotary Club).

Preparing for a conference is similar to preparing for a speakers bureau presentation. A topic must be chosen and an outline written. Speakers should begin with something interactive and attention grabbing, use open-ended questions, and leave the audience with something to take home. Topics for presentations at professional conferences will be different from topics for speakers bureau presentations to the general public. The level of communication should be sophisticated, but the presentation should still entertain. Great teachers learn to say the most complicated ideas in the simplest fashion. Few people want to be lectured nonstop. Audiences like to interact with speakers.

Star Care Managers

Any of these public relations events are best pulled off by someone who is energetic and outgoing—a good speaker and entertainer. Sometimes an agency's owner might not be the right person for the job. In these cases, it is helpful to turn to a star care manager with plenty of charisma and knowledge of the field. Smaller geriatric care management agencies presenting in the local area might select a speaker who is generally known in the community. Larger agencies presenting regionally and nationally might want to use someone who is known throughout the field and might draw a considerable audience. This professional might have published an article, done national work in care management associations, or done a series of presentations at national conferences like CMSA or NAPGCM.

ADVERTISING

The beginning geriatric care management agency is going to need some very basic advertising materials. In designing brochures, print ads, or any other advertising materials, agencies should remember that they are marketing to distinct target markets, including older people, their adult children, and third parties who will refer clients. If any piece of advertising cannot address all groups simultaneously, then separate ads or brochures should be made, and that could be expensive. To address all target markets, materials should list all services, from "help for long-distance caregivers" (which speaks to adult children) to "medication monitoring so that older people can safely remain at home" (which speaks to older people). Photos included in the advertising materials should show a variety of scenes (e.g., an adult child laughing while at dinner with a parent, an older person talking to a smiling GCM).

People starting agencies should collect brochures from many other agencies and decide what they like and dislike about those brochures. CMSA and NAPGCM have information tables at their regional and national conferences where agency brochures are available. People can also ask other agencies directly for copies of their brochures.

Graphics artists and copywriters should help design and write advertising materials. Although this can be expensive, agencies should keep in mind the importance of image. A brochure often provides people with their first impression of an agency.

Agencies should have presentation folders if they plan to make one-on-one marketing calls to accountants, attorneys, and others. Presentation folders are rather expensive customized pocket folders, usually with the agency's name and logo on the cover, that contain a variety of printed information about the agency (e.g., an agency brochure, descriptions of agency products and services, articles about the agency printed in local newspapers, a brochure from CMSA or NAPGCM, articles about geriatric care management generally). Before each marketing call, the agency representatives making the call can select the materials that would most interest the people they will be visiting. For instance, an article about an agency's GCMs working with attorneys would be an appropriate choice for a meeting with an elder-care lawyer. Looking at other agencies' presentation folders can help a new agency get some ideas.

Agencies may advertise in many places, including newspapers, senior magazines, senior directories, and senior newsletters. They can also advertise on the radio and on television. Most new start-up GCM businesses do not have the budget for this type of advertising, however.

A marketing consultant and various advertising professionals can help agencies develop print ads. The marketing consultant will help with developing a concept behind the ad, and advertising professionals can help with graphic design and layout as well as copywriting. Unless an ad is well conceived and looks professional, it is not worth the money to print it. As with brochures and other materials, agencies should take a look at what competitors are doing with their ads.

The ad should be easy to read and have attractive, pleasant illustrations or graphics. People buy hope, not hopelessness. There should not be a photo of a unhappy-looking older person in bed with a GCM leaning over the bed. A smiling older person should appear instead. The picture should look like the end result of the geriatric care management services, not the initial problem. If the agency specializes in serving adult children or long-distance care providers, the ad should state that. The agency's phone number, including any toll-free numbers, should stand out. If the agency is available 24 hours a day, the ad should state that.

A print ad can be a very good beginning to an ad campaign and can even be used for a Yellow Pages ad. It is helpful to use the same ad in different places while the business is still getting its footing; consistency will help people remember the agency.

An agency's advertising can also include a Web site. An agency can link its Web site to those of NAPGCM or CMSA to enhance traffic to the agency's Web site. Many adult children and long-distance caregivers use the Web to search for services. More information about developing a Web site is contained in Chapter 6.

CONCLUSION

The key to marketing a GCM business is offering the best geriatric care management services and treating customers well. Everything should be viewed as an opportunity. There will be problems (ads will not produce a response, people will refuse marketing calls). But any problem is just an opportunity to improve the marketing effort the next time. With this kind of attitude toward marketing, a geriatric care management is bound to thrive.

NOTES

1. Levinson J. *Guerrilla Marketing.* Boston: Houghton Mifflin; 1984.

2. Knutson K, Langer S. Geriatric care managers: A survey in long-term/chronic care. *GCM J.* 1998;8:9–13.

3. Beckwith H. *Selling the Invisible: A Field Guide to Modern Marketing.* New York: Warner Books; 1997.

4. Cress C. Why market? *GCM J.* 1993.

CHAPTER 8

Revenue Sources for Geriatric Care Managers

Robert E. O'Toole

Professional geriatric care management as an independent business enterprise has moved in recent years from its early developmental stages into a more sophisticated but still emerging field of professional practice. While this unique field is expected to see significant growth, along with the growth of the older population, it remains largely a group of small for-profit companies. These small companies are run mainly by entrepreneurs who have positioned their business to serve as an alternative to the publicly funded and nonprofit elder-care system, which has been struggling with severe fiscal constraints for several years.

The independent professional practice of geriatric care management is still very much a developing sector of the larger and rapidly growing long-term care industry. Before setting out on their own to offer a private, fee-based alternative to the existing long-term care service delivery system, many geriatric care managers (GCMs) worked in settings such as nonprofit agencies funded by grants or the United Way, church-supported organizations, and tax-supported public or quasi-public agencies—settings where care recipients and their family members rarely paid for services. When recipients and family members did pay, it was usually on a sliding scale, with fees ranging from as little as a few dollars to perhaps as high as $25 per hour or unit of service.[1]

Other GCMs came from settings such as hospitals, outpatient health clinics, certified home health agencies, and nursing homes. In these set-tings, most, if not all, of the cost of long-term care was paid for by various forms of third-party insurance, most likely from a federal insurance program such as Medicare or the joint state and federal insurance program known as Medicaid (Medi-Cal in California).

The tradition of having most long-term care paid for by third parties has created an expectation that has become firmly established in the American psyche. The prevailing attitude is that long-term care, whether provided in a facility or in a home, should be paid for by somebody else, regardless of income. The resistance to paying privately for care is so strong in this country that even middle- and upper-income people will go to great extremes to avoid paying for their care or the care of a family member.[2]

A booming cottage industry known as "Medicaid planning" has developed over the last two decades. Medicaid planning was developed to take advantage of loopholes in federal and state regulations regarding the financial eligibility requirements of the Medicaid program. By establishing various forms of trusts designed to shelter the assets of a person who might otherwise be expected to pay for long-term care, these legal maneuvers create a financial status that some have termed "artificial poverty."[2] An affluent individual with hundreds of thousands or even millions of dollars can start a Medicaid trust and become eligible for services paid for with public funds.[3] This deeply ingrained "entitlement" mentality, coupled with the legal process that supports and encourages it, makes the move to become an independent provider of long-term care services a risky business venture.

Nonprofit and publicly funded agencies that provide "free" or subsidized elder-care services are overwhelmed by increasing demand and severe budget constraints. Despite the fact that their limitations prevent them from providing the rich package of services that may be affordable to many of those who contact them, employees of these agencies are still reluctant to refer even affluent clients to private practice GCMs. Apparently, working in a climate where services, however limited, are provided without charge makes them skeptical of any professional, no matter how qualified, who charges fees to provide assessment, care planning, and care management services.

As the above text makes clear, GCMs who strike out on their own face many challenges when it comes to funding. This chapter will discuss some of these funding sources, including payment by private individuals and their families, payment through long-term care insurance, and payment through noninsurance third-party sources. It concludes with a section discussing the financial and other benefits that can accrue when GCMs join forces.

PAYMENT BY PRIVATE INDIVIDUALS AND THEIR FAMILIES

When many GCMs are asked why they chose to leave the public and nonprofit sectors to become entrepreneurs, they mention the opportunity to earn more money, to have more autonomy, and to deliver a higher-quality level of service. These GCMs have reported that they felt squeezed by increasingly constrained budgets and an ever-increasing demand for services—factors that led to unwieldy caseloads, unrealistic time demands, and an inability to meet all client needs. Professionals who held themselves to high standards of performance felt they were being asked to lower their standards. Independent practice was the way out for these GCMs.[1]

To survive and thrive as a small independent business, offering a high-quality alternative to the limited services available from nonprofit organizations, home care agencies, and health care facilities requires more than high standards, however. To create a successful business, GCMs must locate the people who are willing to pay for higher-quality services rather than settle for less or be placed on a waiting list by the traditional long-term care provider. No longer supported by the third–party-funded infrastructure that provided them with an office, a predictable salary, supplies, and overhead costs such as reimbursement for travel, independent practice professionals learn very quickly to charge fees to those for whom they provide services.[4]

The traditional long-term care service delivery system as we know it today has developed over the last 35 years—since the inception of the Medicare and Medicaid programs in 1965. The evidence that this publicly financed service delivery system cannot begin to meet the steadily growing demand has been mounting over the last decade.[5] News stories about inadequate care in nursing homes, cutbacks in home health funding, high turnover and chronic understaffing in nursing homes and home health agencies, and abuses in the court-supervised guardianship system have proliferated in recent years.[6] The imminent financial collapse of the Medicare program has been a major concern of the U.S. Congress, which is considering placing further limitations on the amount of services provided to those eligible, in order to keep the program solvent as nearly 80 million Americans between the ages of 35 and 55 reach retirement age over the next 25 to 30 years.[7]

Despite growing awareness of the crisis that is looming in the nation's long-term care service delivery system, GCMs have had difficulty educating the public about the fact that a private sector alternative exists and can be far more effective and desirable. Fifteen years after the formation of the National Association of Professional Geriatric Care Managers, most consumers are still unaware that this alternative exists, nor do they know how to find or utilize the services of a private GCM. GCMs need to spread the word that consumers can obtain services that were previously limited or unavailable and that it is worth paying more to obtain a personalized and highly professional level of service.

Paying privately for highly skilled professional services is nothing new in the American marketplace. When consumers seek the services of an attorney, an architect, an accountant, a financial advisor, a carpenter, a plumber, or a gardener, they are well aware that they will be expected to pay for those services themselves. And yet because of the well-established precedent of elder-care services being paid for by taxpayers, charities, or third-party insurance sources, consumers have different expectations about elder-care services. To succeed, the private GCM must spread a message with three important components:

1. Eventually, you or a member of your family may need specialized professional attention because of aging or disability. Finding the services needed to help can be a difficult, time-consuming, and frustrating process, so planning ahead is a good idea.
2. A high-quality alternative to the traditional long-term care delivery system is available if you are willing to pay for it.
3. The services of a GCM are well worth the price.

If GCMs fail to get this three-part message to consumers, many fledgling businesses will fail.

One way GCMs have found to reach those who need and can benefit from their services is to target specific groups. Private practice professionals have found, for instance, that attorneys who practice elder law and estate planning, bank trust officers, and financial advisors who manage the resources of affluent clients are sources of referrals that can help to build an independent practice.

No matter how hard GCMs try to spread their message and raise awareness about geriatric care management, the consumer who has been conditioned to expect that most, if not all, long-term care services are covered by Medicare or private charity is likely to balk at having to pay for the costs of a GCM. When a national network of professionals in independent practice began to emerge in the mid-1980s, virtually all revenue generated by GCMs was from private fees paid directly by the family seeking professional elder-care assistance. But in recent years, new sources of reimbursement for independent GCMs have emerged. This trend is expected to continue.[8] New sources of third-party revenue for GCMs include but are not limited to managed care organizations, including health maintenance organizations (HMOs); preferred provider organizations (PPOs); private insurance companies; and employers and labor unions, usually by using an independent "work/life" vendor. These new sources of revenue are discussed in greater detail below.

LIMITATIONS OF THIRD-PARTY REIMBURSEMENT AND THE RISE OF LONG-TERM INSURANCE

Limits on traditional third-party reimbursement for consumers and providers are becoming increasingly stringent. Medicare pays for a very limited amount of long-term care services, and the Medicaid program is becoming increasingly restrictive in both the amount and the type of long-term care services paid for if it appears that the individual or family has resources to pay for the care.

Because of the catastrophic costs of long-term care, the risk exposure for older people and their families is enormous. Those with assets ranging from moderate to substantial are required to deplete their assets before receiving publicly subsidized services. Those with few assets are forced into the increasingly unpleasant alternative of Medicaid-funded services.[9]

It is estimated that more than 12 million Americans will need long-term care in the years ahead. Yet to date barely 5% of those over 65 have purchased any long-term care insurance, a private sector product designed to pay for those costs that are not insured under Medicare or other third-party insurance sources.[10]

Reduced government spending for long-term care, coupled with incentives for the purchase of private insurance could result in substantial growth in the private financing of long-term care. Private long-term care insurance policies are now offered by more than 100 companies in the United States. Less than a dozen of these companies control nearly 75% of the market at this time.[10]

Established GCM Roles in Long-Term Care Insurance

Insurance companies have already started to utilize GCMs and other elder-care specialists in several aspects of the long-term care insurance process. During the initial application or underwriting stage, independent professionals are used to help determine whether an applicant is an acceptable risk. Nurses and social workers with experience in long-term care are retained to conduct 30-minute face-to-face interviews with selected applicants. Using a variety of functional assessment instruments, care managers help underwriters get a picture of how independent a potential insured person is prior to approving the application. These interviews are not required for all applicants, usually just those over age 72.

An insured individual is eligible for benefits when he or she meets specific benefit "triggers" (conditions defined in the insurance contract that make the insured person eligible for benefits). While these vary somewhat among companies, the usual benefit triggers consist of two or three activities of daily living (ADLs) such as bathing, eating, dressing, toileting, mobility, and transfer. Simply needing supervision due to a cognitive impairment such as Alzheimer's disease is sufficient to qualify for benefits in any well-designed long-term care policy.

When claims are filed, insurers also use GCMs to expedite the claims process. A growing number of private practice GCMs have integrated participation in regional and national provider networks into their practice. The GCM is asked to go to the home or the facility where the claimant is receiving care. Using an ADL-based functional assessment tool, the GCM prepares a report that helps claims specialists confirm that the claim is valid.

New GCM Role in Long-Term Care Insurance

A third role for GCMs is now beginning to emerge in long-term care insurance: that of care manager or care coordinator for policyholders while they are still healthy. This role includes providing information and referral services for healthy insured persons who have family members in need of long-term care. Also, as those now holding policies get older, the claims activity of insurance companies is expected to grow substantially. This means that the care management/care coordination role in the private insurance market will grow as well.[11]

When long-term care insurance policies were first introduced, there was no provision for care coordinators. By the early 1990s, companies such as CNA Insurance began to offer their applicants the option of using some of their benefits to pay for the services of a nurse or social work care manager.[11]

These professionals could be used to provide assistance in selecting and arranging for care, monitoring the quality of ongoing care, and otherwise helping the insured person to maximize the use of long-term care insurance dollars. The care coordination benefit was initially offered as an option for which the insured person paid an additional premium. In recent years, several long-term care insurance products have included such services as part of the basic benefit package at no additional cost.

Some insurers require that the care manager be a participating member of the insurer's preferred provider network. Companies such as Travelers Insurance of Hartford, Connecticut; Fortis Investors of Milwaukee, Wisconsin; and UNUM Life Insurance of Portland, Maine (three of the major players in the long-term care insurance marketplace) now offer a care coordination benefit that each company claims is "unique in the industry."

Travelers policyholders, for example, can at no extra cost use their benefits to pay for coordination of services using a care coordinator of their own choosing. Other insurers such as CNA prefer to have the policyholder utilize a specific network of providers who are under contract to CNA to manage the care coordination benefit of the long-term care policy.

Once the owner of a long-term care insurance policy needs to use the benefit, policies with care coordination benefits will extend home health care benefits to include a privately hired home health aide. The care coordinator must then arrange for the services of a certified nurse aide/ home health aide who meets the qualifications set out in the policy. Care coordinators are also used to determine what community-based services (e.g., respite care, adult day health programs) might be available to allow the policyholder to get the most cost-effective use of the benefits and receive care in the most appropriate setting.

Most long-term care insurance policies are issued with a deductible or limitation period. This limitation period, during which no benefits are paid, typically ranges from 20 to 100 days, a choice the insured person makes at the time of application. Since care coordination benefits may be used before receiving other benefits, payment for the care coordinator starts immediately after the policyholder meets the ADL triggers. In other words, no limitation period needs to be met to utilize the care coordination benefit.

Services Provided by the Care Coordination Benefit

A review of several of the better-designed long-term care insurance policies available in 1999 indicates that under the care coordination benefit the GCM may perform the following functions for the client:

- complete an initial assessment to certify that the individual meets the benefit triggers (is unable to perform two or more ADLs or needs substantial supervision due to a cognitive disorder)
- develop a care plan with specific recommendations for services to meet the needs identified in the assessment as well as arrange and coordinate nursing, home, and community services or facility care (in conjunction with family members whenever possible)
- ensure that Medicare, other insurance coverage, and/or publicly financed services are used to the extent that the insured person may be eligible for such services

- provide ongoing monitoring and customization of services to accommodate changing needs
- counsel and educate family caregivers and help to maximize informal supports
- serve as the policyholder's care advocate (especially valuable when the person receiving long-term care insurance benefits has no family nearby)

At this time the number of long-term care insurance policies in force remains small. Sales are expected to grow substantially as both federal and state governments continue their efforts to limit benefits and make Americans aware that they have little or no coverage for long-term care.[12]

It is important to note that care coordination benefits vary among insurance companies. What may be a reimbursable expense for care management services under one policy may not be covered by other companies.

GCMs' businesses will benefit from the anticipated growth of private sector financing of long-term care and the increased recognition by insurance companies of the important role care managers can play in the delivery of long-term care.

Obtaining Reimbursement for Services for Long-Term Care Insurance Policyholders

GCMs should ask if the person for whom they are about to provide services owns a long-term care insurance policy. This information should be obtained at intake when asking about other forms of coverage owned by the client, including Medicare, retiree health benefits from an employer or a labor union, and veterans benefits. GCMs should ask for and review a copy of any insurance coverage to determine exactly what benefits may be available and then, if necessary, contact the insurance company or the third-party administrator who has the contract to manage the coordination and payment of claims. Even if the services of a GCM are not specifically defined as reimbursable in the insurance contract, a phone call to the benefits administrator explaining how a GCM's services may be a cost-effective alternative for the insurer may elicit approval for payment of at least some services.

In the case of privately purchased long-term care insurance policies, the specific clauses providing for the services of a "care coordinator" (also referred to in various policies as a "personal care specialist," "case management agency," or "personal care advocate") have become commonplace in policies sold since the mid-1990s. Older policies may not contain a specific clause providing for reimbursement of a care coordinator, but it is worth calling the company that issued the policy and asking if the services of a GCM can be reimbursed under the policy. Some companies, recognizing the value of such services, may approve payment, while others will not.

Some insurance companies offering the care coordination benefit require that the insured person use a GCM who is preapproved by the company. In some cases, the insurance company may have a contract with an agency in the community and insist that the care coordination services be provided by the contracted agency. Other policies leave the choice of the care coordinator up to the insured person.

Coverage for Healthy Policyholders, Too

An encouraging new trend for both GCMs and consumers is the range of services now offered by several leading insurance companies for those who purchase long-term care policies while they are still healthy.

A major objection many consumers have had to purchasing long-term care insurance policies is the fact that they could pay premiums for many years and never use their benefits. To make their policies more attractive, several insurance companies began offering benefits to help their clients plan for the future—both to actively prevent or postpone their need for care and to help them with information and referral services for other family members who may need care. Fortis, CNA, and UNUM are some of the companies offering this coverage.

These companies have developed programs that provide tangible benefits on an ongoing basis that the insured person and family members can use today long before the traditional long-term care benefits are needed. These "added value" programs are available for all policyholders of the companies who offer them, at no extra cost. They are marketed under such names as Productive Aging (Fortis) and LTC Connect (UNUM).

Under the Productive Aging program, for example, Fortis provides an information and referral service (including referrals to GCMs around the country) exclusively to its policyholders. Fortis claims to be the first long-term care insurance company "to take the traditional view of long-term care insurance coverage and bring it to a completely new level" with the Productive Aging program. Services offered under the Fortis Productive Aging program include the following:

- organizing important financial, legal, and insurance documents
- preparing wills, living wills, and other advance directives to ease the burden on family members during stressful times
- organizing family meetings to discuss care preferences
- managing finances
- planning for retirement
- funeral planning

Productive Aging also claims to help policyholders with issues they are facing today:

> With a little help you may even be able to help prevent problems before they occur or Productive Aging can help you learn more about:
> - Healthy living, including information about exercise, nutrition, and other health topics, like dental, vision, hearing, and foot care.
> - Personal safety, including home modifications.
> - Opportunities for enhancing your lifestyle with volunteer work, community programs, and recreation.
> - Consumer fraud.
> - Safe use of prescription and over-the-counter drugs.
> - Stress management.
> And more.[12(pp2–3)]

Productive Aging promises to assist in locating senior citizens centers or retirement communities, home health care services, community programs, and traditional or alternative living facilities. It also offers support in discussing sensitive health care issues with family members, coping with a chronic disease, and managing grief.

Rather than compete with private GCMs, the services offered by companies such as Fortis and CNA provide toll-free numbers for policyholders to call. Callers are either provided answers or resources from a comprehensive database or referred to professionals in the area where they are seeking services. In the case of Fortis, the Productive Aging program is managed by AdultCare, a private company (now owned by Fortis) based in Deerfield Beach, Florida.

AdultCare's founder and president David J. Levy emphasizes that its Productive Aging program does not behave like an HMO or managed care plan, so Fortis policyholders are always free to make their own choices:

> While some companies may offer you a listing of referrals to other groups and organizations, productive aging gives you information to make your own plans and decisions. When you have a question or need advice, help is just a toll-free call away. When you or your family call, our trained advisers will be there to help plan for the future by discussing options, as well as offering guidance to help prevent problems before they occur. That's what Productive Aging is all about.[12(p3)]

As often happens in the constantly changing long-term care insurance market, once one company offers an added benefit, other companies soon follow suit. UNUM is one of the most established long-term care insurance companies in the United States as well as the country's largest disability insurance provider. In 1998, UNUM announced a new program for its insured persons, LTC Connect. LTC Connect offers individuals who own a UNUM long-term care insurance policy many of the same benefits covered under the Fortis Productive Aging program.[13]

UNUM contracts with Ceridian Performance Partners to administer LTC Connect. A Pennsylvania-based corporation and one of the largest providers of employee assistance programs in the United States and Canada, Ceridian uses its Boston subsidiary, Work/Family Directions (WFD), to provide the information and referral portion of LTC Connect. According to Ceridian's Manager of Work/ Life Programs, Jason Robart,

> WFD counselors provide complete and impartial information without requiring callers to use a particular provider or service. Policyholders can get answers to questions about long-term care 24 hours a day simply by calling a toll-free number. This voluntary, confidential service provides callers with access to trained, experienced counselors who will listen, provide objective information about long-term care services, and help callers explore their options.[14]

Robart continued:

> LTC Connect offers UNUM policyholders the opportunity to discuss any topic relating to long-term care, including home care, personal finances, or the demands of caregiving, and receive help from experienced financial counselors with budget planning and managing long-term care costs.[14]

LTC Connect also offers its policyholders substantial discounts on items such as eyeglasses, contact lenses, or prescription drugs—items not often covered under other insurance plans. UNUM's program lets policyholders buy health products at reduced rates.

- Fifty percent discounts on both brand-name and generic prescription drugs through a network of more than 40,000 participating pharmacies, including most major chains
- Sixty percent discounts on prescription eyewear, including glasses, contact lenses, and sunglasses, through more than 7,000 locations nationwide, including major out-

lets such as Sears, Montgomery Ward, J.C. Penney, and Pearl Vision

- Twenty percent discounts on hearing aids and supplies, along with annual cleaning and inspection of hearing aids purchased through the LTC Connect program, with a network of approved audiologists[14]

Future Role in Long-Term Care Insurance

Merrily Orsini, who recently sold the successful independent geriatric care management practice she began in Louisville, Kentucky, served as moderator of a discussion forum entitled "Looking into the Future of Long-Term Care Insurance: Where Does the Geriatric Care Manager Fit In?"[15] Orsini asked all panelists what role they thought GCMs would have in the long-term care insurance industry of the future.

The panelists, seven experts on long-term care insurance trends who were from all around the United States, indicated that long-term care insurance may become a significant source of business for independent GCMs.

Joseph Hancock, MSW, risk manager and manager of claims underwriting and case management at Aetna Life Insurance Company in Hartford, Connecticut, was one panelist. Hancock was asked how long-term care insurance policies have changed over the past 10 years:

> Policies have gotten a lot better. . . . [There has been an] expansion of the types of services that people can use. Ten years ago it was nursing home care only. Now there is respite care, adult day-care, chore services, a variety of services that you can use are now all covered under standard long-term care policies. Newer policies cover an array of services. Competition has led to much better policies.[15(p18)]

Hancock also cited the introduction and usage of care management as a major change over the last 10 years.[15]

William J. Brisk, a Massachusetts-based elder-law attorney who has written extensively on long-term care issues, saw GCMs as a key element in the delivery of services financed by private insurance dollars:

> The need to organize home care for frail people and avoid institutionalization at any cost . . . requires varied skills: monitoring clients' physical and mental status and needs, supervising skilled and unskilled employees, the ability to tap public and private funding for what can be very expensive care, judgment on alternative living arrangements, and tact to lessen family conflicts.
>
> We work with a variety of geriatric care managers who offer very different sets of skills than elder-law specialists. Because of the growing complexity of what they do, future geriatric care managers will either specialize in a particular aspect of their work or consolidate with others to offer "the complete package."[15(p19)]

Joan Quinn, MS, BSM, senior vice president and general manager of government programs and Medicare management at Anthem Blue Cross/Blue Shield of Connecticut, told Orsini that, in her view, the role of GCMs in the future will depend on their knowledge of clinical as well as social support services in the community:

> They will be focused not only on the hospital episode of illness which will consume a small portion of hospital time to the member, but the greater focus will need to be on the medical and social support services available to the individual in the community and how they are coordinated and paid for. The insurer under a Medicare risk contract will pay for the medical needs of the individual but not the chronic care needs. The need for acute and long-term care services will need to be identified by the geriatric care manager. An outstanding issue for the insurer will be whether the care manager

will be an employee of the Company or a contractor with them. The care manager will be responsible for health assessment, disease management and seeing that the meals on wheels are delivered at the same time.[15(p20)]

Donald Charsky, president of LifePlans Inc., played a role in the design of newer long-term care insurance products to replace older, poorly designed products that were widely criticized by consumer advocates when he was working at UNUM's long-term care division. Charsky told Orsini that:

> the trend toward deinstitutionalizing long-term care creates a great opportunity for professional geriatric care managers to fill the role of assuring access to quality care that is appropriate for the need. Financing sources, including private insurance, are embracing the home and community care option. However, these added options tend to require greater care in the initial planning, as well as the ongoing monitoring of service delivery. In addition, care managers may need to play [a] greater role along with consumers in provider management.[15(pp20–21)]

Aetna's Joseph Hancock noted that all companies have adopted some kind of case management system, including eligibility determinations and on-site assessments:

> There will be an increased need for nurses and social workers who have expertise in functional and cognitive assessments and can go into the home and provide care planning. Just giving benefits to individuals is not enough. They need to know how to use the benefits wisely. The Aetna plan is a cash benefit and it makes no sense to just send money to a cognitively impaired person. Clients need to know how to identify services and to use the money wisely.[15(pp20–21)]

Vicki Zoot, RN, manager of group long-term care insurance at CNA in Chicago, saw the future of GCMs in the growth of long-term care insurance as providing five specific functions:

- Maintaining the social model and long-term care.
- Interfacing and collaborating with medical case management, including consulting and training.
- Participating in state programs, especially those not limited to poverty level participants.
- Continuing to work with family systems over extended periods of time, including acting as family advocates.
- Continuing role as private care managers.[15(p20)]

As people stop thinking of long-term care insurance as "nursing home insurance" and start thinking of it as "insurance to keep me out of a nursing home," the role of the GCM will become increasingly visible in long-term care insurance.

NON–INSURANCE-RELATED THIRD-PARTY REVENUE SOURCES FOR GCMs

Other target markets that are beginning to emerge include employer groups, labor unions, and professional organizations. Subcontracting opportunities are also available for GCMs in provider networks operated by employee assistance programs, work/life programs, and relocation services. This section will discuss some of those noninsurance third-party revenue sources.

Obtaining Business from Other Third-Party Sources

Additional opportunities for independent GCMs to grow their business by establishing relationships with third-party sources are beginning to develop. These opportunities range from local and regional contractual arrangements with health systems to participation in national provider networks such as participating professional networks (PPNs), PPOs, and work/life or dependent care networks. All of these models appear likely to grow in size and scope.

Miriam Oliensis-Torres, a clinical social worker who runs Geriatric Support Associates in Milwaukee, discussed how her firm has developed alliances with HMOs in Wisconsin. These collaborations, according to Oliensis-Torres, have yielded positive results and have provided her firm with an additional referral stream as well as the opportunity to serve those who could not, or would not, pay privately for services.

Geriatric Support Associates has contracted with one HMO to provide three levels of service: brief, intermediate, and extensive. Her care management firm receives a flat reimbursement rate for each of these three levels.[16]

A variety of PPNs, which operate somewhat like the better-known PPOs, are being developed by regional and national companies, including a California company called Senior Care Review. Senior Care Review specializes in conducting comprehensive on-site evaluations of senior care facilities such as nursing homes and assisted living facilities. Senior Care Review offers its services to individuals and families who are considering placement in a senior care facility of some type. According to Marjorie Nichols, LMSW, the company's senior vice president, "Many of these individuals and families are looking for assistance in selecting the facility of highest quality for their particular situation in their desired geographical area."[17] Utilizing a nationwide network of independent elder-care professionals, Senior Care Review promises consumers to make the process of screening and selecting a suitable housing alternative less stressful and more successful. While many GCMs provide such services as part of their basic service package, Nichols sees her company's services as a more effective way for the GCM to generate new business, without duplicating service or competing with the local GCM.

"At first glance," Nichols said, "you may perceive of this service as one which you are already providing to your clients based on your familiarity with the various facilities in your area. In many cases, we expect that you have also visited the facilities in your area as well. However, we believe that the services from Senior Care Review are actually complementary to those which you are likely providing." She adds:

> Senior Care Review is not a referral and placement agency, and receives no compensation from any facility. Rather, working directly on behalf of the consumer, our licensed healthcare professionals, utilizing carefully developed evaluation instruments, conduct thorough onsite evaluations of the identified facilities at the time our service is retained by the consumer. Senior Care Review then provides the results of these evaluations to the consumer in the form of a narrative summary report. The evaluations we conduct are timely and contain current information, as opposed to the dated and limited information provided by the various licensure and accreditation agencies. Further, our facility evaluations are also customized to the particular circumstances of the individual.[17]

Senior Care Review's goal is to provide comprehensive, customized, and current information about the facilities to the individual and family seeking placement.

How do independent GCMs become a part of this referral network? "Senior Care Review seeks highly trained professionals interested in evaluating senior care facilities to become part of our evaluator network. Our compensation structure for conducting facility evaluations and the corresponding reports are quite competitive."[17]

Companies such as Senior Care Review often have sufficient start-up capital to build a national marketing campaign to raise brand awareness, but most small GCM businesses do not have that much capital. Senior Care Review, for instance, has developed a well-designed Web site, professionally designed brochures and promotional materials, and a public relations campaign to raise awareness of its professional provider network. Nichols also reported that there are plans to expand Senior Care Review's consumer services to include a national database of GCMs and other elder-care professionals. GCMs wishing to join the network should contact the company or visit its Web site (see Appendix A for contact information).

Another emerging model of contracting for group business is third-party providers to corporations. One such provider is Child and Elder Care Insights (CECI), a work/life or dependent care company based in Cleveland, Ohio. In 1985 current President and Chief Executive Officer Elisabeth A. Breynton started CECI as a child care consulting firm. Breynton wanted to help solve the employer problems that began to emerge as a result of the staggering influx of parents—especially mothers with young children—into the workplace. This change increased stresses and pressures for both employees and employers and made businesses and families more closely entwined. CECI developed new employer strategies and programs to strengthen both the workplace and the family.

According to Breynton, as employers were beginning to feel the effects of their employees' elder-care problems, CECI began to develop innovative strategies to support the full continuum of family concerns. In the late 1980s, CECI began to focus on the development of a national database of elder-care providers and services. The company claims that this database, known as ELDERBASE, is the largest database of elder-care providers and services in the country. CECI continues to focus on expanding its two databases to serve the needs of its clients.

CECI services, says Breynton:

> Are delivered by professional consultants specializing in the identification and location of dependent care resources nationwide. We adhere to internally developed and strictly monitored policies and procedures in the assessment, counseling, and referral of each client. Through this process, CECI continually monitors and balances all levels of service and continually refines our responsibility as a dependent care resource and referral provider.[18]

CECI's standard product offering includes the following:

- an exclusive private-labeled 800 access number
- access alternatives via exclusive Internet, e-mail, and fax
- unlimited phone consultations with dependent care consultants
- a custom-published CareReport with a personalized cover letter
- unlimited referral requests and no limits on the number of referrals provided (i.e., no internal three-referrals limit)
- educational and care-selection materials addressing the referrals requested
- a four-color multiple page "Work/Life" newsletter

ELDERBASE enables consultants to access information on elder-care providers, services, and health and wellness issues. Consultants can also access clearinghouse information, including information on nursing homes, home health agencies, nutrition services, hospices, adult day care centers, legal services, transportation services, self-help organizations and groups, continuing care/retirement communities, senior centers, and many other senior services. ELDERBASE also allows a consultant to access information on health issues often faced by older people (e.g., diabetes, Alzheimer's) and a myriad of other issues older people face (e.g., legal and health insurance issues).

Breynton says that ELDERBASE is unique in its scope,

> enabling our consultants to locate care options in any radius from an employee's home or the home of their older dependent anywhere in the U.S. Thus, employees who live far away from their parents are afforded the ability to locate resources with as much ease as those living nearby.[18]

Ceridian, mentioned earlier in this chapter, offers a similar work/life and dependent care product through its WFD division, based in Boston.[14]

Still another opportunity for GCMs to develop contractual relationships with larger providers while preserving the ownership of their independent business is by entering into contractual relationships with provider organizations that are structured as PPOs. These organizations invite professionals who meet certain standards of experience and hold specific credentials to enroll as participating providers. A membership fee to offset the development costs of the PPO may be required. In return, the participating GCM is included in the select list of providers who receive referrals that are generated by contracts the PPO has established with large group purchasers such as employers, labor unions, government agencies, and health systems.

Peter Belson and Elizabeth Bodie Gross, both former presidents of the National Association of Professional Geriatric Care Managers, are cofounders of InterGenerational Management (IGM), a PPO that is contracting with care managers nationwide. According to Belson, IGM is the first PPO developed by care managers to deliver comprehensive care management services to employers and groups and other large purchasers of services for their constituents.

According to Belson, unlike other networks, IGM is based on each applicant's qualifications, credentials, and ability to deliver services in a specific geographic area. "We strongly believe that our abilities as care managers provide distinct added value and marketability to the GCMs who are participating in our provider network."[7(p11)]

There are some trade-offs that a GCM must consider when entering into a contractual arrangement with a PPO. Membership may place more restrictions on participants than other, more flexible arrangements do.

According to Belson, the terms of IGM's PPO, "while not requiring exclusivity, do bind the participant into a much more structured relationship than an independent contractor. These terms require working on cases under the IGM name, accepting a specific flat fee for a company designated work product, agreeing to giving IGM cases a priority level, and other terms. The value received in return, Belson added, is participation in the success of the PPO in the form of profit sharing or additional equity in IGM."[7(pp11–12)]

Two examples of contractual arrangements with health care provider groups, one in California and one in Georgia, are worth noting as well. Sue Shearer of the Huntington Hospital in Pasadena, California, has developed a growing network of relationships with individual physicians for Huntington's fee-for-service care management program. "Physicians are still largely unfamiliar with fee-based care managers," said Shearer. "Reaching out to them as individuals requires a lot of effort and time, but can pay off in a growing stream of referrals from private physicians."[7(p11)]

Garland Fritts, president of Fry Consultants in Atlanta, described the growth of geriatric centers within health systems as providing two major opportunities for fee-based care managers:

> "First," noted Fritts, "most health systems have neither the resources nor the time to develop a care management service. Independent Care Managers, however, can contract with the health systems geriatric center to develop a care management service. Second, some health system geriatric centers may wish to provide care management as an in-house service, thereby providing care managers the opportunity to sell their practices and then manage them from inside the system."[7(p11)]

Risks and Limitations of New Opportunities

Before jumping on the bandwagon and signing up to be a subcontractor, GCMs should be wary of the risks and limitations involved.

Oliensis-Torres stated that as in any relationship, the success or failure of an HMO contract rests with the specific individuals involved. "We are extremely lucky to be working with a very good group of people within the HMO who are genuinely concerned about their members and will actively encourage their physicians to approve referrals to us when appropriate," she said.[16(p24)]

Belson was asked if signing a formal contractual relationship with a regional or national referral network limits the freedom of independent care managers to practice. He responded that "in the most macro sense, the participation in any endeavor limits one's ability to participate in another." He added, however, that "any network that expects to achieve some measure of business success must offer a participant added value beyond mere remuneration for services rendered."[7(p11)]

FORMATION OF REGIONAL TRADE ASSOCIATIONS AND INFORMAL PROVIDER NETWORKS

By ignoring the growth of provider networks in long-term care, the small independent practitioner runs the risk of becoming a dinosaur. On the other hand, participation in such networks comes at some cost and a degree of risk, not the least of which is giving up the professional autonomy that many GCMs sought when they left the public or nonprofit sectors.

The appeal of operating one's own business, free of oppressive restrictions and compromised standards, is seductive. But at some point in the development of the GCM's small business, the hard realities of managing and growing a small business often become apparent. It is difficult to compete with other companies with more capital. Getting the message out about the availability of high-quality alternatives to the severely strained, publicly funded traditional providers requires mounting a marketing campaign. That requires money and time, two resources that many GCMs find are in short supply when they are struggling to make a profit.

Signing on as an individual subcontractor with existing PPO networks is not the only avenue of affiliation open to GCMs. Realizing that the individual or small group practice has its limitations, some GCMs are beginning to explore the development of regional trade associations or informal "virtual" partnerships by networking or using a concept such as "teaming."[19] Independent GCMs are experimenting with such ideas as pooling their resources to launch a cooperative marketing effort and banding together to form an informal provider network that can offer a wider array of services and cover a larger geographic area.

One example of this is the New England Elder Life Planning Group, a joint effort by six independent GCM practices based in Massachusetts, Maine, and New Hampshire, with plans to grow into Vermont, Rhode Island, and Connecticut. The group describes itself as "a trade organization which promotes and provides competent, principled care management through education, public relations and the development of contractual relationships with other members of the health care industry."[20] Members are experienced professionals who help older people and their families with plans designed to maintain maximum independence and peace of mind. Each member of the group has maintained an independent business identity while jointly developing a series of publications and educational programs to promote the group to a broader audience of potential referral sources. Thus far, the group has developed a brochure, a quarterly newsletter, a speakers bureau, and a Web site. The group also provides peer support both in group meetings and via phone and e-mail. This helps to address one of the drawbacks of owning an independent small business: professional isolation.

The advantages of forming such a professional alliance (similar groups have recently formed in the Chicago and Washington, DC/Virginia regions) are outlined in the book *Teaming Up: The Small Business Guide to Collaborating with Others To Boost Your Earnings and Expand Your Horizons.*[19]

The authors caution that while there are many benefits to alliances, there are drawbacks as well:

> Alliances require a high level of mutual trust, cooperation, and planning. Therefore there's a higher risk of conflicts, disappointments, complications, and even problems affecting your reputation if an associate doesn't deliver top-quality work. . . . There is always a risk that, in the future, a client or customer (or provider network) will have only enough work for one of you and will prefer working with your associate even if their initial contact was with you. That could mean losing a valued customer, client, or referral source.[19(p69)]

Being part of an interdependent alliance also requires keeping additional records and doing more administrative work to track time and expenses, process invoices, and meet tax obligations. Legal liability and financial risk are also potential problems:

> Usually you are truly interdependent in a joint venture. You must depend on someone else to accomplish the joint goals. This added vulnerability creates greater potential for conflicts, disappointments, and disagreements. You're legally liable for actions of your joint venture partner. To protect your legal and financial interests, you need to get all joint venture agreements in writing. This can take time and energy and add complications to your life."[19(p75)]

The authors also caution that the joint venture can drain time, energy, and money from a person's primary business and point out that "it's harder to ask to back out if things don't work out because others are dependent on you and you're legally liable for whatever you've jointly contracted to do."[19(p75)]

While these drawbacks are not insignificant and GCMs should consider them carefully before deciding to develop or participate in a joint venture, the authors clearly endorse the idea of teaming up. The book emphasizes that there is not a "one size fits all" model of partnering or teaming. The authors offer 10 specific models that are worth considering: networking, mutual referrals, cross-promoting, interdependent alliances, joint ventures, satellite subcontracting consortia, family/exposed collaborations, partnerships, virtual organizations, and proactive strategic alliances. The success of such ventures depends on the participants' ability to choose the model that is best suited to their personal and professional styles and personalities.

Finally, the authors offer their "12 Principles for Negotiating Honest, Fair, and Lasting Financial Agreements:"

1. Make Negotiating Fun.
2. Let the "51% Rule" Prevail. (The willingness of each partner to contribute a little more than just 50% to the joint effort.)
3. Don't Procrastinate About Key Points.
4. Work Toward Flexible Agreements.
5. Think Long-Term, Not Short-Term.
6. Aim for Financial Equality.
7. Account for Nonfinancial Contributions, Too.
8. Be Creative and Open in Your Negotiating Positions.
9. Agree That the Party Who Loses Any Ensuing Lawsuit Pays All Court Costs.
10. Don't Just Say It: Ink It.
11. Don't Negotiate with Someone Who Won't Negotiate.
12. Cut Your Losses—Fast.[20(pp176–189)]

CONCLUSION

This chapter has discussed a variety of emerging financing opportunities for GCMs running their own businesses. GCM entrepreneurs must stay abreast of the constant changes in the marketplace, especially changes that can directly or indirectly affect revenue and referral sources. If GCMs continue to believe that our revenue base today will remain a constant source of operating income in the future, they are likely to miss out on emerging opportunities to grow their businesses or discover that their businesses can no longer compete in this rapidly changing marketplace.

NOTES

1. Elkind A. The early development of the geriatric care management movement. *Geri Gazette.* 1987, 1988;1.

2. U.S. Senate Committee on Aging. *Medicaid Estate Planning: Analysis of GAO's Massachusetts Report and*

Senate House Conference Language. Washington, DC: U.S. Government Printing Office; 1993.

3. Moschella A, Nelligan J, Marcus M. *Resource Guide: What You Need To Know about the Medicaid Eligibility and Transfer Rules.* Boston: MedLaw; 1998.

4. Barker RL. *Social Work in Private Practice.* 2nd ed. Baltimore: National Association of Social Workers; 1991.

5. Petersen PG. *Will America Grow Up Before It Grows Old: How the Coming Social Security Crisis Threatens You, Your Family, and Your Country.* New York: Random House; 1997.

6. Collapse of Medicare. *Wall Street Journal.* June 19, 1997: PB1.

7. O'Toole RE. Independent care managers: emerging payment sources for the 21st century. *Inside Case Manage.* 1998;4:10–12.

8. Private geriatric care management: how families are served. *J Case Manage Pract.* 1992;1:108–112.

9. Reschovsky JD. Demand for and access to institutional long term care: the role of Medicaid in nursing home markets. *Inquiry.* 1996;33:15–29.

10. Graham E. Weighing the benefits of buying insurance for extended elder care. *Wall Street J.* 1999;March 31:B1.

11. O'Toole RE. Growth of private long term care insurance will expand the role of case management. *Inside Case Manage.* 1995;2:10–12.

12. Fortis Investors. *Introducing Productive Aging.* Milwaukee: Fortis Investors; 1997.

13. UNUM Life Insurance Corporation. *LTC Connect: Answers to Your Long Term Concerns.* Portland, ME: UNUM Life Insurance Corporation; 1998.

14. Robart J. Interview by author. April 14, 1999, Boston.

15. Orsini M. Q & A: looking into the future of long-term insurance: where does the geriatric care manager fit in? *GCM J.* 1998;8:17–23.

16. O'Toole RE. Independent care managers: emerging payment sources for the 21st century. *Inside Case Manage.* 1998;4.

17. Nichols M. Interview and correspondence with author. April 20, 1999, Boston.

18. Breynton E. Interview with author. April 20, 1999, Boston.

19. Edwards P, Edwards S, Benzel R. *Teaming Up: The Small Business Guide to Collaborating with Others To Boost Your Earnings and Expand Your Horizons.* Berkeley, CA: Tarcher Press; 1997.

20. *Mission Statement.* Dedham, MA: New England Elder Life Planning Group; 1998.

CHAPTER 9

Care Management Credentialing

Rona S. Bartelstone and Monika White

INTRODUCTION

Care management has become a dominant feature in the health and social services delivery systems in response to the continuing fragmentation and increasing complexity of both systems. There has also been a parallel increase in the numbers and types of consumers who need care management services because of the prevalence of chronic illness among many segments of the population. Older people, people with developmental disabilities, people with chronic mental illness, and others benefit from care management. Furthermore, care management has been increasingly encouraged by legislative and funding actions that have included care management as a means of addressing the demographic and medical challenges that create the need for ongoing multiple services.

Significant activities have taken place during the past 20 to 25 years, resulting in current efforts to "professionalize" care management. For example, care management was a specific component of the Developmental Disabilities Act of 1975. During the 1980s, care management became a prominent feature of the Medicaid waiver programs. The 1980s also saw the emergence of care management in workers' compensation and private practice, especially with older people. In the late 1980s and early 1990s, numerous professional associations—including the National Association of Professional Geriatric Care Managers (NAPGCM), the National Council on Aging, and the National Association

of Social Workers—began to promote standards for care managers. The growth of managed care in the 1990s further expanded the care management role in all settings and with all populations. This led to the establishment of standards in 1999 for care management organizations by the American Accreditation HealthCare Commission/URAC. Finally, efforts to certify individual care managers began in the early 1990s, as the demand for care management staff expanded prior to the development of academically-based curricula. All of these developments demonstrate a broad-based consensus that care management has become a useful and important component of the health and social services delivery systems. Despite apparent agreement on the value of care management, there is little to guide individual or corporate purchasers about who should do it, under what circumstances, for whom, and through which funding mechanisms. This has created confusion among consumers, funders, policy makers, and even personnel.

Credentialing is the effort to determine what competent practice is. It is a process that results in licensing, certification, or another form of recognition or acknowledgment of a standard. Included in this process is the body of knowledge and the skill set that allow the practitioner to perform the job tasks of a specific field of practice. Because care management has evolved as a transdisciplinary field, it is important to delineate the functions, roles, values, and ethical perspectives of a competent care manager. Given the fact that each participating discipline and profession has its own definitions, this presents a major challenge.

Mechanisms for credentialing care managers have been actively developed by large professional associations, local agency coalitions, and nonprofit organizations, among others. To date, the majority of these mechanisms focus on specific disciplines or areas of work such as physical therapy or workers' compensation. Rehabilitation, managed care, and acute care increasingly request or require care management certification as a condition of employment, and health care professionals in these settings are obtaining certification by the thousands. At the same time, there has been little demand for care management certification in nonmedical settings. Many care managers from the proprietary and nonprofit community-based service and long-term care arena rely on their educational degrees and professional licenses and do not perceive a need to add another credential. Yet interest in credentialing programs continues to grow, as does the number of programs.

This chapter discusses credentialing for care managers generally, not just geriatric care managers. After a section discussing the motivations behind and history of care management credentialing, the chapter provides an overview of selected credentialing and certification organizations. A discussion of some current and future issues concludes the chapter.

MOTIVATION

In addition to validating education and experience, there are several reasons why people are motivated to establish care management certification. Among them are the following:

- informed consumer choice
- consumer protection
- marketing
- insurability
- education
- research
- self-regulation

The sections below discuss each rationale.

Informed Consumer Choice

One of the primary reasons for the development of a credential is to enable the consumer to make a discriminating choice of the type of care manager who should be hired for a given circumstance. For example, an acute medical setting might warrant the employment of a nurse or other clinical technician with in-depth experience with a particular diagnosis. In a community-based setting, a care manager with a background in social work, psychology, or mental health might better serve the client, such as a grieving widow or individual with chronic mental illness. In other situations an expert with a background in both medical and psychosocial fields might be most appropriate. There might also be differentiating circumstances based upon the specific population whose needs are to be met. An older adult might be better served by a care manager with a gerontological background, just as an individual with human immunodeficiency virus/acquired immune deficiency syndrome would need the expertise of someone knowledgeable about this specific disease process, treatment, services, and emotional impact. Rosen and colleagues note that certification could provide some consensus about expectations for service delivery.[1]

Consumer Protection

The consumer also needs protection from an individual who might call him- or herself a care manager but have no training in the care management process, roles, and functions and no understanding of health and social services systems and psychosocial dynamics. Since no licensing or other regulation currently exists, the consumer has no guidelines from which to "shop" for services except the current certification programs. These certifications, then, are very important mechanisms for guiding the consumer. They provide protection for other well-trained, appropriately experienced care managers who are competing, perhaps unfairly, with individuals, who are of lesser capacity and charge lower fees often for inferior services.

Credentialing can give the consumer confidence that a care manager has, at minimum, qualified to take an exam and possesses core knowledge about care management.

Marketing

Most health care and social services providers today seek a competitive advantage in the individual, corporate, and nonprofit markets. Credentialing of individual employees on the basis of their competency becomes a selling point, especially when providers are looking to broaden their markets and when there is a likelihood of passing along risk. Network providers of all types look to affiliate with organizations and individuals that meet industry standards for practice as part of their marketing approach and for liability reasons. Care managers can use their credential as a marketing tool to distinguish themselves from those who are not certified and as proof of core competency for network affiliation or membership.

Insurability

Another rationale for credentialing is the ability to be covered by malpractice insurance and to receive payments from third-party insurers and other reimbursement sources. While reimbursement for care management is still limited, it will increase as care management is more fully recognized and funded, especially in the social services arena. An insurer who is considering a malpractice policy for care managers or care management organizations needs to be able to identify who it is insuring, for which job functions, within which settings, for what populations, and with what decision-making or fiduciary responsibilities. Without this knowledge, it would be impossible for an insurance company to develop such a liability policy. As of 1999 there were three insurance companies providing malpractice coverage for care managers. With the growth of care management networks that require insurance coverage, there are indications that certification may become the norm in the future.

Education

Educating care managers in a defined body of knowledge is another rationale for providing a credentialing process. As previously stated, care management did not evolve from an academic program within the nation's college or university systems but developed in response to consumer need. In order for a field of practice or a discipline to become professionalized, there must be a defined and determinate body of knowledge so that it can be taught with uniformity and consistency.

In the late 1990s, Anne Reban of the University of North Texas conducted a study of existing academic, continuing education, and agency-based training for care managers. The outcome of this study is expected to further the discipline and the consensus about the job tasks, knowledge base, and skills required of a competent care manager. It is anticipated that broadly accepted curricula for the training of care managers in academic settings will eventually be developed.[2]

Care management degree and certificate programs are being offered or are under development in a number of universities. Many nursing schools already have well-developed care management programs. Others, such as graduate gerontology schools and undergraduate human services departments, have plans to offer courses leading to certification in the near future. Care managers can check with their local university nursing, social work, or gerontology schools for information.

Research

Credentialing of care managers enables research that defines specific outcomes and accountabilities as a result of the process of providing care. Outcomes need to relate to health status, quality of care, cost of care, and efficient use of systems to coordinate services. Outcomes must also be defined in terms of client goals. Such goals might include quality of life, knowledge about needs, increased ability to participate in or maintain care, ability to better use systems of care to meet needs, and better social/emotional functioning of the consumer and the consumer's support system. Again, most outcome measures currently in use come from medical settings. In psychosocial areas, outcomes tend to be anecdotal. Their value is limited because the provider organization determines whether to report, what to report, and when to report it.

Limited empirical research exists in these areas, especially in consumer-defined outcomes, but the body of research is growing. For example, Geron and colleagues have developed client satisfaction measures to determine consumer perceptions of home care and care management services. These measures are already in use by several states and agency programs and provide hope that the quality and success of care management will be more easily quantified in the future.[3]

Self-Regulation

Self-regulation is an essential aspect of any professional field. Just as it is in the best interest of consumers to be involved in defining and creating the systems that work for them, it is in the best interest of care managers to be involved in defining appropriate regulation for their work. Only in this way will accurate expectations for the individual practitioner or system be developed. Government-imposed guidelines often miss the essential ingredients of the value system, nature, and realities of the profession. It is important for care managers to participate in development and implementation of standards and guidelines, in research studies, in legislative or policy activities, and in available and relevant professional associations.

HISTORY

The disability movement of the 1970s spurred the development of several professional organizations focused on the rehabilitation needs of individuals. Two of these organizations, the American Rehabilitation Counseling Association and the National Rehabilitation Counseling Association, formed a Joint Committee on Re-

habilitation Counselor Certification that was reorganized in 1973 to become the Commission on Rehabilitation Counselor Certification (CRCC).

The more specific move toward credentialing of care managers began to gain momentum in the late 1980s and early 1990s with the emergence of a number of professional organizations focused on care management services to various populations in diverse settings. These organizations recognized that they had both competing and mutual interests that could best be served by moving toward a consensus in the role played by care managers in the evolving health and social services environments.

A meeting of these organizations was held in 1991 and was hosted by the Individual Case Management Association. The outcome of this meeting was the formation of a National Case Management Task Force, which appointed a steering committee to address the issues of philosophy, definition, and existing standards of practice. There were 29 organizations involved in this task force. In 1992, the steering committee proposed the development of a voluntary care management credential.

An Interim Commission was incorporated as an independent credentialing organization and in July 1995 was renamed the Commission for Case Manager Certification (CCMC). The CCMC continues to be responsible for the Certified Case Manager (CCM) credentialing process. The CCM eligibility required that an applicant have a:

> minimum educational requirement of a post-secondary program in a field that promotes the physical, psychosocial, or vocational well-being of the persons being served. In addition, the license or certificate awarded upon completion of the educational program must have been obtained by the applicant's having passed an examination in his/her area of specialization."[4(p4)]

This means that the CCM is effectively an advanced practice credential.

Although the Interim Commission included representation from the Certification of Insurance Rehabilitation Specialists Commission, later renamed the Certification of Disability Management Specialists Commission, it is important to note that this group maintained its individual identity. It was instrumental in creating the new certification, and there was apparently no sense that this was a further fragmentation of the care management field.

In 1993, two other organizations began a second set of discussions about credentialing care managers. NAPGCM and the Case Management Institute (CMI) of Connecticut Community Care both felt that the CCM was medically oriented and focused primarily on rehabilitation and acute care management. Furthermore, the eligibility criteria for the CCM excluded most of the staff employed by social services programs in the home- and community-based long-term care social services arena. This excluded most staff from publicly funded programs serving clients through various nonprofit and publicly sponsored programs. It left out many of the front-line staff who provide direct client services through such agencies as the area agencies on aging, vocational and rehabilitation services, substance abuse programs, peer counseling programs, and other grassroots organizations. Such organizations rely upon both formally and informally trained and supervised staff, including those with many years of hands-on care management experience.

Members of NAPGCM and CMI noted that these practicing care managers would be unable to obtain credentialing. In addition, the CCM exam at the time was focused on medical issues, not the core processes and functions of care management. For these reasons, another independent organization was formed called the National Academy of Certified Care Managers (NACCM). The credential offered by NACCM is the Care Manager Certified (CMC), which is also given subsequent to the successful completion of an exam process. The focus of the NACCM exam is the core care management functions of assessment, care planning, care implementation, monitoring/management, reassessment, termination, and professional issues and ethics. NACCM began offering the exam in January 1996.

Throughout the field's history, there have been formal discussions held between the vari-

ous stakeholders in care management. In 1992 and 1993, six professional organizations came together as the National Coalition of Associations for the Advancement of Case Management. These associations represented over 20,000 health and social services professionals and hoped to influence the health care reforms that were part of the President's Task Force on National Health Care Reform, chaired by Hillary Rodham Clinton. Although the health care reform movement was politically hampered, this effort did begin the process of developing consensus about the definitions of the process of care management and the role of care management in ensuring quality care and making efficient use of resources. It also began to point the direction for the future role of care management in defining needs and solutions and acting as a change agent within the system.

In 1997 and 1999, two other meetings were held under the auspices of the Foundation for Rehabilitation Education & Research and NAPGCM. These were identified as the Care and Case Management Summits I & II. This time 16 associations and organizations participated to continue the discussion of care management definitions, review the existing credentialing options and their ethical standards, and compare the knowledge domains of these various definitions and options.

In July 1998, a white paper was published by the sponsoring organizations that presented a summary of the meeting outcomes. The 1999 Summit II outcomes are still in production, as of this writing.[5] However, the organizations and associations that participated in these meetings have agreed to continue discussions in order to promote a unified definition of care management and facilitate a common approach to the issues of credentialing, education, funding, and regulation. The leadership role in this latest effort has been assumed by NAPGCM.

OVERVIEW OF SELECTED CREDENTIALING AND CERTIFICATION ORGANIZATIONS

This section refers to Table 9–1, which lists selected credentialing and certification organi-

Table 9–1 Overview of Eligibility Criteria and Examinations for Selected Credentialing Organizations

	Education	Experience	Prerequisite (license or other)	Exam Content (partial list)	Recertification
American Institute of Outcomes Case Management *Case Manager Certified (CMC)* (562) 945-9990	1. BA, MA, PhD 2. Associate or Diploma RN	1. 36–60 months full-time 2. professional license	License at Associate level	Clinical, customer service, management/ supervision, quality improvement, legal/ risk aspects, payer, utilization review employer and provider organizations, resources	Every 2 years CEU based on scores
Certification of Disability Management Specialists Commission *Certified Disability Management Specialist (CDMS)* (847) 394-2106	1. RN or CRC 2. MA or PhD 3. BA 4. Any degree, BA or higher in other field	1. 12 months full-time 2. 24–36 months 3. 36 months 4. 60 months	License at level 1	Job placement, vocational assessment, case management and disabilities, rehabilitation services and care, disability legislation, forensic rehabilitation	Every 5 years 80 CEU hours total
Commission for Case Manager Certification *Certified Case Manager (CCM)* (847) 818-0292	Postsecondary program in physical, psychosocial, and vocational well-being	12–24 months full-time as case manager or supervisor, 12 months under CCM or 24 without CCM	Valid license or certification	Coordination, service delivery, physical and psychological factors, benefit systems, case management concepts, community resources	Every 5 years 80 CEU hours total
Commission on Rehabilitation Counselor Certification *Certified Rehabilitation Counselor (CRC)* (847) 394-9104	MA or PhD in rehabilitation counseling or related field; includes 600 hours of internship	0–5 years depending on status of other requirements and 12 months of supervision under a CRC	NA	Focus on medical, psychosocial service coordination, client assessment, planning for individuals with disabilities	Every 5 years 80 CEU hours total
Healthcare Quality Certification Board of the National Association for Healthcare Quality *Certified Professional in Healthcare Quality (CPHQ)* (626) 286-9415	Any degree, Associate or higher or RN or LPN license	2 years full-time in health care quality, utilization or risk management	RN or LPN license if no degree	Management leadership and continuum of care and subcategories	Every 2 years 80 CEU hours total

continues

Table 9–1 continued

	Education	Experience	Prerequisite (license or other)	Exam Content (partial list)	Recertification
National Academy of Certified Care Managers *Care Manager, Certified (CMC)* (800) 962-2260	1. MA 2. BA 3. High School Diploma	1. 2 years 2. 4 years 3. 6 years 2 years supervision	NA	Assessment, care planning, coordination, monitoring, termination, ethical and legal issues	Every 3 years 45 CEU hours total 1500 hours practice
National Board for Certification in Continuity of Care *Continuity of Care Certification, Advanced (A-CCC)* (860) 586-7525	BA	2 years full-time	NA	Continuity of care process, health delivery system, clinical, legal, reimbursement, professional issues	Every 5 years 50 CEU hours total or retake exam
Rehabilitation Nursing Certification Board *Certified Rehabilitation Registered Nurse (CCRN)* (800) 229-7530	RN	2 years in rehabilitation nursing	RN license	Rehabilitation, rehabilitation nursing models and theories	Every 5 years 60 CEU hours total or retake exam

Note: CEU = continuing education unit.

zations along with the major criteria that define their requirements and their perspective on care management practice.

CCMC

As noted above, CCMC administers the CCM credential. The CCM designation has been offered since 1993. An applicant to sit for the CCM must meet the requirements quoted earlier in this chapter. In addition, there are employment requirements:

> *Category 1* 12 months of acceptable full-time case management employment or its equivalent under the supervision of a CCM for the 12 months. OR
>
> *Category 2* 24 months of acceptable full-time case management employment or its equivalent. Supervision by a CCM is not required under this category. OR
>
> *Category 3* 12 months of acceptable full-time case management employment or its equivalent as a supervisor, supervising the activities of individuals who provide DIRECT case management services.[4(p5)]

The CCMC has defined care management as an advanced practice area within an already licensed or certified profession. In fact, in a 1994 paper published by the Foundation for Rehabilitation and Research, Michael J. Leahy found that the most frequent settings in which surveyed CCMs worked were:

> independent case management companies (23.8%), followed by hospitals (11.7%), independent rehabilitation/ insurance affiliates (11.0%), and health insurance companies (8.0%). The most frequent job titles of respondents include case manager (45.9%), registered nurse (19.8%), rehabilitation counselor (10.9%), and administrator/manager (7.6%).[6(p3)]

NACCM

As noted earlier in the chapter, NACCM administers the CMC designation. NACCM was founded in 1994 and began offering its examination in 1996. As also discussed above, NACCM founders believed that the CCM exam was so medically oriented that it did not accurately reflect the needs of those working in primarily social services delivery systems. The founders also knew that many practitioners in the social services arena did not have postsecondary degrees and were not trained at the professional level at all. The intention then was to recognize those who were delivering the services as care managers already and to attempt to raise the minimum standards by requiring a credentialing examination and a program of continuing education. For these reasons, candidates for the CMC can qualify to take the exam in one of the following ways:

> *Criteria 1* A minimum of 6 years of paid, full time, direct experience with clients in fields such as social work, nursing, mental health, counseling or care management, two years of which must be supervised (50 hours/year), that includes face-to-face interviewing, assessment, care planning, problem-solving and follow-up. This experience must be subsequent to obtaining a minimum of a high school diploma or any degree unrelated to the field of care management. OR
>
> *Criteria 2* A minimum of 4 years of paid full-time direct experience with clients in fields such as social work, nursing, mental health, counseling or care management, 2 years of which must be supervised (50 hours/year) paid, full time care management experience that includes face-to-face interviewing, assessment, care planning, problem-solving and follow-up. This experience must be subsequent to obtaining a BA/BS degree in a field related to care management (social work,

counseling, nursing, mental health, psychology, and gerontology). OR

Criteria 3 A minimum of 2 years of supervised (50 hours/year), paid, full-time care management experience that includes face-to-face interviewing, assessment, care planning, problem solving and follow-up. This experience must be subsequent to obtaining a Master's degree in a field related to care management (social work, counseling, nursing, mental health, psychology, and gerontology).[7(p7)]

These criteria are more inclusive but raise the issue of the "professionalism" of the practice because individuals with high school diplomas may sit for the exam if they meet experience and employment criteria. A high school diploma is not usually considered a professional/terminal degree. And, while these criteria may be more reflective of the experience of care managers in the social services system, as differentiated from the health delivery system, it is prudent to question the hiring practices of those agencies and organizations that leave the management of consumer lives to staff with such limited training.

National Board for Certification in Continuity of Care

The National Board for Certification in Continuity of Care administers the Continuity of Care Certification, Advanced (A-CCC). This certification is open to people from multiple disciplines, including nurses, social workers, therapists, dietitians, and physicians. The candidate must have a bachelor's degree plus 2 years of full-time experience within the last 5 years in continuity of care, or equivalent part-time experience (4,000 hours) within the past 5 years. This certification evolved from the area of discharge planning within a number of institutional settings.

Given the fact that many hospitals and other inpatient settings have combined their discharge and utilization management departments, often calling them care management divisions, the future demand for Continuity of Care Certification is uncertain.

Rehabilitation Nursing Certification Board

The Rehabilitation Nursing Certification Board administers the Certified Rehabilitation Registered Nurse certification. This certification is solely for those who have an "unrestricted RN license plus at least two years of practice as registered professional nurse in rehabilitation nursing within the last five years."[8(p3)]

This process then is limited to those within the nursing profession and does not address the inter- and transdisciplinary nature of care management.

Healthcare Quality Certification Board

The Healthcare Quality Certification Board of the National Association for Healthcare Quality administers the Certified Professional in Healthcare Quality certification. This is a very broad-based certification with a number of ways to qualify for the examination, as follows:

Criteria 1 Associate's, Bachelor's, Master's or Doctorate degree in any field; OR

Criteria 2 Valid RN or LPN license; OR

Criteria 3 Valid accreditation in medical records technology plus minimum of two years of full-time experience or its part-time equivalent in health care quality management, utilization management, or risk management activities in the last five years.[8(p3)]

The test covers management/leadership activities and the continuum of care with additional subcategories. In this test, care management is conceived of as less of a direct service delivery system and more of a management function.

Certification of Disability Management Specialists Commission

The Certification of Disability Management Specialists Commission administers the CDMS certification. This commission was originally developed in 1984 as the Certification of Insurance Rehabilitation Specialists Commission and was changed to the current name in 1996. This certification has nine different categories within which a candidate may qualify, as follows:

Category 1A Master's in Rehabilitation Counseling granted by a program that was accredited by the Council on Rehabilitation Education, or current certification as a CRC. This also includes a minimum of 12 months of acceptable full-time employment providing direct disability management services to individuals with disabilities receiving benefits from a disability compensation system; OR

Category 1B Master's Degree in Rehabilitation Counseling granted by a program that was not accredited by CORE, plus a minimum of 12 months of acceptable full-time employment providing direct disability management services to individuals receiving benefits from a disability compensation system with the 12 months spent under the supervision of a CDMS or CRC; OR

Category 1C Bachelor's Degree in Rehabilitation Administration or Rehabilitation Service, plus a minimum of 24 months of acceptable full-time employment providing direct disability management services to individuals receiving benefits from a disability compensation system with 12 of the 24 months spent under the supervision of a CDMS or CRC; OR

Category 2A A current license as an RN and a Master's Degree in Nursing, plus a minimum of 12 months of acceptable full-time employment providing direct disability management services to individuals receiving benefits from a disability compensation system with the 12 months spent un-

der the supervision of a CDMS or CRC; OR

Category 2B A current license as an RN and a Bachelor's Degree or Nursing Diploma, plus a minimum of 24 months of acceptable full-time employment providing direct disability management services to individuals receiving benefits from a disability compensation system with 12 of the 24 months spent under the supervision of a CDMS or CRC; OR

Category 2C A current license as an RN and an Associate's Degree in Nursing, plus a minimum of 36 months of acceptable full-time employment providing direct disability management services to individuals receiving benefits from a disability compensation system with 24 of the 36 months spent under the supervision of a CDMS or CRC; OR

Category 3A A master's degree and license in a field that promotes the physical, psychosocial or vocational well being of the persons being served. In addition, the license that is awarded upon completion of the educational program MUST have been obtained by the applicant's having passed an examination in his/her field of specialization. Furthermore, the required employment experience is a minimum of 12 months of acceptable full-time employment providing direct disability management services to individuals receiving benefits from a disability compensation system with the 12 months spent under the supervision of a CDMS or CRC; OR

Category 3B A bachelor's degree and license in a field that promotes the physical, psychosocial or vocational well being of the persons being served. In addition, the license that is awarded upon completion of the educational program MUST have been obtained by the applicant's having passed an examination in his/her field of specialization. Furthermore, the required employment experience is a minimum of 24 months of acceptable full-time employment providing direct disability management services to individuals receiving benefits from a disability compensation system with 12 of the 24 months spent under the supervision of a CDMS or CRC; OR

Category 4A Master's or Doctoral degree that meets specific course requirements, plus a minimum of 36 months of acceptable full-time employment providing direct disability management services to individuals receiving benefits from a disability compensation system with 24 of the 36 months spent under the supervision of a CDMS or CRC.[9(pp4-6)]

Here again, the emphasis does appear to be on the nursing profession; however, the more advanced degrees do allow for other training so long as they include specific courses in disability, vocational/occupational information, counseling, and other direct service training criteria.

CRCC

The CRCC, mentioned earlier in the chapter, administers the Certified Rehabilitation Counselor (CRC) certification. This certification also allows people multiple ways of meeting the eligibility requirements. The first three are presented below. The additional seven categories will be described in a general manner, as they have very specific course requirements. The reader is referred to the Commission for more specific details.

Category A Master's in Rehabilitation Counseling from an education program accredited by CORE that includes an internship/practicum; OR

Category B Master's in Rehabilitation Counseling from a program that was not accredited by CORE, but included a practicum, plus 12 months of acceptable employment under the supervision of a CRC; OR

Category C Master's in Rehabilitation Counseling from a program that was not accredited, and did not require a practicum, plus 24 months of acceptable employment including a minimum of 12 months under the supervision of a CRC; OR

Categories D1, D2, D3, H, I, J, and K All of these categories relate to master or doctoral programs in other than Rehabilitation Counseling, but with very specific course, experiential and supervision requirements.[10(pp5-9)]

This credential defines care management as an advanced practice field, making the credential similar to the CCM.

CURRENT AND FUTURE ISSUES

The first two summit meetings have not resulted in a unified approach to care management; there remain diverse views and even controversy in a number of areas. This section highlights some of the major issues that continue to be discussed:

* philosophical approach
* training and multiple disciplines
* supervision
* specialty credentials and levels of credentials
* organizational versus individual credentialing
* implications for policy development and reimbursement

Philosophical Approach

There are many philosophical questions related to care management. Several are posed here.

Is care management a social, medical, integrated, or coordinated service model? Traditionally, the social and medical models have been considered separate largely because of the diverse funding sources for each. In addition to reimbursement and funding differences, the fragmentation in legislation, authority, and standards in health, mental health, and social services programs have made it nearly impossible to develop a unified holistic or integrated model of care. There is increasing recognition on both health and psychosocial sides of the debate that there is a need for greater crossover and flexibility to allow the integration of these components. However, the structural and financial issues have yet to be resolved. Ideally, future public policy makers will look at the total needs of the population and provide funds to be used for any social service, mental health, or medical service needed by an individual or family at any given moment. Private insurance policies might likewise be integrated. The role of care managers would be to triage clients to help determine the most appropriate level of intervention and to monitor client status and service delivery.

Does the care management process cut across the continuum of care or can it be performed within a single setting? There is growing consensus that care management services cut across settings as evidenced by modifications in the CCM requirements that include work across the continuum of care. This does not change the fact that funding remains tied to particular settings and is not typically portable to other parts of the continuum of care.

Is there a value to maintaining an individual at a level of functioning, or is the goal rehabilitation? There is a growing sense that there is value in ensuring that a level of functioning is maintained. Perry's study concluded that delaying institutional care through a program of maintenance would save the government $5 billion in health care and custodial costs in just 1 month.[11] Other studies suggest similar savings. The National Alzheimer's Association estimated that the annual cost of Alzheimer's to American businesses is at least $33 billion. Families and people with Alzheimer's pay an estimated $3.7 billion to $6.5 billion for the medical costs of Alzheimer's.[12] These costs are not borne by the general public. The implications for empowering caregivers and focusing on the quality of life are enormous.

Is care management considered a profession, a practice field within a primary profession, or a role that does not require professional status? In 1964, Carr-Sanders and Wilson provided a model of professionalization that includes:

> Attracting practitioners on a full-time basis;
> Having acquired support from foundations and large governmental sponsors;
> Having a growing body of literature supported by academic journals;
> Having numerous university training programs;
> Having accreditation of academic programs;
> Practitioners receiving a fee for services;
> Being successful in influencing public policy;
> Having a professional association with conditions for entrance; and
> Having registration or licensure requirements for practice.[13]

According to this definition, care management has not quite reached professional status because of the lack of accredited educational programs to prepare individuals for practice and the lack of regulation to govern the field.

Is the role of the care manager inherently that of a gatekeeper and resource allocator? The care manager's approach to service provision is best addressed in light of the practice setting. There will be major differences in the ability to authorize, distribute, or utilize resources in a health maintenance organization, a state waiver program, and a private practice. While all aspects of care management include some resource allocation, resource allocation is not always the role of the gatekeeper. Furthermore, in times of scarcity, use of resources becomes an ethical matter regardless of the source of funding or reimbursement. It is clear, however, that the way a care manager views this role will impact other decisions.

Training and Multiple Disciplines

Who should do care management and what core knowledge is needed to perform the essential tasks and activities within a given setting or specific population have long been topics of debate and discussion. Since the practice of care management developed from within the field rather than from an academic program, there is no consensus about the body of knowledge needed nor is there a unified set of core skills for care managers. Further complicating this issue is the lack of common standards for continuing education of care managers. The various credentialing organizations listed in Table 9–1 have different criteria for what continuing education credits will be accepted, of what those credits should consist, and who should have provided those credits.

There is great disparity as well among practicing care managers about what their core training should be. The backgrounds and training of social workers, nurses, psychologists, gerontologists, counselors, and therapists vary widely. Increasingly, practitioners are also coming into care management from other fields because of changes in demographics, corporate downsizing, and midlife career decisions. Some come into care management as a result of their own experience in dealing with an aging loved one or other person with a catastrophic or chronic illness. Others enter from such diverse venues as the long-term care insurance field, law, financial planning, life planning, retirement planning, accounting, and recreational therapy. This great diversity helps explain why some of the credentialing organizations require a prior license or certification.

Supervision

As Table 9–1 and the text above make clear, several credentialing organizations require an individual to have been supervised. One reason for this is that the individual care manager's professional training and degree may not require

supervision to practice at the independent level. Another problem is the lack of certified or credentialed individuals to meet the needs of a growing work force.

This raises the question of who is qualified to provide supervision. For some credentialing organizations, the supervisor must be an individual who already holds the care management credential. Other organizations have a broader interpretation to include anyone in a supervisory capacity that can attest to the candidate's work in the successful performance of care management with clients. The desire for supervision in the work setting is largely due to the lack of practicum experience focused on care management, the lack of availability of credentialed supervisors, and the desire to ensure that the knowledge base of the care manager has been successfully transferred to direct client contact.

Specialty Credentials and Levels of Credentials

Another distinction that might be made among the various credentials is a determination of the level of practice and an area of specialization. The credentialing bodies that require another license or certificate might characterize the care management credential as a form of advanced or specialty practice. Several of the credentialing organizations that do not have such prerequisites might also consider this a specialty credential but not an advanced credential. NACCM, for example, characterizes its examination as a test of "core" knowledge of the care management process and anticipates that workers will specialize based upon their work with a specific population or setting. The concept of a specialty or advanced credential would require the distinction of differential skills, interventions, and potentially outcomes. This is a controversial area and one that is only now beginning to come to the forefront of credentialing activities.

Organizational versus Individual Credentialing

With the recent publication of the American Accreditation HealthCare Commission/URAC standards for credentialing care management organizations, a new question appears: Should organizations, individuals, or both be credentialed? As provider organizations have carved out service specialties and the incidence of risk sharing has increased, credentialing of organizations has become important as part of risk management protocols. The question remains whether this credentialing has a tangible impact on quality or is just an additional cost to providers with little or no benefit to the consumer. It would be premature to speculate on the answer at this early stage. However, the burden imposed and the potential for positive outcomes should be carefully examined as organizational credentialing becomes more widespread.

Implications for Policy Development and Reimbursement

The failed attempts to reconfigure the health care delivery system in the early 1990s demonstrated how difficult it is to make revolutionary changes in an established set of services where so many individuals appear to have conflicting interests. Over the past decade there have been dramatic changes in the health care delivery system because of a combination of administrative changes, regulatory modifications, economic changes, and the growing recognition of the needs of populations with chronic conditions. Typically, change has continued to be incremental and, therefore, fragmented. This has hampered the ability to integrate or coordinate the funding and delivery of health, mental health, and social services. While a fully integrated system is a distant vision that may not be shared by the majority of policy makers, it will be necessary to address many emerging issues such as the following:

- how care management will be funded
- under what auspices care management will be provided
- who the care managers will be
- how the impact of particular programs goals will be measured
- what people will be served by care management, how long they will be served, and what level of service they will receive

In addressing these issues, policy makers will need to be cognizant of different approaches and philosophies so that programs can be sculpted to meet the particular needs of each setting and population. This potentially means that there is a need for recognition of different skill sets in different environments that still come within the commonly defined process of care management. It also means that all funded programs need to have a research component so that outcome data can be obtained to answer these questions. Research design will be critically important if it is to enable comparison of different care management models across programs and professions.

CONCLUSION

The growth of care management over the past few decades has been significant. Virtually every human services setting in the country provides some form of care management regardless of the population served. The growth of geriatric care management has also been noteworthy, especially in the private practice arena. The move toward credentialing is an effort to control quality by requiring those who want to do the work to meet established criteria and standards and to set some agreed-upon level of consumer and professional expectations.

NOTES

1. Rosen AL, Bodie-Gross E, Young E, Smolenski M, Howe D. To be or not to be? Case/care management credentialing. In: Applebaum R, White M, eds. *Key Issues in Case Management around the Globe.* San Francisco: American Society on Aging; forthcoming.
2. Anne Reban study.

3. Geron SM. Measuring the quality and success of care management: developments and issues in the United States, England and other countries. In: Applebaum R, White M, eds. *Key Issues in Case Management around the Globe.* San Francisco: American Society on Aging; forthcoming.

4. Commission for Case Manager Certification. *CCM Certification Guide*. Rolling Meadows, IL: 1997.

5. Gross EB, Holt E. Care and case management summit: The White Paper (Sponsored by the Foundation for Rehabilitation Education and Research and the National Association of Professional Geriatric Care Managers). Chicago, IL, October 19–20, 1997 (published July 1998).

6. Leahy MJ. Validation of essential knowledge dimensions in case management. Technical report. Rolling Meadows, IL: Foundation for Rehabilitation and Research. 1994.

7. National Academy of Certified Care Managers. *Handbook and Application for Candidates for Certification Examination*. Colchester, CT: 1999.

8. Compare and contrast: Here's basic information for 6 popular CM Credentials. *Case Management Advisor*, January 1997.

9. Certification of Disability Management Specialists Commission. *CDMS Certification Guide*. Rolling Meadows, IL: 1997.

10. Commission on Rehabilitation Counselor Certification. *CRC Certification Guide*. Rolling Meadows, IL: 1997.

11. Perry, D. *Aging Research: Keeping Older Americans Healthy, Health & Aging*. 1977.

12. Koppel R. Alzheimer's disease costs business $33 billion a year in caregiver loss, medical expenses. Paper presented at the Washington National Press Club for the Alzheimer's Association. Washington, DC, September 1998.

13. Peterson DA, Wendt PF. A Draft Proposal for the Certification of Professionals in Gerontology. University of Southern California, September 1992. Unpublished paper.

PART IV

Clinical

CHAPTER 10

Geriatric Care Management with Families

Anne Rosenthal

INTRODUCTION

This chapter discusses the work that geriatric care managers (GCMs) do with adult children, spouses, and other family members caring for older people. It addresses many pertinent issues for GCMs, including helping long-distance caregivers, identifying and relieving caregiver overload, working as part of a team of people helping the older person, and helping caregivers make the decision to place their older relative in a care facility.

GERIATRIC CARE MANAGEMENT WITH FAMILIES

A recent survey by the National Alliance for Caregiving and the American Association of Retired Persons found that 22.4 million U.S. households, nearly one in four, are providing care to a relative or friend aged 50 or older or have provided care during the previous 12 months.[1]

GCMs often find themselves assisting family caregivers. What are these caregivers providing? Typically, they spend 18 hours a week taking the person they care for to physicians, managing the older person's finances, helping with grocery shopping, and providing hands-on personal care. Two-thirds of the caregivers also are employed. Of these, slightly more than half have had to make workplace accommodations, such as coming in late, leaving early, dropping back to part-time work, or even passing up promotions, to

provide elder care. How can GCMs assist families in dealing with the conflicting demands of jobs, families, and caregiving?

There is much GCMs can do to offer families direct and indirect assistance. It behooves GCMs not only to be experts on community resources but to be adept at understanding and communicating effectively with many different types of families, especially families that are in crisis.

In other words, GCMs are experts in knowing how to save families' time and money and prevent situations from taking an emotional toll on family members. Some of the areas where these resources can be conserved are home care services, community-based programs, and facilities. GCMs can also help families keep their finances in good shape through options such as long-term care insurance and publicly funded programs.

From GCMs, families also learn more about the illnesses with which their family members cope. GCMs are familiar with the symptoms and course of chronic diseases such as Alzheimer's and vascular dementia as well as stroke, Parkinson's disease, and arthritis. Families will benefit from GCMs' suggestions about what adaptive equipment can make the older person safer; the most effective ways to communicate with a distressed, demented individual; and other matters.

Frequently, families contact a GCM during a point of crisis. For instance, Mrs. L came with her adult son and daughter to the office of a GCM to discuss a possible placement for Mr. L.

Mr. L had been recently hospitalized for a debilitating stroke and was ready to be discharged from the hospital.

The daughter and son wanted to see their father cared for at a skilled nursing facility, but their mother wanted to care for her husband of nearly 50 years at home. The adult children expressed an objection to the home arrangement primarily because their mother had always been extremely dependent on her husband.

Mr. L had been a successful businessman, active in the community and civic affairs. His wife, coming from an earlier generation of women, knew little of managing anything outside the home, let alone managing the team of home health staff—nurses, a physical therapist, an occupational therapist, and a speech therapist—who would be caring for her husband. Mrs. L could not arrange for the durable medical equipment (e.g., a hospital bed, a wheelchair, and a commode) that he would need to remain at home. In fact, Mrs. L had never even written out a check!

The GCM met with the family together to discuss each member's concerns. The GCM assessed Mr. L's aptitude for making judgments, his reasoning ability, his memory, his orientation, his cognition, and his motor skills. The GCM also assessed whether the home was safe for someone with limited mobility who was using a wheelchair.

The GCM was able to assure the family that it was feasible to have Mr. L remain at home. Although he had some recent memory deficits, he seemed to be able to make sound judgments on his own behalf. He clearly expressed his desire to remain in his own home. Because the house had stairs, the GCM recommended that a ramp and strategically placed grab bars be put in and some area rugs be removed.

Together, the GCM and family were able to agree on a plan of care. The home care agency best equipped to care for Mr. L was contacted. It was Medicare certified, and Mr. L qualified for services at home that would not have to be paid for out of pocket.

The family members were grateful for the savings in time and cost. A coordinated schedule of care that supported Mr. L at home was established. His wife was pleased with the experienced help.

The adult children were able to return home to their jobs and families, knowing that the GCM would be monitoring the home care, following up with any additional matters that arose, contacting them regarding any change in their parent's status, and keeping them current on the situation at home.

The physician was able to obtain details from the home health staff, which helped him in treating Mr. L.

Although Mr. L eventually died peacefully at home in his sleep, the story does not end there. His wife continued to live in the same home. The GCM counseled the wife regarding her grief over the loss of her husband. After a period of mourning, she became interested in becoming more independent. She was supported and assisted in learning how to write out checks and take more control of her daily life. She has taken three cruises and regularly travels to see her family.

Recently Mrs. L was hospitalized. The adult children, all of whom have busy professional schedules, contacted the GCM to assist with their mother's care. The GCM visited Mrs. L in the hospital. The GCM offered assurances that she would take care of whatever was necessary to settle Mrs. L back in at home. In addition, the care manager met with the hospital nurses and discharge planner to understand more fully Mrs. L's recovery care. The GCM remained in close contact with Mrs. L's family members to ensure that they agreed to the recommendations made for the assistance Mrs. L would need once she returned home.

The family saved time and money. The GCM was able to identify services for which Mrs. L would qualify under her insurance program. Mrs. L, who always prided herself on her cooking skills, reluctantly agreed to receive home-delivered meals. Later she admitted to being grateful for the nutritious meal and for the friendly volunteer who brightened her day. An attendant came during the week to do light housekeeping, to stand by while Mrs. L took a bath, and to run errands until Mrs. L's strength returned. Mrs. L was able to resume her visits to her family, enjoying new grandchildren. The family members know that when Mrs. L returns home, the GCM will be only be a phone call away.

There are many problems commonly faced by adult children. Three examples are given below. In each case, a GCM stepped in to help the adult children solve the problems:

Problem Situation 1. An older woman fell and broke her hip. She was hospitalized for hip replacement surgery, and the hospital says she is now ready to return home. The woman's daughter is panicking because she is scheduled to leave for a trip to Europe in 2 days and she doesn't know how her mother can manage without her. She calls a GCM to ask for help.

The GCM would want to ask the following questions:

- Does the mother want to return to her home or go to a care facility to recuperate?
- Can the mother complete activities of daily living (e.g., dressing, eating, toileting, bathing) on her own?
- How are the mother's cognitive functions? Is she oriented to time, place, and person?
- How is the mother's judgment and reasoning ability?
- What is the mother's living environment like? Are there obstacles (e.g., stairs, bathroom adaptive equipment, rugs) that should be dealt with?

The GCM should talk to the hospital discharge planner regarding the following matters:

- What will Medicare cover if the mother is at home? What will Medicare cover if the mother is at a care facility?
- What will the GCM do if the mother returns home? Determine the amount of home care required and recruit the home care worker?
- What will the GCM do if the mother transfers to a care facility? Locate the facility and arrange for admission?
- How will the GCM help the mother to deal with her questions, anxiety, and planning during her daughter's absence?

- What support system can be put in place during the daughter's absence? Is there a local family who can offer support? What will the GCM do if the daughter would like to retain ongoing care management services?
- What will the GCM do to communicate with the daughter, monitor the mother, and communicate with the mother's hired caregivers during the daughter's absence?

Problem Situation 2. A working professor has concerns about his mother, who lives out of state. The mother is in an assisted living facility, appears quite depressed, and is now displaying some paranoid ideations. He is the only relative and is 3,000 miles away. He thinks he should relocate his mother to live with him, but he is not sure. He asks for the advice of a GCM.

The GCM would want to explore with the son the quality of his mother's living situation. Is she happy where she is? What is the quality of the care she is receiving? Are there other levels of care available in the facility should she require a higher or lower level of care?

The care manager should visit the mother in her facility and have more discussion with the son to determine answers to the following:

- Who visits the mother now?
- What is the son's home situation like? What kind of social stimulation is available for the mother there?
- What has been the quality of her visits to his home in the past?
- If the mother moves to his home, what modifications would be necessary for her safety?
- What are the financial aspects of the two options being considered (i.e., relocation to the son's home, remaining in the care facility)?
- Are there facilities to be considered in the son's area should the home arrangement not be feasible?
- What about the mother's paranoid ideations? Does she have a history of emotional disturbance? What is the nature of the psychiatric intervention she has received at the care facility? Could that inter-

vention be improved? If the mother relocates to the son's residence, can the mother's emotional problems be adequately addressed?

- How does the mother feel about her son's wish to relocate her to his home? Is she comfortable with the idea?
- What are the son's motivations for wanting to initiate the move? Are there other family members to consider?
- If the mother remains where she is, what could be done to improve the quality of her life?

Problem Situation 3. An older divorced woman with a history of dementia secondary to alcoholism is addicted to buying items from a home shopping channel. The older woman is indiscriminately ordering hundreds of dollars of items each week. She has a live-in attendant who helps with personal care. The older woman's sister calls a GCM because she is concerned there will be no money left to use for the older woman's long-term care.

The GCM should ask the following questions:

- What is the attendant's role with regard to the impulsive shopping? Can she be enlisted to intervene?
- What seems to trigger the older woman's impulse to make phone purchases?
- Can the older woman be diverted?
- Is the older woman cooperative?
- Does the older woman lack the capacity to consider the consequences of her actions? If she does lack this capacity, should a conservatorship or a guardianship be considered?

What do these three problem situations have in common? In all three, families are facing problems and GCMs provide assistance using their problem-solving skills and understanding of short- and long-term planning. All three families benefit from a GCM's assistance. In all three cases, the GCMs assess the situation, learn what the family's preferences are, make appropriate recommendations based on what is feasible, implement the recommendations once the family members approve them, follow up and moni-

tor the situation, and adjust services and GCM involvement as the family's needs change.

The assessment tool shown in Exhibit 10–1 may help GCMs identify problem behaviors.

WORKING WITH LONG-DISTANCE CAREGIVERS

Adult children living at a distance from their older relatives face complex emotional and logistical issues. How do they know what to look for if they suspect that their parents are having problems? Here are some warning signs:

- unpaid bills
- missed appointments
- clutter in a home that was once always neat
- weight loss
- memory loss
- poor grooming by a person who was once meticulous
- getting lost
- wandering

Families living far away from their older relatives should take the following steps:

- know the older person's important emergency contacts, keeping handy a Yellow Pages from the area where the older person lives
- keep complete information on the older person's physicians
- know where the older person has prescriptions filled
- look at the dates on medication bottles, the dosage, and the amount of medication left in the bottles to figure out whether the older person is taking the correct amount of medication
- find a GCM in their town through the National Association of Professional Geriatric Care Managers, area agencies on aging, Eldercare Locator, or www.careguide.com

Many long-distance caregivers perceive themselves to be at a logistical disadvantage as they attempt to assess an older person's needs, locate appropriate resources, and stay in touch with other family members. In addition to rou-

Exhibit 10–1 Checklist of Brain Impairment Problems

Please check one box for each problem, indicating how often these problems have occurred *in the past week.*

Problem	Very Often	Somewhat Often	Never	Comments
1. Asking the same question over and over				
2. Having trouble remembering recent events (e.g., items in the newspaper or on TV)				
3. Having trouble remembering significant past events				
4. Losing or misplacing things				
5. Forgetting what day it is				
6. Starting but not finishing things				
7. Having difficulty concentrating on a task				
8. Destroying property				
9. Doing embarrassing things				
10. Waking up others at night				
11. Talking loudly and rapidly				
12. Appearing anxious or worried				
13. Engaging in behavior that is potentially dangerous to him- or herself or others				
14. Threatening to hurt him- or herself				
15. Threatening to hurt others				
16. Being verbally aggressive toward others				
17. Appearing sad or depressed				
18. Expressing feelings of hopelessness or sadness about the future (e.g., "Nothing worthwhile ever happens," "I never do anything right.")				
19. Crying and being tearful				
20. Commenting about the death of him- or herself or others (e.g., "Life isn't worth living; I'd be better off dead.")				
21. Talking about feeling lonely				
22. Commenting about feeling worthless or being a burden to others				
23. Commenting about feeling like a failure or about not having worthwhile accomplishments in life				
24. Arguing, being irritable, and complaining				
25. Being unable to communicate				

tine caregiving expenses, the long-distance caregiver also faces enormous outlays for telephone and travel. The combination of these pressures can create extraordinary stress. In an attempt to alleviate this stress, many long-distance caregivers have contacted GCMs who live near their older relatives. The following case illustrates the problems that can arise in long-distance caregiving.

A working daughter became concerned because her mother, who lives across the country, began phoning her frequently through the day and night, sometimes up to 15 times per day. The daughter suggested that her mother come live with her or have a companion, but the mother refused to discuss the subject. The worried daughter contacted the employee assistance division of her company and was given the name of a GCM in her city as well as the names of several GCMs in her mother's town.

The daughter first contacted the GCM in her own city. That GCM gave the daughter information about the nature, depth, and scope of geriatric care management services. The GCM also provided the daughter with a guideline statement called "How To Find a Qualified Geriatric Care Manager" (Appendix 10–A).

Shortly thereafter, the daughter flew out to see her mother. She had made appointments to interview four GCMs using the guidelines she had been given. She met with each GCM at her mother's residence, introducing the GCM as someone who specialized in helping older people live as independently as possible.

The daughter hired the GCM who responded to the guideline questions most thoughtfully and competently and to whom her mother responded most favorably. This GCM was also the most proactive. For instance, the hired GCM was the only one who asked the mother what she thought she needed to make her life better. The mother was able to state that she would like to have someone live in a spare bedroom. The GCM assessed the mother and her home and made recommendations for household adaptations such as a railing, improved lighting, and an address that was clearly marked outside the house. Additionally, the GCM recruited an attendant, who

was sensitive to the mother's habit of calling her daughter. The incessant calls to the daughter gradually ceased as her mother became comfortable with the new companion. The GCM visited the client on a regular basis, offering activity suggestions to the companion. For instance, the mother was very fond of dogs. At the GCM's suggestion, the mother and her companion visited the local dog park, got books from the library on dogs, and got a subscription to a dog magazine. The GCM was even able to arrange visits on a regular basis from a GCM assistant with a calm and responsive dog.

Other tasks provided by the GCM to this long-distance family on a direct and indirect basis included the following:

- phoning the daughter regularly to provide status reports and to respond to the daughter's ongoing concerns about her mother
- arranging for weekend relief help and relief help when the regular attendant needed time off
- making appointments to meet with medical specialists, dentists, optometrists, and psychiatrists as needed
- replacing a broken washing machine and torn window dressing
- locating a bill-paying service
- locating an audiologist and reputable hearing aid specialist
- arranging for plumbing and gardening services
- arranging for volunteers to call regularly and arrange for intervention should the situation warrant follow-up
- arranging for the installation of devices that help older persons better manage in their homes
- arranging for an emergency response system to allow an older person who falls and is injured to push a button, leading an automatic dialer to contact a central system that can then contact the person or responsible parties

Some public utilities and the U.S. Postal Service offer gatekeeper/home observation programs in which servicepeople who visit the home regularly are trained to notice anything unusual or any indication of need and report it so that someone may investigate and take action.

It is not uncommon for a GCM to contact a GCM in another town (where either the out-of-town relative or the older person lives) to coordinate efforts or to provide background information (with the permission of all parties) so that the other GCM can provide services.

HELPING ADULT CHILDREN AND FAMILIES MANAGE THE OVERWHELMING DEMANDS OF CAREGIVING

Middle-aged people, usually women, who are balancing family, work, and caregiving responsibilities are likely to report feeling stressed, frustrated, and sometimes even angry. Because they often care for children and parents simultaneously, these adult children have sometimes been referred to as the "sandwich generation." They feel squeezed between the needs of so many people that they are vulnerable to anxiety, depression, and weakened immune responses. Caregiving can stress even the happiest of marriages.

GCMs are able to help with practical suggestions regarding placement, referrals, and medical needs as well as some very specific recommendations that can assist caregivers in reducing their stress. For instance, GCMs may recommend that caregivers join support groups or otherwise alleviate caregiver overload.

Joining Support Groups

Support groups can be of help if the participants are focused on a particular problem. The following is one family's experience with a support group.

Mrs. R's husband was away on business when he suffered a debilitating stroke. Until this time the Rs were actively enjoying their "golden years." Mr. R's stroke rendered him unable to speak. He could still manage most of his daily living activities, attending speech therapy three times per week at a local rehabilitation center.

However, his inability to communicate placed a tremendous burden on Mrs. R, who continued to work outside the home.

Mr. R continued to be as good-natured as ever, but Mrs. R was exhausted from worry and on the verge of mental collapse. The hospital social worker recognized the wife's fragile mental state and referred her to a private GCM. The GCM met with the wife in the hospital and after recognizing her overwhelming situation, recommended that she join a support group for spouses of stroke victims. Mrs. R reluctantly joined the group and was immediately relieved to know that there were others who shared her experience. Through the support group, she made new friends and learned about new resources to help her.

In addition to the sense of camaraderie found in support groups, there is a cathartic effect that frequently takes place because it is only in a milieu of peers that some people can share their feelings. Support groups have been developed for various kinds of geriatric problems. There are support groups for spouses, adult children, those who have family members with an Alzheimer's diagnosis, those who have a diagnosis of early Alzheimer's, dementia, stroke, diabetes, Parkinson's, and the like. Support groups are frequently organized through nonprofit entities such as family service agencies (Jewish Family Services, Catholic Family Services) and religious affiliations such as synagogues and churches. Hospitals and long-term care facilities also frequently offer support groups to the community at large. The local area agency on aging, county department on aging, and senior centers offer support groups directly or will be able to recommend support groups. Academic institutions, especially universities with medical and gerontological programs, offer support services. The Alzheimer's Association and Family Caregiver Alliance are also excellent sources for group support. GCMs should develop a list of these support groups for use in their practice.

Alleviating Caregiver Overload

Because many adult children take the "I can do it all" approach, they frequently become overwhelmed with unrealistic caregiving expectations. GCMs are in a position to point out the need to make compromises and assist adult caregivers with adjusting their expectations when they are distressed over the burden of caregiving. One helpful approach is to assist caring family members in setting limits on their time and energy—to assist them in knowing to what extent they are able to be directly involved and when they can rely on hired help or services to ease the burden of caregiving. Even after family members set limits on their time, they may tend to push these limits further. If this occurs, the family members need to be encouraged to look at why they are uncomfortable with the limits they have established. Family members may be advised to be alert for signals that they have overextended themselves. The following are signs of caregiver overload:

- *Sleep disorder.* Depression, overexertion, and nighttime caregiving may prevent caregivers from getting adequate sleep.
- *Marital problems.* Marriages can be strained due to caregiving responsibilities.
- *Reduced employment.* Caregiving demands may force family members to curtail their hours or quit a job, adding financial stress.
- *Social withdrawal.* Family caregivers may become lonely, lamenting diminished contacts with friends and fewer social activities.
- *Depression.* Caring for a physically or cognitively impaired individual may leave the caregiver feeling helpless and hopeless.
- *Guilt.* Caregivers may begin to wish the care recipient was the way he or she used to be or that someone else would take some of the responsibility. They may feel guilty about having these thoughts.
- *Anxiety.* Family caregivers may begin to feel edgy or nervous. Regardless of their efforts, they may have a sense of falling behind.
- *Physical problems.* Increased physical and emotional stress may decrease the body's resistance to sickness. Family caregivers may complain about frequent colds, headaches, or backaches.

- *Fatigue.* Caregiving is physical and emotional hard work and may lead to exhaustion.

Following are some strategies that a GCM can suggest to family caregivers experiencing caregiver overload:

- The GCM can help family members to begin setting realistic expectations of themselves as caregivers.
- The GCM can encourage family members to explain to employers that flexible scheduling at certain times may be needed to help parents keep physicians' appointments. The GCM can also offer suggestions for making up the work. If comprehensive caregiving is required, the GCM can suggest that the Family Leave Act may be used.
- The GCM can encourage caregivers to talk with other family members about feelings and ask family members for their suggestions. Caregivers can ask children what they need (e.g., help with homework, a special shopping trip) and ask for their help in making it happen. Caregivers can also try to include children in caregiving responsibilities by asking them to run errands, fix a meal, or simply sit and visit with the older person.
- The GCM can encourage caregivers to plan some time for spouses, explaining personal stressors and asking the spouse to share personal stressors as well. Spouses can work together to make some changes in the partnership that will help accommodate the caregiving responsibilities.
- The GCM can encourage caregivers to seek out and use community resources. Most people are surprised at the wealth of community resources that are available at no cost. Public libraries, area agencies on aging, and local senior centers have information about community resources.
- Most important, the GCM can encourage family caregivers to make time for themselves. Unless caregivers stay physically and mentally healthy, they will not be any good to themselves or others.

Frequently, family members will express a sense of relief that they have found a GCM, someone whom they can call on to help with problem solving and listen to frustrations.

WORKING WITH DYSFUNCTIONAL FAMILY SYSTEMS

It is inevitable that a GCM will assist some families that are dysfunctional. These family systems may be the most challenging situations a GCM experiences. It is rare to find a genuinely despicable human being, yet it is not rare at all to find human beings acting despicably to members of their family, particularly older people. A professional GCM can help to alter the conditions that make people act abusively. If the older person's well-being is threatened or suspected to be threatened, either physically, emotionally, or financially, due to actions or neglect, the county adult protective service agency should be contacted.

Many times families require help in finding ways to manage their stress and frustration. They need to understand positive models that can frame the situations for them, positive modes of communication, and channels to express their frustrations in ways that do not harm the family.

In order to be useful to clients, GCMs must have some clinical skills. Frequently, the most difficult skill GCMs must learn involves their own self-discipline. Indeed, skilled counselors and care managers are differentiated from well-intentioned laypersons by what counselors and care managers do not do. In other words, clinicians learn from their training that there are certain interactional traps that must be avoided in order for clinicians to be useful to their clients. Inexperienced care managers often fall into these traps and end up feeling angry and frustrated. There are some basic tenets to follow (although every rule has its exceptions):

- GCMs should avoid arguments. Their set of values will not win over another's. Their clients will believe that they are being reasonable.

- GCMs should maintain rapport, empathizing and showing support.
- GCMs should avoid overinvolvement (taking sides, making accusations, letting the family's problem become the GCM's problem). The family is coming to the GCM for a larger perspective and not looking for a new family member. Any good GCM is honestly concerned about the problems of clients and their family members. Through discussing important practical and emotional issues, the care manager will establish rapport. Trust will develop, enabling the care manager to work effectively. Yet this process must not lead to overinvolvement.

For example, a GCM was helping a client complete an application for an adult day program and during the process discovered materials from the Hemlock Society. The Hemlock Society is known for its philosophy of euthanasia for individuals who believe that ending their life is preferable to living. The GCM explored with the older gentleman why he would have such materials in his possession. He assured the GCM that he had no intention of ending his life. The GCM was not satisfied and phoned his physician. The physician was not concerned based on his conversation with his patient, yet the GCM pursued this issue with every professional her client encountered, including the adult day program director. A seasoned GCM would have respected her client's right to self-determination after the appropriate discussion with the patient's physician.

The following are signs that a GCM is overinvolved:

- making accusations
- making threats
- taking sides
- feeling the family's problem to be his or her own problem
- being more worried about the situation than the client
- sympathizing, not empathizing
- not offering unconditional positive regard

The GCM may need to set limits with the family sometimes. The family members may want to engage the GCM in their arguments or want the GCM to share information that he or she is not comfortable sharing. The GCM should model ways of showing concern without rejecting.

What should GCMs do when they find themselves helplessly entrapped in a mistake, such as getting involved in a family's argument? One approach might be to say "You know, I realize that I have been trying to change your mind on something that you have some definite feelings about. Could you excuse me for this and explain the situation to me once more?" Another approach might be, "Although I didn't mean to, I think I've been arguing with you instead of listening to you. Could you help me out by explaining it to me again, while I pay better attention?"

Families who are having difficulties working as a cohesive family system may benefit from guidance from a GCM. Family caregivers can be helped to recognize and prioritize their problems so they can become empowered to develop their own solutions.

Some things for the GCM to consider are how the family seems to be functioning. What is the family caregiver's own attitude toward aging and an older person's particular illness (e.g., Alzheimer's disease)? If the caregiver has the attitude that older people are supposed to become demented, then the older person's behavior will not be seen as a problem to be considered. What motivates the family to care? If a caregiver has a full load with a job, marriage, and children, he or she may not be looking for additional problems. How does the family work? Do the family members address problems together, or do problems split them? Is there domination from a single family member? Are abuse and threats, implied or real, used to control others? What is valued by the family? Will the family be receptive to suggestions?

If the family is receptive to suggestions, a GCM can help improve how a family communicates.

- The GCM should not interrupt family members until they have finished speaking.

- The GCM should show each member that he or she has value in the family.
- The GCM should show each member that his or her views are valid.
- The GCM should show each member that his or her experience of a situation is valid.
- The GCM should help family members work together to make the load easier for all.
- The GCM should realize that family members will make mistakes and that mistakes are okay as long as the family members learn from them.
- The GCM should remember that it is okay for a family member to state that he or she has reached his or her limit of time, emotion, or stress.
- The GCM should encourage family members to ask each other for help.
- The GCM should allow family members to decide whether they can be helpful.

HELPING FAMILIES DEVELOP SOLUTIONS FOR THEIR NEEDS

Professionals should look beyond actual medical care and understand the caregiving dynamic of an older person's family to help ensure that both the older person and the caregiver have an adequate support system. Two older people can have exactly the same needs, but two caregivers will perceive the degree of burden very differently.

The following strategies can help GCMs to assess the needs of family caregivers and counsel them to develop appropriate solutions for their individual needs.

Dealing with a Caregiver's Denial

Denial is a common defense mechanism that individuals use, especially when they are under stress. To deny or ignore a problem allows the individual time to temporarily adjust to the idea of the problem or may serve to permanently keep the troubled thought or problem out of consciousness. Caregivers wait an average of 3 years from the onset of symptoms of Alzheimer's disease or vascular dementia before bringing an older person to be evaluated, usually following a dramatic event such as setting the stove on fire. Caregivers in denial are restless and inattentive. Their ability to process information may be impaired. They are controlling but may be very tired. They may report that they do not have time to exercise, or they may overeat. The coping strategies are not to think, not to feel, not to do. Professionals need to repeat information, perhaps over a period of a year or more, until they know caregivers are assimilating it.

Dealing with a Caregiver's Emotions

Caregivers frequently attempt to control their emotions, particularly anger and anxiety, so they are not overwhelmed by them. That anger surfaces when an adult daughter looks at a mother who is falling apart physically and sees herself or when she looks at someone she has never really liked very much, such as an alcoholic and abusive father, and realizes she has to care for him or her. What motivates the caregiver may not be love but rather a sense of responsibility, ethics, and morality. Caregivers facing such predicaments struggle with a complex array of emotions. There may be a desire to be absolved from responsibility, but the family caregiver feels bound to the parent because he or she is a moral human being. A GCM can help with this by sorting out the emotions, clarifying feelings, and finding support for those feelings, including psychotherapy.

Helping Caregivers Build a Partnership

GCMs should encourage caregivers to talk with older relatives without controlling the older relatives. Caregivers should work with the older person to develop a list of questions before a physician's appointment, for example, rather than monopolizing the discussion with the physician during the appointment. Partnerships are difficult to achieve when individuals have not always had a caring, loving relationship. When older people do not want to go along with the program, caregivers should be accepting without attacking them or becoming hostile. Caregivers must be helped to recognize that they cannot al-

ways be the most effective change agents. Perhaps someone else within the family system can be the catalyst. GCMs can work with the family physician, neighbors, or clergy as individuals who can get the older person to see the world differently. The following story illustrates how a GCM can help a family build a partnership.

Mrs. D was always, according to her four children, a controlling mother. As a result, all of her children became successful professionals in their fields; Mrs. D would not have it any other way. However, when Mrs. D turned 87, she suffered a series of strokes that would have incapacitated most individuals. Mrs. D's determination overrode her frailty. Her adult children finally convinced her to stop driving, with the help of her physician, who they believed was one of the few people in her life for whom she had high regard. Her life at home was quite marginal because it could not be adapted to meet all of her disabilities, including disabilities in vision, hearing, and mobility. Her children were convinced that the only solution was for her to move to a care facility, but Mrs. D refused to discuss it. The GCM helped Mrs. D's children form a partnership with her physician, who fully agreed with her children that it was not safe for her to be in her home. It took several months of medical visits; each time Mrs. D's physician brought up the subject of relocation Mrs. D would agree to consider it, and the discussion progressed at each medical visit. When Mrs. D asked her physician where he thought she should move, he suggested her children be included in the discussion of relocation. Mrs. D finally agreed to make the move, especially since she convinced her physician to make her his only home-visit patient.

BUILDING PARTNERSHIPS WITH PROFESSIONALS

The GCM works as part of a professional team. GCMs can offer a full-service package to their client families by developing alliances with allied professionals such as elder-law attorneys, certified public accountants, fiduciaries, trust officers, nurses, and geriatric psychiatrists and psychologists. This team approach is advantageous for several reasons: It streamlines the services offered to older clients, ensuring continuity of care; it makes for a more efficient services delivery pathway; and it avoids duplication of services.

The GCM can be at the fulcrum of the service matrix, recommending the types of services and the extent of service required based on an initial evaluation of the client and adjusting the recommended services as the client's needs change. For example, the chronically ill single son of an older client contacted a GCM to assist with concerns he had for his mother, Mrs. H. Mrs. H was living alone and seemed to the son to be losing weight, forgetting medical appointments, and unable to keep track of bills that needed to be paid. Mrs. H had several falls but no resulting injuries. The son stated that his mother had always been a private and self-sufficient woman and that this new behavior was very much out of character. He had had a recent medical emergency and was concerned who could look after his mother in the event he was unable. He said his mother had not yet drawn up a will.

The GCM arranged to meet with the son and his mother at the mother's residence the following week. The GCM wanted to assess Mrs. H in her home. During the course of this first meeting the GCM was sensitive to Mrs. H's need for privacy and independence and yet was able to establish enough rapport with her that Mrs. H confessed to the GCM that she was worried about herself. She was aware that she wasn't managing as well as she once had. The GCM used this time as an opportunity to ask the mother if she was at all concerned about her memory. "Oh, yes, indeed," she replied. "I know my memory isn't what it once was because I can no longer do my *New York Times* crossword puzzles." The GCM asked Mrs. H whether she would like to know how her memory was, that perhaps it was not as poor as she thought. The GCM explained that she could administer a short memory quiz and they could determine in just a few minutes whether there should be further concern about her memory. The GCM used the Short Portable Mental Status Questionnaire (see Exhibit 11–5).

Mrs. H scored 7 out of 10, missing the questions related to the presidents and the math calculation. The GCM also noted that the home was quite cluttered and dusty. As a result of the first meeting with Mrs. H, the GCM identified several areas where Mrs. H's quality of life could be improved. With her son's and Mrs. H's approval, she would proceed with the following suggestions:

- Although Mrs. H's memory showed only mild impairment, the GCM recommended that she see a neurologist for further testing to rule out any treatable conditions such as thyroid disorder, diabetes, dementia, or depression. The GCM offered to be available for these appointments.
- The GCM recommended a bill payer to organize Mrs. H's statements and set up a system for having bills paid on an automatic basis as much as possible.
- The GCM recommended having a home attendant see that Mrs. H's house was cleaned up and keep track of medical appointments. The GCM would recruit an attendant through the best home care agency. She would introduce the attendant to Mrs. H and her son, explain Mrs. H's needs to the attendant, supervise the attendant, and follow up with any necessary adjustment in the care provided.
- For some appointments, the GCM would herself see that Mrs. H got to the appointment, accompanying her on occasion if there was important information that should be relayed to the physician. On other occasions, the son would transport his mother for routine appointments, such as dental exams, or the attendant would accompany Mrs. H using public paratransit or transportation for the disabled.
- The GCM recommended a physical therapy evaluation to determine the reason for the recent falls.
- The GCM recommended finding a bank trust officer to handle the estate in the event Mrs. H's son was not able to manage his mother's financial affairs at a later date.

- The GCM recommended having an elder-law attorney draw up a current will and help Mrs. H identify an individual who could act as a surrogate executor in the event the son was incapacitated.
- The GCM would make regular visits to Mrs. H, address any new needs that arise, and make referrals and adjustments as required.
- The GCM would be in regular contact with the son, apprising him of the results of her efforts and noting any change in his mother's condition. Likewise, the son would advise the GCM of any progression or other changes in his mother's symptoms.

As the above example illustrates, the GCM can be at the fulcrum of the service matrix, recommending the types of services and the extent of service required based on an initial evaluation of the client and adjusting the recommended services as the client's needs change.

HELPING CAREGIVERS DIFFUSE CONFLICT

The GCM can help caregivers to manage conflict. Creative resolutions emerge out of conflict. Caregivers can be made aware of their conflict management style. They must learn to think before they talk or act. Instead of escalating conflict, they can practice deflecting the negative emotions that stir conflict. Family caregivers can be reminded that an aging person with dementia may not be aware of what he or she says to a caregiver. The following story illustrates how a GCM helped a caregiver diffuse conflict.

A demented woman with a history of psychiatric disturbance was very hostile to her daughter-in-law, and criticized how she dressed, prepared meals, and kept the house. The couple came to the GCM for assistance regarding managing the mother but also disclosed during the course of the assessment that their marriage was under considerable strain due to the husband's mother's interference and criticism. The GCM was able to help the daughter-in-law deflect the criticism by framing it in the context of her mother-in-law's history of mental difficulties. The son was able to set limits with his mother. The daughter-in-law was gradually able to disregard the criticism and tolerate her mother-in-law to a greater extent.

HELPING CAREGIVERS ESTABLISH GOOD COMMUNICATIONS

Some families work well together and develop a kind of partnership, where each member assumes a certain role. Other families do not want to work together at all. If two siblings were not a close part of each other's early life, it is understandable that they may not care to work together to help with the care of an aging parent. For example, a 45-year-old son relocated from Delaware to assist his mother in Oregon who was becoming increasingly withdrawn, depressed, and confused. He contacted a GCM, who assessed the mother, found psychiatric assistance for the mother, and offered support to the son, who was a recovered alcoholic and substance abuser. The son had not abused alcohol or drugs for 10 years. The mother had another son who lived in California but expressed resentment toward his mother and chose not to become involved in her care. However, when the brother from Delaware assisted his mother with her financial and estate planning, the brother in California was outraged and asserted that his brother could not be trusted with their mother's estate matters due to his former alcohol and drug habit. The brother in California could not bring himself to become constructively engaged in his mother's care. Blaming his brother for his history seemed to be the only way he could remain involved, albeit negatively. The GCM worked with the brothers to help build trust and establish a working alliance where the division of labor was comfortably defined. For example, the brother in California managed the finances for their mother while the brother in Oregon took care of her instrumental activities of daily living, such as transportation to medical appointments and meal shopping and preparation. The brothers did not develop a close relationship but were able to work together for the benefit of their mother.

ENCOURAGING FAMILIES TO COMMUNICATE THEIR NEEDS

The caregiving situation should be assessed by the GCM from the perspective of each family member. The GCM should solicit opinions from each family member, from youngest to oldest. Tasks should be identified and plans formulated. Caregivers can become overwhelmed when there is one problem after another. Breaking caregiving into manageable tasks is important. For instance, can spouses or teens in the family help with errands or phone calls? Can out-of-area siblings offer monetary support? The following story illustrates how a GCM encouraged one family's members to communicate their needs.

One son and two daughters were concerned about their widowed mother, who was becoming increasingly forgetful. The mother had remained in the home where she had raised her family. One local daughter lived close enough to check in on her mother, do grocery shopping, and stand by when the mother took a bath, but this daughter was facing surgery and had a chronically ill husband. The other two adult children lived out of town.

The adult children came to see the GCM for guidance. The local daughter was inclined to have her mother placed in a local assisted living facility. However, the other two siblings did not like the idea. The mother was willing to be placed to relieve her daughter of "the burden of my care."

The GCM helped the family organize a system that would help the mother remain at home and not overburden the local daughter. The GCM helped the family caregivers strike a balance by making several suggestions for manageable tasks the adult children could handle.

- The GCM was told that the son was financially solvent. She therefore suggested that the son finance home care so that the chore work and personal care would be done by attendants. The son agreed.
- The daughter who lived out of state arranged to have her mother's mail sent to her address and engaged her teenage son to sort the mail. Bills to be paid were forwarded to the brother. The daughter maintained close contact with her mother and attendants and ordered groceries and household items on the Internet, arranging for their delivery to her mother's home.
- The local daughter was able to visit her mother when she felt up to the task. Her visits were primarily social. The older mother was most pleased with this new arrangement and lived in her home until she died 2 years later.

HELPING CAREGIVERS STRIKE A BALANCE

Juggling the demands of an aging parent, a spouse, children, and a job is at the heart of the caregiving dilemma. Professionals are in a position to provide caregivers with models of balance. What is a well-balanced caregiver? According to Donna Cohen, PhD, director of the Institute on Aging at the University of South Florida in Tampa, and C. Eisendorfer, "It's someone who knows herself—what she can and cannot do. She's aware of the impact she has on others, can accept weakness in herself and others, and can identify strengths in others."[2(p130)] A happy caregiver can live with imperfections in him- or herself, his or her home, and his or her loved ones.

One of the single greatest challenges of caregiving is resisting doing everything. It is preferable to be a coach and delegate responsibility; professionals and caregivers alike can benefit from this advice. GCMs can assist family caregivers in striking a balance between doing it all and feeling guilty that they are not doing enough. Most family members are receptive to suggestions that they consider other individuals and service providers who can lighten their burden. For example, a GCM who is working with a caregiver who has siblings in other states can suggest a family meeting or conference call where each adult child and possibly older grandchild is able to offer a way to lighten the load of the local family caregiver. Some family members might offer to come into town to stay with the older parent on a scheduled basis to give respite to the local family caregiver. Other family members may be in a position to send financial support to hire help at the parent's home. Older grandchildren may be able to provide visits or household help themselves. Some older people are stable enough to split their residence, living part of the year with one relative and then returning to live with another relative. This option is feasible only if the older person likes the arrangement and is well enough to do so. Caregivers might consult with a family physician if a change of residence is being considered.

ASSISTING SPOUSAL CAREGIVERS AND WORKING WITH COUPLES

The institution of marriage is here to stay. If people are married long enough, one spouse is likely to have to care for the other eventually. Spouses of the chronically ill are constantly reminded of a relationship that is no longer the same. They have stated that their needs are often overlooked by health care providers. Almost all cultures place great value on caring for the sick, and yet caregiving can now continue for more decades than many marriages used to last—and without the benefit of an extended family.

A spousal caregiver may be a depressed, lonely, isolated, fatigued, anxious individual who may have physical problems, a sleep disorder, and reduced employment. Spousal caregivers experience feelings they view as negative or unacceptable: they feel anger and resentment at the partner for being sick, they feel jealousy at always being second, and they feel deprived of pleasure because they have to do too much work. GCMs can help spousal caregivers considerably. Many of the suggestions discussed in the sections above also apply to spousal caregivers. Spousal caregivers face many of the issues that other caregivers face, but spouses also have some special issues of their own.

Principles of Intervention with Spousal Caregivers

How can GCMs assist couples in managing the often overwhelming demands of spousal caregiving? Experts say that spousal caregivers need both the lifeboat and the oars—both the

support and the skills to do the job. These experts believe that caregivers are driven by five primary forces: love, morality, equity, ethics, and greed. Other factors affecting the caregiving process include family dynamics, divided loyalties, an understanding of age-related medical and psychological problems, physical endurance, the marital relationship, and the ability to communicate.

In *The Good Marriage,* Judith Wallerstein and Sandra Blakeslee cite four basic types of marriage: romantic, rescue, companionate, and traditional.[3] Although some may argue that this paradigm oversimplifies a most complex union, for the sake of examining caregiving styles, it may be useful.

Wallerstein gives case examples of couples who develop patterns that she deems good. For example, partners in a successful romantic marriage have at their core a lasting, passionately sexual relationship. The common bond the couple in a romantic marriage share is the sense that they were destined to be together.

Partners in a successful rescue marriage had early experiences that were traumatic. The comfort and healing that take place during their life together become the central theme of their relationship. Should one partner become frail and require caregiving, it might not upset the equilibrium as much as it might in another type of marriage, such as a companionate or traditional one.

A companionate marriage, which may be the most common form of marriage among younger couples, has at its core friendship, equality, and the value system of the woman's movement, with its corollary that the male role, too, needs to change. A major factor in the companionate marriage is the attempt to balance the partners' serious emotional investment in the workplace with their emotional investment in the relationship and the children.

The fourth type is the traditional marriage, where the stronger, more dominant spouse (usually the husband) is the breadwinner. Should the breadwinner become incapacitated and aphasic due to a stroke, for example, the system in this type of marriage would be profoundly upset. Changing dependencies, hostility, and the unspoken wish for escape all redefine the nature of affection in this relationship.

The style of spousal caregiving is determined in large part by a person's coping style, practical abilities, and marital relationship. GCMs should consider the following examples:

- A husband devotes himself for years to caring for his wife, who has Alzheimer's. Then he murders her. What might a GCM have done to prevent this tragedy?
- A wife cares for her chronically ill husband, quits her job, and neglects herself. Her adult children want her to spend more time with her grandchildren and have a more normal life. She says it is her choice and she would not have it any other way. How would a GCM counsel the family?
- A husband who is caring for his wife with Alzheimer's states that she instructed him to call Dr. Kevorkian when she no longer recognizes him. He has told a GCM of this directive. How should the GCM react?

How can GCMs help emotionally vulnerable clients to develop the new coping styles that will be necessary to spare them further stress? How much preventive intervention can care managers offer? Is it possible to prepare spouses for the often inevitable spousal caregiving responsibilities they will face? Can advance directives or a durable power of attorney for health care play a role in this?

Mr. and Mrs. H believed so. They had been married for 50 years and were grateful for their many blessings. They had good, open communication and agreed to state in the advance directives that under no circumstance would one spouse be expected to sacrifice their physical or emotional health at the expense of the other. Both had experience with chronically ill parents and recognized the toll caregiving can take.

They agreed to purchase long-term care policies that included home health care as well as institutional care and to implement these policies as necessary at the discretion of the well spouse. The couple said that it was a tremendous relief to know that each of them could be cared for, not necessarily by the other, and still feel that the spousal devotion was intact.

This couple, of course, was very enlightened, but they can serve as a model for couples who may wish to communicate about this most delicate subject.

Problematic Relationships

What about a situation in which a couple has not openly discussed caregiving preferences and one spouse becomes chronically impaired both cognitively and physically? How can a care manager help the well spouse achieve a relatively satisfying life while caring for the ill spouse? A case in point occurred when a GCM was facilitating a support group for well spouses of the chronically impaired. Two of the well spouses approached the GCM for her opinion. They were interested in dating each other but were very conflicted. Both members of the support group had been caring for chronically ill spouses. Both of the ill spouses were impaired to the extent that they no longer recognized their spouses.

The GCM counseled the two group members separately and together over a period of several weeks. They both expressed an overwhelming sense of devotion and guilt. Through counseling, the care manager was able to help the couple resolve the conflict. The result was that the well couple was able to define the parameters of the relationship in a way that would not conflict with the marriage vows and was comfortable. They shared a meaningful relationship and offered tremendous emotional support to one another.

What does the codependent caregiver look like? According to Melodie Beattie, the guru of codependency issues, that person is taking responsibility for others—too often not taking responsibility for him- or herself.[4] Codependent caregivers take inappropriate responsibility for the feelings, thoughts, behaviors, problems, choices, and life course of others. Codependent caring makes people feel used, victimized, unappreciated, and unsuccessful in their efforts. Codependent caring makes them feel controlled by the others' needs while simultaneously feeling that the caregivers' own needs are not getting met.

In the context of clinical intervention for codependent spousal caregivers, GCMs might ask themselves the following questions:

- What is the caregiver's own attitude toward aging?
- What is the motivation to care?
- Is the caregiver denying the spouse's issues and his or her own?
- Can the caregiver be helped to deal with his or her emotions?
- Can the GCM help the caregiver build a partnership with the spouse and helping professionals?
- Can the GCM help the caregiver manage conflict?
- Is it possible to help the caregiver to establish good family communication?
- Can the caregiver be helped to strike a balance between the need to care and his or her own needs?

General Principles for All Types of Spousal Caregivers

True helping and healthy giving are good, and they are different from caretaking. The following guidelines are summarized from the National Council on Aging "Caregiving Tips" series.[5] They may be useful for a GCM to suggest to stressed spousal caregivers.

- Encourage spousal caregivers to admit their feelings. Feeling tired, isolated, helpless, angry, or scared can be an indication that they are trying to handle too much without the help and information they need. Such feelings, though difficult, are natural.
- Encourage spousal caregivers to talk to their family and friends about what they feel rather than keeping everything inside.
- Encourage spousal caregivers to set reasonable expectations and not to reproach themselves for failing to be a superwoman or superman.
- Encourage spousal caregivers to admit to themselves and their friends what they want and need and what they can and cannot do for themselves. Knowing their limits is an important part of taking care of themselves.
- Encourage spousal caregivers to seek help when they need it, looking to professionals and service agencies as partners who can provide guidance and counseling. Help caregivers realize that there is nothing wrong with asking for help.
- Encourage spousal caregivers to ask questions. If they do not find the answers right away, they should continue to search for people who can answer the questions.
- Suggest that spousal caregivers take care of themselves physically; eat regular, balanced meals; exercise as part of their daily routine to maintain fitness and ease tension; use relaxation techniques such as meditation, deep breathing, and massage; and maintain a sense of humor.
- Remind spousal caregivers not to forget to take care of themselves when things are tough. This is the most important time for them to be good to themselves.
- Suggest that spousal caregivers avoid destructive ways of coping such as overeating, abusing alcohol or drugs, and neglecting or taking out their stress on others.
- Encourage spousal caregivers to maintain activities and social contacts that they enjoy and plan occasions for their own pleasure and renewal.

Sometimes the most helpful counseling is based on good listening and empathic responding. GCMs should help caregivers give themselves permission to take care of themselves, emphasizing that this is not selfish or uncaring but part of surviving. Caregiving is difficult work that involves not only doing but coping.

Expressions of Sexuality

The need for closeness and intimacy does not diminish with age. But despite the sexual revolution, our culture still views some types of sexual behavior as inappropriate.

One of the greatest fears is that older people will develop inappropriate sexual behavior. Inappropriate sexual behavior is an infrequent problem with individuals with dementia. More common than actual inappropriate behavior is the myth that confused older people will develop inappropriate sexual behavior. However, should such an unfortunate incident occur, a matter-of-fact reaction without any more fuss than is absolutely necessary is what is called for. The caregiver's reaction may have more impact on the observer or the victim than the actual incident. For example, removing the person from the situation and explaining simply that "He forgets where he is" may be all that is needed.

Some people with dementing illness have an increased sex drive, while others have a decreased sex drive. If the individual has an increased sex drive, remember that it is a factor of the brain injury, not a reflection on the relationship. The GCM can assist the couple in finding a balance of sexual activity that is comfortable for both. Referral to a clinician who specializes in dementia problems might be helpful. A university-based clinic could be a good resource.

Inappropriate Behavior

Occasionally confused people will expose themselves in public or fidget in such a way that reminds others of sexual behaviors. This can be upsetting, especially to family members. Family members may benefit from knowing that the problem will probably not worsen as the dementing illness progresses.

There may be reasonable explanations for seemingly sexual behaviors such as disrobing or handling the genital area. The GCM may suggest a family meeting to identify some of the triggers, suggest explanations, and allow family members the opportunity to vent their feelings. Solutions may arise during the process. Here is a list of behaviors with possible explanations and interventions.

- unbuckling belt buckle: feels clothing is too tight
- unzipping trousers: needs to urinate, forgets where bathroom is
- fidgeting with buttons on blouse: is too warm
- making sexual advances to attendant: confuses the attendant with a spouse
- making frequent requests for sexual relations: forgets the sexual relations that do take place
- handling genital area: has a urinary tract infection (should be checked with a physician)

- pulling off pants: feels uncomfortable in clothing, needs to use bathroom
- disrobing: is too warm, is uncomfortable in clothing

Differential Diagnosis: Sexual Acting Out versus Medical Problem

An older woman was placed in a care facility's unit for people with dementia. Her family received a call from the nurse on the unit that the older woman was wandering into the beds of other residents, disrobing, and touching her genital area. After a thorough medical examination and a family meeting, it was revealed that the woman had a urinary tract infection; she also came from a large family and was recently widowed. After her urinary tract infection was treated and she was more regularly taken to social activities, the wandering and genital handling subsided. The staff of the care facility was asked to provide more evening one-on-one attention, which seemed to address this woman's need for companionship at night.

CONTINUUM OF CARE RESOURCES— WORKING AS PART OF A TEAM

Just as no person is an island, no GCM stands alone. A good GCM will know about a staggering array of experts who can assist clients in areas where the GCM's expertise is lacking or where there could be a conflict of interest. For example, a middle-aged son came to see a GCM because his father, with whom the son lived, was beginning to require more care than the son could provide. The father was falling on occasion and appeared to be confused at times. The son traveled regularly on business. As the consultation progressed, it became apparent that the home was held in joint tenancy by the son and his father. There was another sibling who lived out of state who had a physical disability and was receiving public assistance. The father was beginning to show signs of dementia and had not yet developed a will or a general durable power of attorney, or one for health care.

The GCM suggested that the son contact an elder-law attorney to advise him regarding estate matters. A neurologist was recommended to evaluate the nature of the father's dementia and possible interventions. In addition, the father's physician was contacted to see about an order for home health care, physical therapy, and occupational therapy that would include an evaluation of the need for adaptive equipment and equipment to make the home environment safer.

The GCM asked about the father's typical day, and the son explained that his father was alone all day, ate poorly during the day, and "waited" for his son to arrive home from work, which was sometimes not until 7 PM. The GCM suggested an adult day program that provided transportation, meals, and socialization. The father responded favorably to the social stimulation and improved diet.

While developing a will with the father, the attorney also set up a trust for the estate and a special needs trust for the son with a disability. The special needs trust would allow that son to receive an inheritance and monthly stipend without disqualifying him from receiving public assistance. The neurologist diagnosed the father with a pseudo-dementia that abated after regular participation in a social day program and an improved diet. Many of these kinds of dementia have as their underlying problem depression and nutritional deficiencies, both easily reversed conditions, if treated early. The father now resides in a local retirement facility recommended by the GCM, who assisted in his acclimation. The facility has several levels of care so that as the father's needs change, he can receive assistance without relocating. The local son visits his father regularly and knows that he can rely on the GCM to advocate for his father, especially during his frequent out-of-town business trips.

GCMs should think of the following additional professionals and service providers when assisting families with identifying resources:

- services that may be covered by Medicare
  1. adult day health care
  2. assessment services
  3. home health aide services
  4. homemaker services
  5. hospice services
  6. medical social work
  7. mental health services

8. occupational therapy
9. personal care
10. physical therapy
11. physician care
12. protective services
13. respite care
14. speech therapy
15. transportation
- services that may be covered at no cost through a public agency
  1. care management
  2. chore services
  3. health insurance counseling
  4. information and referral
  5. legal services
  6. supervision
  7. telephone reassurance
- other services
  1. emergency response systems
  2. home-delivered meals
  3. paid companions and sitters

HELPING FAMILIES MAKE THE DECISION TO PLACE

The decision to place an older person in a care facility usually occurs when all attempts to keep the person at home have been tried and have failed. The decision to place becomes inevitable.

Lately, some older people have been planning ahead and deciding to move to a facility before a crisis occurs. This type of vision for the future is the best approach, but many seniors and their family members wait for a crisis before facing the often daunting task of relocating to a care facility.

The decision can be overwhelming. One must think about the geographical area where one should be looking, any budgetary constraints, the quality of care that is provided, and the level of care that is needed. There are psychosocial issues to consider, such as loss of role, loss of privacy, loss of control, change in status, and other adjustment issues. All in all, making the decision to relocate can be one of life's major challenges.

GCMs are sensitive to these issues and help family members cope with the turmoil that may occur before, during, and after the placement process. The older person faces issues such as coping with letting go of material possessions and familiar surroundings. The adult children may have quite different issues, such as the speed with which the older person is willing to make the change and how a busy working professional will find the time to tour facilities, visit, and assist in the adjustment of a parent who may be living farther away from the adult children than he or she was before. Both the older person and the adult child also realize that the older person does not have that many years of life left, a realization that can be difficult for both.

In most cities, there can be a staggering array of institutional choices with various levels of care, pricing options, and reputations. In rural areas, there may be few choices, so the search may need to include a wider geographic area. Many families find facility directories through a chamber of commerce or an area agency on aging. Directories can be useful unless there are just too many facilities from which to choose. This is where a GCM who stays abreast of the quality of care in a range of facilities in a geographic locale can save families time, money, and emotional difficulty.

It is important that a GCM remain current on the quality of care facilities in an area. There are several ways to acquire this information, the most common being experience working with families who have used the facilities. Other ways are through the local ombudsman, the county department on aging, the information and referral agency of the area agency on aging, and private registries that specialize in placement services. The local department of health and social services will have survey results available to the public. Survey results help consumers make decisions about choosing licensed skilled nursing or residential care facilities.

Some family members may consider having their older relatives live with them. This can be a short- or long-term arrangement. Its success depends on several factors. There are many issues to consider in coming to this decision, and GCMs can help families consider the issues.

It is often painful for adult children to admit that they cannot ask their mother or father to live with them. They may have practical reasons (e.g., inadequate living space, poor health, no settled home) or more personal reasons (e.g., personality clashes, adolescents who require emotional attention, marital strain). But how much more difficult it is to take such an irrevocable step, inviting a parent to live in one's home, and then find out that it does not work. The ensuing aftermath and responsibility the adult child will feel for disrupting the parent's life is even more painful.

Sons and daughters who are considering inviting an older parent to live with them even though they are reluctant to do so may be comforted to know that other people share that reluctance. National surveys consistently show that the majority of young and old adults in the United States think it is a bad idea for older parents and their children to live together. One might assume that the strongest opposition to such living arrangements comes from the younger generation, but that is not true; the surveys show that the older the parents, the less likely they are to favor living with their children. Older people particularly do not want to be burdens.

Even if the older mother or father directly or indirectly suggests a common living arrangement, sentiment should not dictate the decision. Instead, the decision should be based on a careful analysis of the situation, the wishes of the other members of the immediate family, and the history of the relationship between the parent and the adult child. GCMs can aid the family in considering these questions:

- How does the spouse of the adult child feel about the common living arrangement?
- What kind of financial arrangements are being considered?
- What kind of living space will be available for everyone?
- Will the older person depend completely on the son or daughter's family for companionship and entertainment?

What about other friends, relatives, and contemporaries? What about recreational, cultural, and religious needs?

- Can the family honestly expect to live comfortably together? Do the personalities clash? How have previous visits been?

How often did family members have a migraine headache, ulcer flare-up, or other stress-related symptom during these visits?

- When the older person visited in the past, were the family members counting the days until the older person left?
- Can the older person allow the adult child to run his or her own household?
- Would the older person—because of temperament—feel comfortable in the home and with having friends visit there?
- Will the adult children be able to make sure the older person has ongoing, accessible, competent medical care?
- Will having the older person in the house violate anyone's sense of privacy?

While some of these questions are difficult, they are important in determining whether living together can be a viable solution.

Placement: Levels of Care

It is estimated that by the year 2023, 21% of the U.S. population will be 65 or older. Census figures show that nearly one-third of all older adults—more than half of them over 75—live alone.[2] While this is a good option for many seniors, for others it means living in isolation, perhaps failing to eat a proper diet or get any exercise. Simple day-to-day activities can become stressful if physical frailty provokes a fear of falling or of not being able to call for help in a medical emergency. Many older adults are afraid to walk alone in their own neighborhoods, even in the daytime. Increasing difficulty with maintaining a large home and maneuvering on stairways is another common problem. The concerns can be even greater if family members live a significant distance away. Almost half of all older adults do not live near their families.

There are several different levels of care available to older persons. Sometimes these levels are housed together on the same site, and other times the levels are provided separately in a single location. The concept of "aging in place" has been appealing for many older people and their families who choose to plan ahead and make one major move to a senior residence while they are relatively well, receiving assistance within the same facility as their needs change. This type of facility, commonly known as a continuing care facility, may cost more, but if one can afford it, savings in time and mental anguish can more than make up for the increased financial cost. If the individual lives for a very long time, there may be a financial benefit to residing in a continuing care facility that has a buy-in fee. Studies even indicate that living at a retirement community can prolong one's life by 5 to 7 years. That is because communities offer good nutrition, exercise and fitness programs, and an active lifestyle, all of which contribute to a more positive frame of mind and a better state of health.

The number of options in retirement living has grown enormously in recent years. The following are descriptions of the types of retirement communities that are available. The costs vary according to the level of service, the type of care, and the size and location of the facility.

- *The planned adult community for people 55 and over.* These are large residential developments with a country club atmosphere. Many offer lots of social and recreational activities (e.g., golf, swimming) as well as the benefits of homeownership (e.g., appreciation, tax advantages). Although medical services are not provided, they are generally located nearby.
- *Independent living/congregate housing—full-service rental communities for older adults.* This type of community stressing an independent lifestyle may appeal to those who want to hold on to their assets or who cannot afford to purchase a home or pay a substantial entrance fee. The monthly rental fee covers living accommodations and services. Many such communities provide assisted living for residents who require help with daily living activities such as dressing and bathing. The monthly rate may even include long-term care insurance for skilled off-site nursing care.
- *Continuing care retirement community for those 65 and over.* This type of community

offers an independent lifestyle with graduated levels of care (e.g., independent living, assisted living, rehabilitation services, dementia units, skilled nursing care). There is frequently an entrance fee and a monthly fee. The monthly fee can change based on the level of service provided.

- *Continuing care retirement community with equity preservation, for those who want to combine homeownership with a comprehensive health care program.* Most of these facilities provide on-site assisted living and skilled nursing care. Health care may be included in the monthly fee.

- *Assisted living communities and board and care facilities.* These facilities provide personalized care for those who require assistance in daily living activities such as dressing, bathing, and taking medication. Some facilities are licensed to care for older people who are nonambulatory and will also provide assistance with toileting and grooming. The new assisted living programs allow older adults to live an independent lifestyle in the privacy of their own apartments while receiving the care they need. Some also provide dementia care.

- *Skilled nursing facilities.* These facilities provide the highest level of nursing and medical care. Some facilities offer rehabilitation services and Alzheimer's and dementia care.

Many factors should be considered by a GCM in helping families evaluate the choices in retirement communities and care facilities. What is the older person's financial picture? What are the older person's health requirements? What location and type of housing does the older person prefer? Many older adults prefer to stay in familiar territory, near their friends and neighborhood activities. Some are more comfortable in a casual country setting, while others prefer a sophisticated city lifestyle.

It is always advisable to encourage the families to visit a few facilities, taking a tour, joining some residents for lunch or dinner, and attending a social event or activity. Some facilities have guest accommodations and will arrange an overnight stay. It is not uncommon for people to visit a community six or eight times before making a decision. Some facilities offer the option of a temporary placement or rental option for 6 months or a year.

Most people do not realize that many retirement communities have long waiting lists, especially for the larger units. Many have age restrictions, and entrance requirements vary. For instance, one must be ambulatory to enter a life care or continuing care retirement community, which will not accept people confined to a wheelchair or on constant oxygen. Applicants are required to provide a complete medical history and to pass a physical examination. It is important that applicants understand the conditions attached to long-term care insurance or a community's health-care plan. There could be exclusions for a preexisting condition; for example, in continuing care retirement communities, it is mandatory for residents to participate in the community's lifetime health care plan. Others honor a resident's private long-term care insurance, which could decrease the monthly fee. The longer one waits, the fewer the choices.

Conducting Evaluations: Questions and Guidelines

This section offers lists of guidelines and questions for GCMs and family members to use when evaluating different types of facilities and different aspects of each facility. GCMs should consider the following general questions when helping families evaluate all retirement communities, assisted living facilities, and skilled nursing facilities:

- What is the availability? Are there waiting lists for certain units?
- What is included in the basic entrance charge?
- Are many of the residents in the community employed?
- Are there climate or weather considerations?

- What kinds of recreational and social activities are available? Are there additional charges for these activities?
- Is transportation service available?
- How close are medical clinics and hospitals?
- How are complaints about the facility handled?
- How much can the monthly fee be increased?
- Are refunds or rate reductions possible?
- Who decides when a resident may be moved to the nursing care facility?

Evaluating Assisted Living Facilities

- Use common sense in assessing the environment; does the facility smell clean and is it well lighted?
- Look at whether the staff members treat the residents in a dignified manner that is natural or in a manner that seems stuffy and patronizing.
- Listen to how the facility managers talk about the facility's residents. Do they appear to have a genuine affection for older people and see them as independent, or do they seem to think of older people as dependent and helpless, requiring constant care?
- Evaluate whether the facility seems to have a sense of community. Is there a resident's council? Does it simply plan activities, or is it influential in determining policy?
- Talk with residents; ask what they like and dislike about the facility. Are staff responsive to their suggestions and complaints? Observe whether residents feel free to discuss their opinions. Are managers hovering nearby? Ask managers what residents object to about the facility. If the managers say the residents do not have any objections, they are out of touch with the residents or just not telling the truth.
- Consider the types of activities offered. Is it just the proverbial bingo, birthday parties, and crafts, or are there intellectually stimulating activities and volunteer opportunities?
- Ask about the demographics of the population. Are most of the residents from the area, or have they moved there to be nearby adult children or other family members?
- Ask about the credentials, training, experience, and turnover of the staff. Are there psychiatry, psychology, and social work consultants or staff members?
- Ask whether the facility has relationships with any home health care company or community service agencies.
- Check with local ombudsmen, GCMs, and social workers who may have followed clients through the facility and can offer their opinion about the facility.
- Check the facility's finances. How long has the company that operates the facility been in business? Who are the investors? How many other facilities are operated by the company, and where are they located?

Evaluating Skilled Nursing Facilities

- Ask to see the entire facility, not just the nicely decorated lobby and one floor or wing. Although the physical environment is important, try to get an impression of the type of care that is provided and how the residents are treated by staff.
- Look into state licensing through the local department of health to see what citations the facility has received in recent surveys.

Evaluating Residents

- Are residents up and dressed by 9 or 10 AM? Are they well groomed—shaved, wearing clean clothes, with hair combed and nails trimmed and clean?
- Do residents appear alert, content, and occupied? Or are they lethargic, listless, and dazed?
- Are residents restrained in chairs or beds?

Evaluating Staff Members

- Is the number of staff members adequate? What is the staff-to-resident ratio?
- Are call bells and resident requests responded to in a timely manner (within 5 minutes)?
- Are the staff courteous to residents? Do they treat residents with dignity and re-

spect? Is the staff attitude condescending? Are childish or otherwise inappropriate nicknames used when speaking with residents? Do staff members talk about residents as if they were not present or as if they were children?

- Do the administrator/manager and director of nurses appear to know the residents?
- Do staff members take measures to respect residents' privacy (e.g., knocking on doors before entering rooms, keeping privacy curtains drawn while care is being given)?
- Do staff members wear name tags?
- Is the administrator licensed?
- Are there therapists on staff, or does the facility contract out for therapy?
- Is there a qualified social worker on staff full-time? Is that social worker licensed with a degree in social work, gerontology, care management, or marriage and family counseling? How long has he or she been on staff?
- Does the facility have permanent, full-time nurses and certified nurse assistants, or are registry nurses and aides frequently used?

Evaluating the Facility's Overall Environment

- Is there an obvious odor in the facility? Strong urine and body odors may indicate poor personal care or poor housekeeping. Heavy "air fresheners" and other temporary chemical coverups may be used to hide a lack of conscientious care and maintenance.
- Is the facility clean, well lighted, and free of hazards?
- Is soiled linen lying about, or is it properly disposed of? Is there adequate linen?
- Are floors clean and not slippery?

Evaluating Resident Rooms

- In which area of the facility would the resident's room be located?
- How many residents share a room? Generally, rooms should have no more than four beds, at least 3 feet apart, with privacy curtains around each bed.

- Is there a bedside stand, reading light, chest of drawers, and at least one comfortable chair for each resident? Is there adequate storage space and is it separate from that of other roommates?
- Are the beds easy to reach? Is there room to maneuver a wheelchair or Gerichair easily?
- Are call bells accessible to residents?
- Is there fresh drinking water at each bedside?
- Are residents allowed and encouraged to bring any of their own furniture? Have residents personalized their rooms?

Evaluating Hallways, Stairs, and Lounges

- Are halls wide enough to accommodate wheelchairs? Are they free of obstacles and debris? Are stairways and exits clearly marked?
- Are there handrails in all corridors?
- Are fire extinguishers visible? Is there a disaster plan posted, and does the facility have drills?
- How many lounge areas are available for residents and visitors? Are they clean and comfortably furnished? Is there sufficient room for visiting and watching television?

Evaluating Bathrooms and Shower Rooms

- Are bathrooms conveniently located?
- How many residents share a bathroom?
- Do bathrooms have handgrips or rails near all toilet and bathing areas?
- Is there a call button near all toilets?
- Are residents allowed to choose their preference of a shower or a bath, and what is the frequency of this care?

Evaluating Kitchen and Dining Areas

- Is the kitchen clean and well organized?
- Is the food handled and stored in a safe and sanitary manner?
- Is the dining area pleasant, clean, and comfortable?
- How many residents eat in the dining area? Is it large enough to accommodate most of the residents? Are there shifts for meals?

- Do chairs fit under the table so that residents are comfortably close to their food?

Evaluating Menus and Food

- Try to visit the facility during a meal. Observe the way the food is served, how residents are assisted with eating, and what their reaction is to the food. You can probably buy a meal to sample the food.
- A menu for the current and following week should be posted. If a menu is not posted, ask to see one. Is the food listed on the menu actually what is being served?
- How often are meals repeated? Are alternatives available, as required by law?
- Does the food appear and smell appetizing? Is it nutritious? Are fresh foods used, or is it mostly canned or frozen? Do residents appear to enjoy the food?
- Are dishes and silverware used, or are disposable plates and utensils used?
- Are those residents who need assistance with eating and who are being fed by nurse's aides eating at their own pace and finishing their meals? Are assistive devices available to those who may be able to feed themselves with a little help?
- Are meals served at appropriate temperatures?
- What provisions are made for residents who are unable to eat in the dining room?
- Who plans the meals? Is a professional dietitian on staff? How are special dietary needs met?

Evaluating Activities

- Are activity calendars posted? If not, ask for a description of the activity program. Meet the activity director, if possible.
- Do the activities cover a broad range of interests?
- Are activities tailored to individual preferences?
- What activities are available to residents confined to their rooms?
- Do volunteers visit the facility?

- What arrangements are made for residents to participate in religious services of their choice?
- What is done for holidays and birthdays?
- Is there a resident council? When does it meet, and what is its function?

Miscellaneous

- Is there a family council? When does it meet, and who coordinates it?
- How long has the facility been operating under the present management? Are there any plans to change in the near future?
- What hospital is used in emergencies?
- What is the billing procedure?
- Who should be contacted when there is a problem?
- How does the facility notify the resident and family members of the time and place of the quarterly care planning meetings?
- Is the ombudsman program's phone number posted?
- Are the results from the last inspection by the department of social services posted?
- What is the admission agreement like? Ask to review a copy.
- What is included in the basic costs and what is extra?
- What makes the Alzheimer's unit different from the rest of the facility (especially if it costs more)?
- How is transportation provided for trips to the hospital, medical offices, or community functions? Is there a charge?
- What provisions are made for podiatry and dental care?
- How is personal laundry handled?
- How many residents are in restraints?
- Is there a system to protect wanderers?
- Are visiting hours convenient for residents and visitors?
- How are costs covered? Does the facility accept public assistance?

The long-term care industry is becoming increasingly regulated by governing bodies such as departments of health and social services. The skilled nursing industry is second only to the airline industry in its mandatory regulation process. It is important to research facilities carefully before making commitments. GCMs and family members should speak with other family members who have had residents in a facility, health care providers, local area agencies on aging, departments on aging, and licensing bureaus to learn about the facility's compliance records and quality of care.

CONCLUSION

This chapter focuses on how a GCM can effectively work with adult children, spouses, and other family members to improve the quality of life for older people and ease the burden of caregiving in various situations. GCMs can help all types of families, including long-distance families, dysfunctional families, overwhelmed families, and families who are considering facility placement. GCMs can also work with couples and work as part of a professional team.

The future of geriatric care management work with families will increasingly be tied to the Internet. The Internet will allow family caregivers to identify GCMs in their community as well as GCMs in their older relative's region. The Internet will also enable family members to identify resources, services, and products that will improve the quality of their lives. However, there will never be an electronic replacement for responsive, clinically astute, and empathetic GCMs who can be instrumental in improving a challenging family circumstance.

NOTES

1. *Tomorrow's Choices: Preparing Now for Future Legal, Financial, and Health Care Decisions.* Washington, DC: American Association of Retired Persons; 1992.

2. Eisendorfer C, Cohen D. *Care for the Elderly: Reshaping Health Policy.* Baltimore: Johns Hopkins University Press; 1989.

3. Wallerstein J, Blakeslee S. *The Good Marriage: How and Why Love Lasts.* New York: Houghton Mifflin; 1995.

4. Beattie M. *Co-Dependent No More.* New York: Fine Communications; 1997.

5. Cassel C, ed. *The Practical Guide to Aging.* New York: New York University Press; 1999.

How To Find a Qualified Geriatric Care Manager

Caregivers should be aware that a growing number of geriatric care managers (GCMs) are now certified and known as "Care Managers Certified," or CMCs. They are professionals, usually social workers or nurses, who are capable of conducting assessments and providing short- and long-term care plans for clients.

It is recommended that some or all of the following questions be asked by consumers who are considering retaining a GCM.

1. What are your credentials? A GCM should have an advanced degree in social work, psychology, or gerontology or should be a registered nurse with public health experience.
2. Do you have certification as a GCM?
3. How long have you worked with the frail elderly? How long in private practice? Care managers with more years of experience are likely to be better choices than care managers with fewer years of experience. Public agency experience working with the frail elderly helps.
4. Do you belong to the National Association of Professional Geriatric Care Managers? This association has ethics codes and standards of practice.
5. Are you available 24 hours a day, 7 days a week? If you get sick or go out of town, who backs you up?

6. How do you charge? If by the hour, do you charge for telephone calls? Travel time? What else? GCMs do much of their business by phone and legitimately charge for that time. Most ask half their usual fee for travel. Charges for other services should be spelled out in contracts or fee schedules.
7. If a service you recommended does not work out, what will you do about it? The GCM should promise in advance to correct any problem, and if that fails should arrange something new.
8. Can you provide references from clients as well as local organizations such as hospitals and senior centers?
9. Do you arrange for free, low-cost, or medically insured services when available and appropriate?
10. Do you personally provide any of the needed services?
11. Who screens the home-care providers and what methods are used? Do you run a background check, and does it include criminal records?
12. Are you bonded, and do you carry professional liability insurance?
13. How often and by whom is each service monitored?
14. How frequently can I expect to hear from you? Are your reports written or phoned?

The recipients of care management service should feel comfortable with the GCM.

How do you find a GCM? The National Association of Professional Geriatric Care Managers in Tucson, Arizona, publishes a list of its members. Contact information for this association appears in Appendix A at the end of the book.

CHAPTER 11

Geriatric Assessment

Carolyn Barber

INTRODUCTION

The process of geriatric assessment is much like the process detectives go through to solve a crime. Just as detectives slowly and meticulously sift through clues, leaving no stone unturned in their efforts to ensure that all evidence has been taken into account before reaching conclusions and announcing them, geriatric care managers (GCMs) performing a geriatric assessment must make sure that all facts have been gathered and examined both individually and in combination with one another before writing a report and developing a care plan. Comprehensive geriatric assessment has been defined as a "multidisciplinary evaluation in which the multiple problems of older people are uncovered, described, and explained, if possible, and in which the resources and strengths of the person are catalogued, need for services assessed, and a coordinated care plan developed to focus on interventions of the person's problems."[1] Additionally, the resources and strengths of the older person must be ascertained and evaluated so that they can be tapped into as part of development of a care plan and as a means of recognition of the uniqueness and individuality of that person. Assessment of the impact of illnesses and the aging process upon an older person's physical, emotional, spiritual, and social functioning is a critical component of the provision of appropriate health care. Doing comprehensive geriatric assessment and care planning is a challenge to GCMs.

The Comprehensive Geriatric Assessment Position Statement of the American Geriatrics Society includes the following statements: "Comprehensive geriatric assessment has demonstrated usefulness in improving the health status of frail, older patients. Therefore, elements of Comprehensive Geriatric Assessment should be incorporated into the acute and long-term care provided to these elderly individuals"; and "Medicare and other insurers should recognize as a reimbursable service or procedure: (1) periodic assessment of patients and (2) the support services required for effective application on Comprehensive Geriatric Assessment."[2]

A comprehensive assessment is essential in order to provide the right services at the right time. Older people often have complex health problems with atypical presentations, have cognitive and affective problems that make history taking difficult, react strongly to medication, and are socially isolated and may be economically compromised. If a comprehensive assessment is not done, older people may be at risk for premature or inappropriate institutionalization. Problems often involve more than one domain of the assessment. Treatment of a medical problem or living condition can sometimes affect cognitive or functional status; on the other hand, the client's cognitive and functional status and values must often be taken into account before deciding how aggressively medical problems should be approached. The assessment should be carried out by an experienced GCM. This person is usually either a registered nurse (RN) or a human services professional who has had special training and passed a certification exam in geriatric care management. A team approach involving an RN and a social worker can be very effective. Each team member can evaluate different aspects of the assessment. The RN would be responsible for the nursing assessment, which is usually made up of a physical systems review, medication history, and physical examination, and the social worker or counselor would perform the psychosocial portion of the assessment, which includes assessment of affect, coping styles, family dynamics, and related topics with which the social worker should be familiar. Every effort should be made to pair RNs and social workers so that the assessment can be as comprehensive as possible. If an agency does not employ both disciplines, or the GCM works alone, every effort should be made to contract with an RN or human services professional in the community. There are sources included in Appendix A for both disciplines.

The assessment process begins with a case-finding approach and employs screening instruments and techniques. Based on initial findings, a more detailed assessment is frequently undertaken. The in-depth assessment may require the participation of persons from a number of professional disciplines, such as audiology, psychology, nutrition, physical therapy, occupational therapy, pharmacy, and speech therapy. The assessment should take account of the older person's physical, emotional, and spiritual health; finances; and support systems so that realistic plans for long-term care can be made if necessary. The older person's own goals and wishes should be taken into account in the planning as much as possible.

ELEMENTS OF THE ASSESSMENT

The components of a basic geriatric assessment are discussed below.

Physical Health

A physical examination is performed, with emphasis on identification of specific diseases or symptoms for which curative, restorative, palliative, or preventative treatment may be available. Special attention is directed toward visual or hearing impairment, nutritional status, incontinence, and conditions that may contribute to falling or difficulty in ambulation.

Mental Health

Cognitive, behavioral, and emotional status are evaluated. Identification of dementia, delirium, and depression is particularly important. A range of assessment instruments is available for screening and differentiating among these conditions. Following screening, some clients will be referred for psychiatric interviewing or neurological consultation.

Social, Spiritual, and Economic Status

Identification of present and potential caregivers and assessment of their willingness, competence, and acceptability to the older person are determined through interviews with those parties. Caregiver stress and the support network of the client are also evaluated. Included in the evaluation are the older person's cultural, ethnic, and spiritual values. The older person's concept of what constitutes quality of life should be ascertained. End-of-life decisions and verification of written advance directives should be included as well.

This can be accomplished by doing a spiritual assessment, as discussed in Chapter 14. The assessment should be done not only when the client has spiritual concerns but any time that the client's alienation, hostility, loneliness, or depression seem to be affecting his or her condition or inhibiting him or her from making life-enhancing changes.

Economic resources are evaluated since they are crucial for planning for the provision of personal care and the living arrangements of the client, and can be a factor in compliance with medical treatment.

Functional Status

Physical functioning is measured by the person's ability to adequately and safely perform basic activities of daily living (ADLs) including bathing, dressing, toileting, transferring, and feeding. Instrumental activities of daily living (IADLs) such as meal preparation, shopping, housework, financial management, medication management, and use of the telephone are evaluated by direct observation in the home, interview of the client and family, and administration of standardized questionnaires.

Environment

Evaluation of the physical environment is essential. Home safety must be evaluated. Problem areas must be identified and corrected if the client is to remain in the home environment. What type of environment the client needs at this stage of life and in keeping with the client's functional capacity must be determined. If necessary, the client may need to be moved to another environment.

In 1987 the Consensus Development Conference on Geriatric Assessment Methods for Clinical Decision Making established the following goals of comprehensive geriatric assessment: (1) to improve diagnostic accuracy, (2) to guide the selection of interventions to restore or preserve health, (3) to recommend an optimal environment for care, (4) to predict outcomes, and (5) to monitor clinical change over time.[3] The effectiveness of geriatric assessment has been demonstrated most convincingly with clients in geriatric assessment and rehabilitation units and inpatient geriatric units. Less evidence is available regarding home and ambulatory settings.[4] Outcomes demonstrated included improved diagnostic accuracy, prolonged survival, reduced medical care costs, reduced use of acute hospitals, and reduced use of nursing.

Care Plan

After the initial assessment is completed, a comprehensive list of the client's needs and strengths should be generated, ideally at a multidisciplinary team conference. Recommendations are integrated into a plan of care as interventions. The goal is to achieve the outcomes that the team has determined are desired. Recommendations are then communicated to appropriate care providers and to the client if possible. Periodic reassessment and modification of the care plan are critical to the success of the plan (see Table 1–1 and Table 11–1, page 204). Assessment tools are included in Appendix B.

CASE STUDY IN ASSESSMENT

This section introduces a case that will be referred to again at other points in the chapter. Lena Jones is 83 years old and lives alone. She has spent the last 5 years of her life nursing her husband, who died recently. She has no children. Lena has been a housewife all her life. Her husband left her with an ample retirement income and assets, but she has never managed money or handled finances and she is unclear about what she has and how far the money will go to meet her needs. Lena has arthritis and heart problems. Her health declined during the last year or two of her husband's life and taking care of him became extremely difficult, but she did it without assistance. Now she does not have enough energy to maintain her home and herself. She has pain and difficulty walking due to a bad hip. She also has some hearing loss, which makes it difficult for her to converse with others. She has lost 10 to 15 pounds in the last year. She has bruises on her arms and legs.

Lena lives in a two-story home that she has lived in for 40 years. Although she has difficulty getting up and down the stairs to her bedroom and sometimes has to spend the night on the couch in the living room, she has not considered moving her bedroom to a downstairs room that served for years as her husband's office. Lena does not drive and relies on a neighbor for obtaining groceries and other necessities. The neighbor has been helping out for several years and now has some health problems herself. The neighbor's family is urging her to cut back on her assistance to Lena and, although Lena states she will be able to manage just fine without her assistance, the neighbor calls a GCM to find out what other assistance is available.

NURSING ASSESSMENT

Because of their training and experience, RNs are well prepared for the role of GCM. Having nurses perform assessment and care management across a continuum of care settings is currently being researched as a means of reducing fragmentation of care, reducing the risk of re-hospitalization, improving client outcomes, and reducing costs. RNs with special interest and training in geriatrics are in a position to contribute much to geriatric care management in both the clinical and research settings.

The geriatric nursing assessment may make up one portion of a comprehensive multidisciplinary assessment, or it may stand alone as the only assessment completed for a given client. It may take place during a one-time encounter with the client or may be part of ongoing nursing care. The approach used will vary depending upon the purpose of the assessment, the identified urgent needs of the client or caregivers, the work setting, and the participation of other disciplines in the assessment process. Often the initial assessment is performed on a reluctant client who is apprehensive regarding the possibility of the initiation of care and loss of independence. The responses the client gives in the initial interview may be influenced by feeling out of control, angry at the circumstances necessitating the assessment, anxious, or too sick to fully comprehend and respond appropriately. If the client indicates verbally, with body language, or in any other way that he or she is resistant to the assessment, the RN GCM must remain calm and avoid taking personally anything the client may say or do.

GCMs must convey to the client the feeling that he or she is in control of the situation and can relax and answer questions honestly and completely. The RN GCM can set the tone of the encounter by being calm and not rushing. Asking nonthreatening questions or comments about the client's home, family composition, and pets may help the client feel more secure and valued as a person. Any feelings expressed by the client must be acknowledged and supported. If the assessment is the first step in initiation of home care for the client and he or she does not express concern about giving up independence, the GCM should provide an opening for discussion by acknowledging that giving up independence concerns many older people.

It is crucial that the RN GCM make sure that the client is physically comfortable and as free of distractions as possible so that he or she is able to concentrate on the interview. If the client is cold, is sitting in an uncomfortable position, is hungry, or needs to go to the bathroom, he or she will not want to spend the necessary time to complete the initial assessment visit. Additionally, GCMs must consider common handicaps of older persons. Before starting interviews, GCMs should inquire if they are sitting close enough to the client to be seen and heard. Client deficits may interfere with the gathering of accurate information and will make it difficult for the GCM to develop rapport with the client. If deficits are present, the GCM will need to address them in the care plan.

Due to the complications of communicating with some older persons, the interview process should not be used as the only means of gathering information about the client. GCMs should use their senses of sight, hearing, touch, and smell to evaluate older persons' responses to questions, ability to articulate concerns, affective mood, sensory-perceptual function, comfort level, overall body integrity, and grooming.[5] Having gathered data on any deficits in the sensory-perceptual realm, GCMs should modify their approach to maximize the client's ability to comprehend what they are attempting to communicate. To ensure accuracy, the assessment should be done using a variety of modalities.

Conclusions based on inferences and subjective information should be considered tentative and subject to change as more information is gathered. Modalities used include the history, physical assessment, demonstration of abilities or deficits, and validation interviews with other appropriate persons. The client should be screened for problems that are highly prevalent in the age group and affect functioning (e.g., arthritis and other chronic illnesses, dementia, depression). Many tools are available, and decisions regarding their use must be based on the client and the purpose of the assessment. Besides language, educational, and cultural factors that must be considered, the GCM must take into account the client's perceptual-sensory deficits, energy level, and comfort. GCMs should also remember that clients are not usually familiar with the interview process and with seeing an RN or social worker operate in a nontraditional role as a GCM.

The RN has been trained to perform physical assessment and can screen for a number of conditions common to the age group. It is always wise to remember that in older persons, presenting symptoms may involve the most poorly compensated organ system. A physical condition may present as confusion or dementia rather than the symptoms commonly seen in the younger age groups. For this reason, no matter what the presentation, a head-to-toe systems approach is necessary when physically assessing older persons. The RN GCM can also perform a medication review. He or she can check for medication side effects, the use of outdated medications, interaction of over-the-counter medications, or prescriptions from multiple physicians. The GCM should ascertain if medications are being taken as prescribed or if the client or caregivers are forgetting to administer or making changes in the frequency of the medication because they do not understand the directions, because the medication is expensive, or because the medication has side effects. Communication should be initiated with the treating physician to verify which medications are currently prescribed and to alert the physician to any possible use of medications, prescription or over-the-counter, that might be inappropriate. The RN GCM can review and assess the level of understanding and compliance by the client and caregivers with any prescribed treatment protocol. In addition to medications, this could include special diets, exercise therapy, use of special equipment, follow-up medical appointments, and repeat lab work.

Information obtained while investigating the above areas will provide the GCM with much additional information regarding the mental status of the client, family support, comprehension and compliance with medical instructions, finances, values, spiritual beliefs, outlook on life, potential for health education, and receptivity to care planning.

In the case of Lena, an RN GCM would first ascertain that he or she was sitting close enough and speaking loud enough for Lena to hear the questions asked. He or she would also make sure that Lena was sitting in a comfortable position, taking into account her painful hip and arthritic status so that pain and the need to change position would not interfere with or shorten the interview. While the physical assessment of Lena would be comprehensive and involve all systems, the GCM would focus on heart sounds and vital signs, history of falls and the circumstances surrounding them (e.g., blackouts, tripping over obstacles, unexpected malfunction of joints), areas and levels of pain, possible causes of bruising, medications, diet, and the history of her hearing loss. Lena should be interviewed regarding any measures she may have taken to correct or control her problems, and the GCM should ask which problems Lena perceives to have the greatest impact on her quality of life.

Nursing research has contributed to the growing body of knowledge regarding common problems of geriatric functioning, such as falls, incontinence, and confusion. The findings of that research have been incorporated into nursing practice through assessment tools developed by nurses and people in other disciplines.

Programs have been developed for the frail elderly that are nurse managed and are based on the client's presence at an adult day health center or clinic setting. The Collaborative Assessment and Rehabilitation for Elders program is one example of this type of project.[6] The program was conceived as a link between hospitalization and community-based care and is a joint project of the University of Pennsylvania Health System and the University of Pennsylvania Schools of Medicine and Nursing. Clinical services and operations are managed by a master's prepared gerontologic nurse practitioner (GNP). A GNP is assigned to each client as a care manager. This manager coordinates not only with the multidisciplinary team of the program but also with the client's primary care physician. Clients are those needing very comprehensive assessment and complex interventions. They are a frail, elderly group not usually served by rehabilitation programs. Assessment tools that measure areas of function expected to show improvement while in the program are used. Assessment is done upon admission and at discharge. Postdischarge outcomes are obtained by telephone survey. Investigators at the University of Pennsylvania School of Nursing are studying the program to determine overall outcomes and hope to show cost savings that would make the program appealing, especially in the Medicare managed care marketplace, as a means of combining cost containment with acceptable standards of care.[7]

FUNCTIONAL ASSESSMENT

The functional assessment should be done either by an RN GCM or, ideally, by an RN–social worker team of GCMs. Functional ability is assessed through the measurement of the basic skills of role function. This includes measurement of the performance of basic ADLs (e.g., bathing, eating, transferring) and more advanced IADLs (e.g., handling financial matters appropriately, finding one's way away from home and back). Evaluation of the older person's functional abilities is a critical component of the geriatric assessment. "One of the goals of a responsive health care system is to assist clients in maintaining their functional well-being. Functional status in the older person is characterized by the gradual decreases in organ function that accompany normal aging and the more rapid declines associated with acute and chronic illness."[8(p13)] Medical review of symptoms and diagnosis does not by itself predict an individual's functional impairments. These impairments may be the determining factor in deciding on the living situation that person will require. Together, the medical diagnosis and a description and appraisal of the client's function provide the most accurate assessment. Functional impairment cannot be predicted by the number or severity of medical diagnoses. Impairments in ADLs have been identified as risk factors for falls, injuries, and institutionalization.

As stated by Gallo, functional assessment helps set priorities around which the available medical, social, and economic resources can be rallied. Changes in function signal a problem whose source should be addressed and whose solution may be not in a medical response but in a realignment of the social situation.[9]

In older persons, functional assessment is critical for use with ongoing clients as well as at the time of initial assessment, since functional assessment is a barometer of health status in this age group. Loss of functional ability is the most sensitive indicator for identifying new disease and monitoring the progress of treatment.[10] According to Fretwell, most older persons have one "most vulnerable function" (e.g., cognition, memory, continence, ability to walk).[11] Disorders such as pneumonia, urinary tract infection, myocardial infarction, and heart failure may present initially as confusion, incontinence, and other function-related symptoms in certain older adults. Having knowledge of a person's baseline functional status allows early detection of disease, and the subsequent improvement of that functional impairment is a sensitive indicator of recovery. Some impairments can be identified by interview or observation of the older person performing common everyday functions. Others require the use of screening tools and methods to differentiate them from other impairments and conditions and to determine their severity. Functional impairment of ADLs and IADLs can often be identified by history taking and by demonstration and observation. When questioning the older person, it is more effective to ask about recent activities such as "Did you drive here today?" rather than "Are you still driving?"; and "Did you dress yourself this morning?" rather than "Do you dress yourself?" Asking questions in this manner helps focus the older person on what is possible right now and minimizes the reporting of inaccurate information. If the older person is cognitively impaired, responses should be confirmed with a caregiver. Observation of the client's behavior and abilities at the time of the assessment meeting, such as ability to rise from a chair, ambulate, and respond appropriately when speaking, can provide much valuable information. It is also critical to note whether any activities performed are done slowly, with difficulty, unsafely, or only partially.

If deficits in ADLs are identified, it is important to try to determine the underlying cause of the loss of function and how long ago it occurred. This information will help the GCM determine if the condition is permanent or is potentially reversible, perhaps a symptom of an illness that can be treated, restoring function. Many factors affect the ability to perform ADLs safely and completely. No matter what the determination, it is usually wise to involve the client in treatment to alter the dysfunction, since with the proper treatment, many clients have the ability to regain at least partial function. Living with a growing loss of function has a major impact on the quality of life of older people and their caregivers.

Mobility

The first factor influencing ADL performance is mobility. An RN GCM is best trained to assess mobility. Direct observation can identify problems in gait, balance, ability to transfer, and joint function. Early detection of deficits in function in these areas can identify those clients with reduced mobility, deconditioning, and risk of injury. Whenever possible, rehabilitation can then assist in restoring functional losses and reduce the risk of falls and injury. For those deficits that cannot be rehabilitated, assistive equipment can be provided.

One in five older adults has disorders in gait or transferring ability.[12] Older adults commonly show changes in gait that result in imbalance, increased energy expenditure, muscular weakness, and falls. Besides being affected by joint mobility and muscular strength, gait is influenced by proprioceptive, vestibular, and visual sensory input.[5] As will be discussed below, vision should be tested and balance checked as part of the assessment. For clients who are nonambulatory or demonstrate gait impairments, assessment of ability to transfer from one surface or level to another is important.

Approximately 30% of older adults living at home fall each year. Deconditioning can lead to the older person becoming chair or bed bound.

These older persons often go on to develop edema, contractures, incontinence, or pressure sores. These complications place them at increased risk of falls and nursing home placement. It is important to inquire about recent falls and the circumstances under which they occurred and to test gait performance in all older adults. Factors putting older persons at high risk for falls have been identified. Those at high risk can be identified so that preventative measures can be taken as part of care planning. Factors increasing risk include confusion, incontinence, impaired mobility, generalized weakness, use of sedating medications and alcohol, postural hypotension, and history of previous falls.

Balance

All clients' balance should be assessed by an RN GCM as part of a geriatric assessment. For those who are nonambulatory or are determined to have gait impairments, direct observation of ability to transfer from one surface or level to another is very important. The GCM should observe sitting balance; transfers from a supine to a sitting position; and sit-to-chair, sit-to-stand, and pivoting maneuvers.

Shoulder Function

Shoulder function is a critical, but often uninvestigated, component of ability to perform ADLs. At least one adult in four has shoulder pain, but most complaints are not reported to health care professionals. Age-related changes and clinical conditions are common and can come on insidiously. Reduced shoulder range of motion (ROM) can affect ability to drive, dress, groom, or retrieve items from overhead cabinets. The long-term results of disuse can include muscle weakness, chronic pain, and severely reduced ROM. Shoulder or other upper extremity joint dysfunction is a predictor of reduced grip strength as well as inability to perform ADLs. The RN GCM can inquire about shoulder pain and request that the client demonstrate ability to lift and rotate each arm from the shoulder. Pain or inability to rotate the arm at the shoulder will indicate inability to perform ADLs requiring shoulder movement.

Hand Function

Impairments in hand function also place the older person at increased risk for use of more health resources and institutionalization. Loss of strength to grasp and pinch due to arthritis, neuralgic impairments, vascular disease, and trauma may result in decreased ability to dress, groom, toilet, and feed themselves. The standard medical test of asking the client to squeeze two of the examiner's fingers with each hand provides a simple although somewhat subjective measure of grasp strength. For a test of dexterity, the RN GCM or social worker GCM can ask the client to pick up small objects used in daily functioning such as a penny, a spoon, or a toothbrush. Inability to pick up or failure to hold the item and use it will indicate a need for assistance in ADLs involving these or similar items.

THOUGHT PROCESSES

Alterations in thought process come in many forms and may be caused by a wide variety of metabolic and environmental conditions. The client's behavior may exhibit some or all of the following characteristics:

- disorientation to time, place, or person
- altered ability to think abstractly
- disorders of memory
- misinterpretation of environmental stimuli
- changes in problem-solving abilities
- changes in behavior patterns, including regression
- irritability
- expression of fear of others or of losing control
- hallucinations
- delusional thought
- inappropriate responses to commands
- inaccurate interpretation of the environment[13]

Data must be considered from neurological, functional, and mental status examinations be-fore a diagnosis can be made. The presence of one or more of these characteristics will affect the functioning of the older person as assessment information is being gathered. Information obtained regarding altered thought patterns must be sorted, categorized, and addressed in the care plan for that client.

The assessment can be done by either an RN GCM or a social worker GCM. The assessment and sorting process begins with the assessment of level of consciousness and ability to communicate. The client may be comatose, alert but verbally unresponsive, or alert and able to verbally interact. Comatose individuals should be assessed through the use of a history and physical examination. Those who are alert but unable to communicate may have physical conditions such as aphasia, laryngectomy, extreme hearing loss, psychiatric disorders, or language barriers. Cultural and language differences must always be taken into account. Those clients who are alert and able to communicate should have a mental status exam performed. Before using the formal assessment tool, the GCM should assess the client's ability to follow commands. A simple command such as "Tell me your name" or "Squeeze my hand" can be followed by a multistep command such as "Pick up the pencil and write on this paper." This "mini-assessment" will provide information on the client's ability to perform complex cognitive functions. If the client is unable to perform these requests, he or she may be strongly influenced by illness, environment, or fear that he or she is cognitively impaired and unable to follow instructions and complete a mental status exam.

Cognitive decline becomes increasingly common with advancing age. Between 5% and 15% of persons over 65 and 20% to 50% of persons over 85 are reported to be affected.[11] Mental impairment, including depression and dementia, is frequently underdiagnosed in the geriatric population.

Identification of deficits early on in an assessment is critical since, depending on the severity of the cognitive deficit, responses to interview questions may not be accurate in the cognitively impaired person. Unless a screening tool is used as part of the assessment, early or mild dementia may go unrecognized. Clients with dementia may retain conversational skills and are often able to respond appropriately during a conversation. Unless a mental screening tool is used, deficits may go undetected and clients will not be evaluated for possible reversible causes of the dementia. If reversible causes were found, treatment could begin, improving quality of life for that person. Additionally, plans and decisions may be made based on information provided by the client alone, with resulting potential for inaccuracy. It is especially critical in the case of cognitively impaired clients that the GCM gather information from other sources such as caregivers and family members rather than relying solely on the verbal responses of the older client.

Cognitive decline affects every aspect of a client's life and imposes major psychosocial and economic burdens on family and caregivers. Cognitive decline may produce an overlay of depressive symptoms, or depression may be misdiagnosed as cognitive impairment. Major depression is present in 20% to 40% of older persons with Alzheimer's disease.[14] Since depression may be treatable and reversible, it is important to make every attempt to determine correctly whether the client is suffering from depression that manifests as cognitive impairment. Multiple "I don't know" answers should be a clue that the older person may be depressed. Tests that differentiate between cognitive impairment and depression should then be administered. Inconsistent performance on mental exams also suggests that depression may be present. GCMs must use screening tools that have demonstrated reliability in screening for each condition. The common practice of assessing orientation by inquiring about name, place, and date is ineffective as a screening tool.

When cognitive impairment is detected by screening, the GCM should obtain a history of the duration and progress of the decline from the client and caregivers. Progression can be determined by IADL and ADL functional losses, memory problems, personality changes, and dysfunction at work or in social situations. Cognitive screening is recommended for hospitalized patients; people over 80 years of age; people being moved into new living situations; and older adults with

a history of confusion, changes in level of consciousness, diabetes, Parkinson's disease, or unexplained functional losses.

Once symptoms have been categorized, an attempt can be made to determine if the client suffers from cognitive impairment, emotional problems related to physical illness, or mental or emotional problems due to other causes. The presence of physical illness in later life increases the likelihood of emotional problems. The more serious the physical illness, the more severe the accompanying emotional problem. Severe emotional problems can be found in 10% to 25% of hospitalized older patients.[11] Emotional reactions to illness include depression, anxiety, problems in regard to pain, and decline in body function secondary to physical illness. A physical illness can manifest itself directly as an emotional problem. An example is the manifestation of decreased thyroid hormone as a mood disorder with depression and inactivity. Physical illness can also activate an emotional disorder by means of a maladaptive interpretation of the illness by the older adult. The older adult may exacerbate the use of his or her major coping mechanism (e.g., control, dependency) over and above the needs of his or her physical condition in an attempt to control anxiety about the illness. Impaired coping may also manifest itself by exaggeration of a personality style, undermining adaptation to the illness. Physical illnesses also increase stress and the risk for other problems in the older person's life. Reaction to the illness may thus be over and above what would be experienced by a younger person with the same diagnosis. The older person is more apt to be suffering from attempting to cope with multiple changes and stresses. Each of these changes and stresses plays a part in undermining the older person's coping ability and changing how the person presents him- or herself to the world.

VISION

Visual impairment is very common in older persons and has a major impact on performance of daily activities. More than 90% of older persons wear glasses. Sixteen percent of those between 75 to 84 and 27% of those older than 85 are blind in both eyes.[5] Age-related illnesses resulting in progressive vision loss include macular degeneration, cataracts, glaucoma, and diabetic retinopathy. Acute vision loss can be caused by stroke or giant cell arteritis. Many older people are unaware of losses in peripheral vision and central acuity.

Visual acuity information pertaining to the ability to function in the environment can be gathered by observing the client walking, shaking hands, and completing forms. The client can be asked by either the RN GCM or the social worker GCM to read a headline and a sentence from the newspaper. Ability to read both denotes normal visual acuity. Ability to read only the headline signifies moderate impairment, and inability to read either indicates severe impairment. Visual fields should be assessed using the standard confrontation method of having the client follow the examiner's finger. This method will detect gross defect only.

HEARING

Hearing loss affects one-third of 65-year-olds, two-thirds of those over age 70, and three-fourths of those 80 years of age and older.[5] Screening is important since many older adults do not realize that they have a hearing impairment and do not report it to the GCM. Clients with presbycusis, the most common form of loss, have difficulty hearing the higher-frequency consonants of speech while continuing to hear the lower-frequency vowel ranges. Loss of ability to hear consonants leaves much of the message unrecognizable. As hearing loss progresses, the ability to hear and the ability to understand are lost. To assess hearing, the RN GCM or social worker GCM should ask the client to identify the sound of a ticking watch or the presence of two fingers rubbing together by the ear. Speech comprehension difficulties can be evaluated by whispering 10 words while standing 6 inches behind the client. Inability to repeat 50% of the words can indicate hearing loss. Those with suspected or identified loss should be referred to an audiologist for more definitive testing.

URINARY INCONTINENCE

Fifteen percent to 30% of adults living in the community and almost 50% of nursing home residents are affected by urinary incontinence.[15] The prevalence in older women is twice that of older men. Despite the fact that incontinence is common in aging, it should never be considered a normal condition of aging. Various methods of managing and reducing incontinence have been developed, and many older persons have been assisted with incontinence so that the quality of their life is not so greatly affected.

Due to embarrassment and worry about appearance and odor, clients may not report incontinence unless asked directly. Incontinence increases the risk of falls in older persons. It is isolating and has a major impact on quality of life. Often the development of incontinence is the final factor influencing family caregivers to institutionalize those they care for. Few older people realize that incontinence is often treatable. A number of specialized medical tests can help pinpoint the cause of the incontinence. Older persons assessed by the RN GCM to be incontinent should be referred to their primary physicians. Treatment modalities and client education are often implemented and monitored by nurse practitioners with special training in incontinence.

NUTRITION

Maintenance of adequate nutrition and fluid intake is essential to healing and prevention of disease and functional decline. Fifteen percent of older persons living at home and nearly half of all hospitalized older persons are thought to be malnourished.[16] These figures may be low since determining whether an older person is malnourished can be difficult. Nutrition guidelines for older clients have not been clearly defined. Also, standard assessment methods used on the younger population (e.g., height-weight tables, body mass index tables) are not accurate predictors of the nutritional status of older persons. Skeletal height decreases with age. The proportion of lean body mass decreases and the proportion of adipose tissue increases. Dietary intake, activity level, gastrointestinal changes, metabolic changes, drug-nutrient interactions, and chronic diseases all contribute to older persons' nutritional status.

Causes of poor nutritional intake include major illnesses, surgeries, reflux, constipation, dental problems, dysphagia, alcoholism, multiple medications, poverty, social isolation, depression, dementia, pain, immobility, alterations in hunger or thirst recognition, and impaired taste. Dehydration can be the forerunner of constipation, electrolyte imbalance, weight loss, and confusion. Undernutrition is linked to increased morbidity and mortality; prolonged, more frequent hospital stays; and increased prevalence of pressure ulcers.

The RN GCM is better qualified to evaluate nutritional status since disease is often a factor in both poor intake and decreased ability of the body to utilize the food it has available. In certain circumstances it may be appropriate to contract with a dietitian in order to obtain a more complete analysis of a nutritional problem and to do care planning to address that problem.

No reliable laboratory tests have been validated as effective tools for screening for malnutrition in older persons. Loss of weight is presently the most useful indicator of compromised nutritional status. If possible, reports of weight loss should be verified by obtaining a weight history from a physician or family member of the older person. Reports by the older person of changes in the way clothes fit can also be useful. The older person should be weighed at the time of assessment and routinely thereafter so that nutritional status can be monitored.

The client's intake can be assessed by a 24-hour diet diary. However, since many older persons do not have dependable recall, this method is not likely to be highly accurate unless the person has family or caregivers who supplement information provided by the client. It is helpful for a GCM to observe the client eating a meal because the GCM will note any eating difficulties, the client's appetite, and the mealtime social situation. Observation can also provide valuable information for the care plan since the assessor will have the opportunity to formulate interventions based on the information gathered during the observation.

HEIGHT

Height should be measured by the RN GCM or social worker GCM at the time of assessment and, if possible, a reliable source should verify the height of the older person during his or her earlier years. Height loss of 2 inches or more is an indicator of osteoporosis.[17] While more common in women, either sex can be affected by osteoporosis, which creates an increased risk of fractures both at the time of a fall or spontaneously due to compromised bone density. A referral should be made to a physician for bone density testing.

ASSESSMENT TOOLS

Although some components of geriatric assessment can be done without the use of specific scales or tools, using reliable tools will assist GCMs in the quantification of characteristics and behaviors, will enhance the accuracy of the assessment, and will increase the early detection of moderate impairments, some of which may be treatable. In a study comparing the use of standard functional assessment instruments with the use of clinical judgment alone, it was found that while clinicians accurately identified severe impairments, the sensitivity of their clinical judgment was poor in detecting moderate impairment in four categories: mental status sensitivity (28%), nutrition (54%), vision (27%), and continence (42%).[18]

According to the authors of a recent extensive literature review and evaluation of health assessment instruments, despite widespread searching, a true "gold standard" of functional assessment instruments does not yet exist.[19] GCMs should evaluate any assessment instrument prior to using it, just as they would before referring a client to a senior living facility, for instance. GCMs should be familiar with the strengths, weaknesses, and accuracy of any tool used and understand how to best use the tool to enhance their clinical practice. On a practical basis the instruments chosen must either be short enough to be administered within a reasonable time frame or be able to be administered over multiple visits with a client.

Prior to choosing which instrument to use, it is necessary to determine what the goals of the assessment are. Structured functional assessment instruments can detect impairments in physical function, mental status, emotional status, vision, gait, and continence—impairments that may not be detected by standard physical exams. The information obtained through the use of instruments is then coupled with clinical information from the physical exam. If the findings disagree, the final decision regarding status should be determined by clinical judgment.

For some categories of functional testing, such as mental status, multiple instruments are available. For other categories, such as visual acuity, the choices are very limited. Instruments chosen, whenever possible, should be validated by clinical research. Scientific literature should be available providing information on test-retest reliability. The basic design of an instrument and the method of administration can affect information collected. Instruments must be administered in full and read as written in order to collect accurate information. If the instrument is to be used over time with the same client, as a monitoring tool, it must be sensitive to clinically important changes. Many instruments are summaries of scores of individual items or variables and will not show progressive changes in one individual. Scores of many testing instruments can be influenced by educational level, language, or cultural variables.

Functional Assessment

Measurable dimensions of physical and functional status include the traditional problem list, disease severity indicators, the amount of services used, disease-specific scales such as those measuring gait and dementia, ADL scales, and IADL scales. The problem list is typically compiled by GCMs as part of a physical or social/ emotional assessment. Disease severity indexes are available for only a few conditions, such as heart disease. Quantifying the number of days of hospitalization and disability as well as the amount of services used is helpful in determining the severity of health problems.

The instrument most familiar to researchers and clinicians for performing functional assessment is the Katz Index of ADL (Exhibit 11–1). This instrument measures independence of function and is widely used for assessing treatment outcomes of older persons and the chronically ill. It provides a standardized measure of biological and psychological function and a framework for assessing the ability to live independently. When deficiencies are found, it provides guidelines for care planning for correction of those deficiencies. The client is ideally witnessed by the GCM while performing the ADLs and rated either independent or dependent based on the definitions for performance of each ADL as established by Katz.[20] Caregiver report is often used in situations where it is not practical for the GCM to witness ADL activities. The need for assistance is further broken down into categories for supervision, direction, or personal assistance so that subjectivity of the clinician is minimized. A client refusing to perform any function is categorized as not performing the function even though it might be obvious to the tester that, based on the overall functional abilities, the client is capable of performing the particular ADL. A combined measure of the six ADL functions can be used to quantify changes over time. While this instrument is easy to use in a home or facility environment, it is somewhat time-consuming to administer and might be of more use to the GCM who is assessing the client on an ongoing basis rather than one performing a one-time assessment.

The Rapid Disability Rating Scale (Exhibit 11–2) rates individuals' performance of ADLs and their degree of disability on a four-point scale going from "None" (needing no assistance) to "Total" (needing total assistance). It includes a selection of both ADL and IADL tasks and has sections for "degree of disability" and "degree of special problems." As with other

Exhibit 11–1 Katz Index of ADL

Independence means without supervision, direction, or active personal assistance, except as specifically noted below. This is based on actual status and not ability. A patient who refuses to perform a function is considered as not performing the function, even though he or she is deemed able.

Bathing (Sponge, shower, or tub)

Independent: assistance only in bathing a single part (back or disabled extremity) or bathes self completely

Dependent: Assistance in bathing more than one part of body; assistance in getting in or out of tub; does not bathe self

Dressing

Independent: gets clothes from closets and drawers; puts on clothes, outer garments, braces; manages fasteners; act of tying shoes is excluded

Dependent: does not dress self or remains partly undressed

Going to Toilet

Independent: gets to toilet; gets on and off toilet; arranges clothes, cleans organs of excretion (may manage own bedpan used at night only and may or may not be using mechanical supports)

Dependent: uses bedpan or commode or receives assistance in getting to and using toilet

Transfer

Independent: moves in and out of bed and in and out of chair independently (may or may not be using mechanical supports)

Dependent: assistance in moving in or out of bed and/or chair; does not perform one or more transfers

Continence

Independent: urination and defecation entirely self-controlled

Dependent: partial or total incontinence in urination or defecation; partial or total control by enemas, catheters, or regulated use of urinals and/or bedpans

Feeding

Independent: gets food from plate or its equivalent into mouth (precutting of meat and preparation of food, as buttering bread, are excluded from evaluation)

Dependent: assistance in act of feeding (see above); does not eat at all or parenteral feeding

Evaluation Form

Name _____

Date of Evaluation_____

For each area of functioning listed below, circle description that applies (the word "assistance" means supervision, direction, or personal assistance).

Bathing—either sponge bath, tub bath, or shower

| Receives no assistance (gets in and out of tub by self if tub is usual means of bathing) | Receives assistance in bathing only one part of body (such as back or a leg) | Receives assistance in bathing more than one part of body (or does not bathe self) |

Dressing—gets clothes from closets and drawers; puts on clothes, including underclothes, outer garments; manages fasteners (including braces, if worn)

| Gets clothes and gets completely dressed without assistance | Gets clothes and gets dressed without assistance except for tying shoes | Receives assistance in getting clothes or in getting dressed or stays partly or completely undressed |

continues

Exhibit 11–1 continued

Toileting—going to the "toilet room" for bowel and urine elimination; cleaning self after elimination and arranging clothes		
Goes to "toilet room," cleans self, and arranges clothes without assistance (may use object for support such as cane, walker, or wheelchair and may manage night bedpan or commode, emptying same in morning)	Receives assistance in going to "toilet room" or in cleansing self or in arranging clothes after elimination or in use of night bedpan or commode	Does not go to room termed "toilet" for the elimination process
Transfer		
Moves in and out of bed and in and out of chair without assistance (may use object for support such as cane or walker)	Moves in or out of bed or chair with assistance	Does not get out of bed
Continence		
Controls urination and bowel movement completely by self	Has occasional "accidents"	Supervision helps keep urine or bowel control; catheter is used or is incontinent
Feeding		
Feeds self without assistance	Feeds self except for getting assistance in cutting meat or buttering bread	Receives assistance in feeding or is fed partly or completely by tubes or intravenous fluids

scales, it is important to rate the client on what the client does, not what the client says he or she does. This scale is useful for monitoring changes in clients' condition over time.

Other comprehensive assessment tools that include the functional domain along with other components identified as determining factors of ability to live independently are useful in assessment and care planning. The most widely mentioned in the literature are the Barthel Index, which rates 10 different items;[21] the Older American Rehabilitation Services (OARS), which includes the same items as the Katz within its extensive format of many health parameters but relies on self-reports of clients;[22] and the PULSES (physical, upper limbs, lower limbs, sensory, and social factors) Profile. The PULSES Profile measures wider dimensions of functions but includes ADLs.[23] One of the most

widely used instruments, mainly used in nursing homes, is the Minimum Data Set (MDS). The MDS is based on direct observations made by professionals and a review of clinical records.[19] The Minimum Data Set for Home Care (MDS-HC) is now required by several states. It is a multidimensional assessment instrument similar to the long-term care MDS and is used in combination with the Clinical Assessment Protocols (CAPs) to form the Resident Assessment Instrument-Home Care. CAPs provide guidelines for individualized care planning of triggered problems.[24]

Not originally developed as a comprehensive assessment tool, the Outcome and Assessment Information Set (OASIS) is nevertheless widely used as such in both long-term care facilities and home care. This tool represents core items of a comprehensive assessment and forms the basis

Exhibit 11–2 Rapid Disability Rating Scale-2 (RDRS-2)

Directions: Rate what the person *does* to reflect current behavior. Circle one of the four choices for each item. Consider rating with any aids or prostheses normally used. None = completely independent or normal behavior. Total = that person cannot, will not, or may not (because of medical restriction) perform a behavior or has the most severe form of disability or problem.

Assistance with Activities of Daily Living

Eating	None	A little	A lot	Spoon-fed; intravenous tube
Walking (with cane or walker if used)	None	A little	A lot	Does not walk
Mobility (going outside and getting about with wheelchair, etc., if used)	None	A little	A lot	Is housebound
Bathing (include getting supplies, supervising)	None	A little	A lot	Must be bathed
Dressing (include help in selecting clothes)	None	A little	A lot	Must be dressed
Toileting (include help with clothes, cleaning, or help with ostomy/catheter)	None	A little	A lot	Uses bedpan or unable to care for ostomy/catheter
Grooming (shaving for men, hairdressing for women, nails, teeth)	None	A little	A lot	Must be groomed
Adaptive tasks (managing money/possessions; telephoning; buying newspaper, toilet articles, snacks)	None	A little	A lot	Cannot manage

Degree of Disability

Communication (expressing self)	None	A little	A lot	Does not communicate
Hearing (with aid, if used)	None	A little	A lot	Does not seem to hear
Sight (with glasses, if used)	None	A little	A lot	Does not see
Diet (deviation from normal)	None	A little	A lot	Fed by intravenous tube
In bed during day (ordered or self-initiated)	None	A little (<3 hr)	A lot	Most/all of the time
Incontinence (urine/feces, with catheter or prosthesis, if used)	None	Sometimes	Frequently (weekly +)	Does not control
Medication	None	Sometimes	Daily, taken orally	Daily; injection (+oral if used)

Degree of Special Problems

Mental confusion	None	A little	A lot	Extreme
Uncooperativeness (combats efforts to help with care)	None	A little	A lot	Extreme
Depression	None	A little	A lot	Extreme

for measuring client outcomes for purposes of outcome-based quality improvement. It was developed for use by the Health Care Financing Administration (HCFA). Most data items were derived from HCFA-funded research programs to develop a system of outcome measures for home health care. OASIS items include sociodemographic characteristics, environment, support system, health status, and functional status. Data items included are found in many other home care assessment tools, but due to the fact that the primary purpose of the tool is to measure outcomes, many of the items are very precise, with detailed descriptions. While many clinicians state that the OASIS is lengthy to administer, with its use more precise assessments should result, leading to more effective care planning.

Disease-related assessment scales are available for some conditions, such as gait and balance dysfunction. The Tinetti Balance and Gait Evaluation (Exhibit 11–3) is a 28-point assessment tool that is performed by a trained evaluator.[25]

A condensed version of the Tinetti is available. This test, the Get Up and Go Test, is simple to administer, requires no special equipment, and can be carried out in a brief amount of time.[26] The test begins with the client sitting up straight in a high-seat chair, which allows the

Exhibit 11–3 Tinetti Balance and Gait Evaluation

Balance

Instructions: Subject is seated in hard, armless chair. The following maneuvers are tested.

1. Sitting balance

Leans or slides in chair	=	0
Steady, safe	=	1 _____

2. Arises

Unable without help	=	0
Able but uses arms to help	=	1
Able without use of arms	=	2 _____

3. Attempts to arise

Unable without help	=	0
Able but requires more than 1 attempt	=	1
Able to arise with 1 attempt	=	2 _____

4. Immediate standing balance (first 5 sec)

Unsteady (staggers, moves feet, marked trunk sway)	=	0
Steady but uses walker or cane or grabs other objects for support	=	1 _____
Steady without walker or cane or other support	=	2 _____

5. Standing balance

Unsteady	=	0
Steady but wide stance (medial heels more than 4 in. apart) or uses cane, walker, or other support	=	1
Narrow stance without support	=	2 _____

6. Nudged (subject at maximum position with feet as close together as possible, examiner pushes lightly on subject's sternum with palm of hand 3 times)

Begins to fall	=	0
Staggers, grabs, but catches self	=	1
Steady	=	2 _____

7. Eyes closed (at maximum position No. 6)

Unsteady	=	0
Steady	=	1 _____

8. Turning 360°

Discontinuous steps	=	0
Continuous	=	1
Unsteady (grabs, staggers)	=	0
Steady	=	1 _____

continues

Exhibit 11–3 continued

9. Sitting down

Unsafe (misjudged distance, falls into chair)	=	0	
Uses arms or not a smooth motion	=	1	
Safe, smooth motion	=	2	_____

Balance score: _____/16

Gait

Instructions: Subject stands with examiner; walks down hallway or across room, first at his "usual" pace, then back at "rapid, but safe" pace (using usual walking aid such as cane, walker).

10. Initiation of gait (immediately after told to "go")

Any hesitancy or multiple attempts to start	=	0	
No hesitancy	=	1	_____

11. Step length and height
    a. Right swing foot

Does not pass left stance foot with step	=	0	
Passes left stance foot	=	1	
Right foot does *not* clear floor completely with step	=	0	
Right foot completely clears floor	=	1	_____

    b. Left swing foot

Does not pass right stance foot with step	=	0	
Passes right stance foot	=	1	
Left foot does *not* clear floor completely with step	=	0	
Left foot completely clears floor	=	1	_____

12. Step symmetry

Right and left step length not equal (estimate)	=	0	
Right and left step appear equal	=	1	_____

13. Step continuity

Stopping or discontinuity between steps	=	0	
Steps appear continuous	=	1	_____

14. Path (estimated in relation to floor tiles, 12-in. diameter; observe excursion of 1 foot over about 10 ft of the course)

Marked deviation	=	0	
Mild/moderate deviation *or* uses walking aid	=	1	
Straight without walking aid	=	2	_____

15. Trunk

Marked sway or uses walking aid	=	0	
No sway but flexion of knees or back or spreads arms out while walking	=	1	
No sway, no flexion, no use of arms, and no use of walking aid	=	2	_____

16. Walking stance

Heels apart	=	0	
Heels almost touching while walking	=	1	_____

Gait score: _____/12
Total score: _____/28

person to sit with hips at a 90-degree angle to knees. The client is then instructed to (1) get up (without using armrests if possible), (2) stand still, (3) walk forward 10 feet, (4) turn around and walk back to the chair, and (5) turn and be seated. The evaluator notes sitting balance, transfers from sitting to standing, pace and stability of walking, and ability to turn without staggering. Statistical verification of the test by the developers showed good correlation between test scores and other measures of gait, which in some cases involved more sophisticated laboratory-based measures of balance and gait.

The wide range of abilities involved in IADLs (not only physical but mental and social variables) and the complexity and variation of interpretations of the test results mean that there are more problems with IADL instruments than ADL instruments. IADL scales may result in falsely low scores for men and women who have not performed certain food preparation and laundry tasks during their lifetime but are perfectly capable of performing other IADL functions. The scale most widely used, with reliability and validity with the older population well documented, is the IADL Scale (Exhibit 11–4).[27] The scale measures eight aspects of living that are critical to those living independently.

Cognitive Assessment

The most commonly used and most thoroughly researched screening test for dementia is the Mini Mental State Examination (MMSE).[28] It is used by 90% of physicians and is recommended by the National Institute of Neurological and Communicative Disorders and Stroke and by the Alzheimer's Disease Centers, funded by the National Institute on Aging.[29] It is the test against which other cognitive assessment tools are compared in validation tests. It is a screening tool. It is not expected to replace a complete diagnostic workup, and its results should not be used as a diagnosis. It is relatively quick to administer and requires no special equipment other than a pencil and paper. A score of 23 or lower out of a possible 30 has been defined as indicating cognitive impairment. Test-retest reliability ranges from 0.80 to 0.90. Interrater reliability is above 0.80. The MMSE has been found to have convergent validity with other cognitive tests and with functional measures. Clinically, a sensitivity of 85% or better has been found with clients with dementia. The sensitivity decreases with mild dementia and with the screening of clients in the community versus hospital or clinic setting. Multiple studies indicate that MMSE scores are positively related to the edu-

cational level of impaired and intact adults. Race and ethnicity have also been shown to affect the distribution of MMSE scores.[30] Research has shown that the MMSE can distinguish between depressed clients, clients with dementia, and clients with both dementia and depression.

The Short Portable Mental Status Questionnaire (SPMSQ; Exhibit 11–5) asks 10 questions with each error scored as one point. Intact mental function is indicated by less than 2 errors and severe mental impairment by 8 to 10 errors. The scoring is adjusted for educational level. It is part of the OARS instrument and has been used extensively with the older population. When used as a screen for dementia in persons older than 60 years, the questionnaire has a sensitivity of 95% and a specificity of 88%. Reliability studies performed upon 59 subjects showed test-retest correlations of 0.82 when carried out at 4-week intervals.[31] According to some research, the test does not distinguish between those persons who are mildly impaired and those who are intact or moderately impaired.[32]

In addition to providing valuable information, the Clock Test is used for screening cognitive impairment in clients with Alzheimer's disease.[33] It has the advantage of being very simple to administer. The client is given a blank sheet of paper with the instructions to draw a clock and indicate a specific time. Since the task requires the client to follow an oral command, remember a clock, and perform higher-order mental functions, the test can provide more information than is provided by the performance of verbal memory tasks. Correlations of scores with other measures of dementia are in the 0.50 range.[34] Several scoring systems have been developed based on multiple criteria such as the following: Is there a totally closed figure without gaps? Are the symbols ordered in a clockwise direction? Are the hands of the clock within the closed figure? Good interrater reliability on the scoring systems and good test-retest reliability for the scores have been reported. Sensitivity as a screening tool has been found to be at 86% to 93%.[35] Studies caution against using the Clock Test in the place of more cognitively based screening tools.

Exhibit 11–4 IADL Scale

Male Score		Female Score
	A. Ability to use telephone	
1	1. Operates telephone on own initiative; looks up and dials numbers, etc.	1
1	2. Dials a few well-known numbers	1
1	3. Answers telephone but does not dial	1
0	4. Does not use telephone at all	0
	B. Shopping	
1	1. Takes care of all shopping needs independently	1
0	2. Shops independently for small purchases	0
0	3. Needs to be accompanied on any shopping trip	0
0	4. Completely unable to shop	0
	C. Food Preparation	
	1. Plans, prepares, and serves adequate meals independently	1
	2. Prepares adequate meals if supplied with ingredients	0
	3. Heats and serves prepared meals, or prepares meals but does not maintain adequate diet	0
	4. Needs to have meals prepared and served	0
	D. Housekeeping	
	1. Maintains house alone or with occasional assistance (e.g., heavy-work domestic help)	1
	2. Performs light daily tasks such as dish washing and bed making	1
	3. Performs light daily tasks but cannot maintain acceptable level of cleanliness	1
	4. Needs help with all home maintenance tasks	1
	5. Does not participate in any housekeeping tasks	0
	E. Laundry	
	1. Does personal laundry completely	1
	2. Launders small items; rinses socks, stockings, etc.	1
	3. All laundry must be done by others	0
	F. Mode of transportation	
1	1. Travels independently on public transportation or drives own car	1
1	2. Arranges own travel via taxi, but does not otherwise use public transportation	1
0	3. Travels on public transportation when assisted or accompanied by another	1
0	4. Travel limited to taxi or automobile, with assistance of another	0
0	5. Does not travel at all	0
	G. Responsibility for own medication	
1	1. Is responsible for taking medication in correct dosages at correct time	1
0	2. Takes responsibility if medication is prepared in advance in separate dosages	0
0	3. Is not capable of dispensing own medication	0
	H. Ability to handle finances	
1	1. Manages financial matters independently (budgets, writes checks, pays rent and bills, goes to bank); collects and keeps track of income	1
1	2. Manages day-to-day purchases, but needs help with bank for managing purchases, etc.	1
0	3. Incapable of handling money	0

Exhibit 11–5 Short Portable Mental Status Questionnaire (SPMSQ)

Instructions: Ask questions 1 through 10 in this list and record all answers. Ask question 4A only if patient does not have a telephone. Record total number of errors based on ten questions.

+	–	
_____	_____	1. What is the date today? _____
		Month Day Year
_____	_____	2. What day of the week is it? _____
_____	_____	3. What is the name of this place? _____
_____	_____	4. What is your telephone number? _____
_____	_____	4A. What is your street address? _____
		(Ask only if patient does not have a telephone)
_____	_____	5. How old are you? _____
_____	_____	6. When were you born? _____
_____	_____	7. Who is the President of the U.S. now? _____
_____	_____	8. Who was President just before him? _____
_____	_____	9. What was your mother's maiden name? _____
_____	_____	10. Subtract 3 from 20 and keep subtracting 3 from each new number, all the way down.
_____		Total Number of Errors

Scoring: 0–2 errors = intact mental function
3–4 errors = mild intellectual impairment
5–7 errors = moderate intellectual impairment
8–10 errors = severe intellectual impairment
Allow one more error if subject had only grade school education.
Allow one fewer error if subject has had education beyond high school.

Home Environment Assessment

One-fifth of all households are maintained by a person or persons aged 65 and over. Many older persons choose to live alone if health and finances permit. With advancing age, solitary living increases. In 1990, 47% of those age 85 and over lived alone. Forty-five percent of those over 85 years are projected to be living alone by 2020. The majority of those over 75 living alone are women.[36]

The living situations of this group are diverse. Older persons are more vulnerable to the problems of inadequate, unsafe housing due to other problems such as poverty, lack of social support, reduced physical reserves or disabilities, and cognitive impairment. The three most common housing-related problems of older persons are adequacy of housing for the individual's needs, suitability of the neighborhood, and cost.[5] The majority of older persons own their own homes, but the homes may not be adequate or in good repair. In a study done in 1979, Lawton found that 53% of homes owned by older persons were built 40 or more years ago.[37] These homes are more likely to have physical defects due to age than homes lived in by younger persons. Some of these defects, such as inadequate insulation, may actually increase the costs of day-to-day living of older persons, who often live on fixed incomes.

Other vital components of the home (e.g., wiring, roofing) may need repairs and upgrades that the older person cannot afford. Due to the factors listed above and the reluctance of some older persons to consider making any changes to accommodate physical disabilities, such as the installation of grab bars in bathrooms, relocation to a downstairs area for sleeping, and the addition of ramps for safe entry and exit, some older persons are living in unsafe conditions. This group is at increased risk for falls and fractures and the institutionalization that frequently follows those events.

It is very important and necessary to perform a home assessment as part of the geriatric assessment process. The social worker GCM may have more training in home assessment. The RN GCM can perform the assessment if necessary. The assessment should include the evaluation of safety factors (e.g., smoke alarms, adequate wiring) and how effectively the older person is able to function within the floor plan and room arrangement of his or her home. While the home might be safe for a person without disabilities or cognitive impairments, if there are features (e.g., a second story, sunken rooms or hallways, tiny bathrooms) that are obstacles or potential dangers to a person needing assistive devices or forgetful of steps, that home is not safe for that person. Observation of the client as he or she performs ADLs is invaluable for assessment of the client's home safety and environmental needs as well as functional abilities.

Using a checklist is a time-efficient and comprehensive method for ascertaining the safety of a home. The Home Safety Checklist (Exhibit 11–6) is one tool that can be used to identify fall hazards in the home.[38] Its detailed questions provide some education to the older person in practices that can be initiated to minimize the likelihood of falling. As part of the assessment, caregivers can be educated to be alert for hazards and to evaluate the need for added safety features (e.g., alarms on outside doors, grab bars, raised toilet seats) that the older person may need as the condition progresses.

Exhibit 11–6 Home Safety Checklist

This checklist is used to identify fall hazards in the home. After identification, hazards should be eliminated or reduced. One point is allowed for every *no* answer. A score of 1 to 7 is excellent, 8 to 14 is good, 15 or higher is hazardous.

Housekeeping   Yes   No
 1. Do you clean up spills as soon as they occur?
 2. Do you keep floors and stairways clean and free of clutter?
 3. Do you put away books, magazines, sewing supplies, and other objects as soon as you're through with them and never leave them on floors or stairways?
 4. Do you store frequently used items on shelves that are within easy reach?

Floors
 5. Do you keep everyone from walking on freshly washed floors before they're dry?
 6. If you wax floors, do you apply 2 thin coats and buff each thoroughly or else use self-polishing, nonskid wax?
 7. Do all small rugs have nonskid backings?
 8. Have you eliminated small rugs at the tops and bottoms of stairways?
 9. Are all carpet edges tacked down?
10. Are rugs and carpets free of curled edges, worn spots, and rips?
11. Have you chosen rugs and carpets with short, dense pile?
12. Are rugs and carpets installed over good-quality, medium-thick pads?

continues

Exhibit 11–6 continued

	Yes	No
Bathroom		
13. Do you use a rubber mat or nonslip decals in the tub or shower?		
14. Do you have a grab bar securely anchored over the tub or on the shower wall?		
15. Do you have a nonskid rug on bathroom floor?		
16. Do you keep soap in an easy-to-reach receptacle?		
Traffic lanes		
17. Can you walk across every room in your home, and from one room to another, without detouring around furniture?		
18. Is the traffic lane from your bedroom to the bathroom free of obstacles?		
19. Are telephone and appliance cords kept away from areas where people walk?		
Lighting		
20. Do you have light switches near every doorway?		
21. Do you have enough good lighting to eliminate shadowy areas?		
22. Do you have a lamp or light switch within easy reach from your bed?		
23. Do you have night lights in your bathroom and in the hallway leading from your bedroom to the bathroom?		
24. Are all stairways well lighted?		
25. Do you have light switches at both the tops and bottoms of stairways?		
Stairways		
26. Do securely fastened handrails extend the full length of the stairs on each side of stairways?		
27. Do rails stand out from the walls so you can get a good grip?		
28. Are rails distinctly shaped so you're alerted when you reach the end of a stairway?		
29. Are all stairways in good condition, with no broken, sagging, or sloping steps?		
30. Are all stairway carpeting and metal edges securely fastened and in good condition?		
31. Have you replaced any single-level steps with gradually rising ramps or made sure such steps are well lighted?		
Ladders and step stools		
32. Do you have a sturdy step stool that you use to reach high cupboard and closet shelves?		
33. Are all ladders and step stools in good condition?		
34. Do you always use a step stool or ladder that's tall enough for the job?		
35. Do you always set up your ladder or step stool on a firm, level base that's free of clutter?		
36. Before you climb a ladder or step stool, do you always make sure it's fully open and that the stepladder spreaders are locked?		

continues

Exhibit 11–6 continued

	Yes	No
37. When you use a ladder or step stool, do you face the steps and keep your body between the side rails?	_____	_____
38. Do you avoid standing on stop of a step stool or climbing beyond the second step from the top on a stepladder?	_____	_____

Outdoor areas

	Yes	No
39. Are walks and driveways in your yard and other areas free of breaks?	_____	_____
40. Are lawns and gardens free of holes?	_____	_____
41. Do you put away garden tools and hoses when they're not in use?	_____	_____
42. Are outdoor areas kept free of rocks, loose boards, and other tripping hazards?	_____	_____
43. Do you keep outdoor walkways, steps, and porches free of wet leaves and snow?	_____	_____
44. Do you sprinkle icy outdoor areas with deicers as soon as possible after a snowfall or freeze?	_____	_____
45. Do you have mats at doorways for people to wipe their feet on?	_____	_____
46. Do you know the safest way of walking when you can't avoid walking on a slippery surface?	_____	_____

Footwear

	Yes	No
47. Do your shoes have soles and heels that provide good traction?	_____	_____
48. Do you wear house slippers that fit well and don't fall off?	_____	_____
49. Do you avoid walking in stocking feet?	_____	_____
50. Do you wear low-heeled oxfords, loafers, or good-quality sneakers when you work in your house or yard?		
51. Do you replace boots or galoshes when their soles or heels are worn too smooth to keep you from slipping on wet or icy surfaces?	_____	_____

Personal precautions

	Yes	No
52. Are you always alert for unexpected hazards, such as out-of-place furniture?	_____	_____
53. If young grandchildren visit, are you alert for children playing on the floor and toys left in your path?	_____	_____
54. If you have pets, are you alert for sudden movements across your path and pets getting underfoot?		
55. When you carry bulky packages, do you make sure they don't obstruct your vision?		
56. Do you divide large loads into smaller loads whenever possible?	_____	_____
57. When you reach or bend, do you hold onto a firm support and avoid throwing your head back or turning it too far?	_____	_____
58. Do you always use a ladder or step stool to reach high places and never stand on a chair?	_____	_____
59. Do you always move deliberately and avoid rushing to answer the phone or doorbell?	_____	_____
60. Do you take time to get your balance when you change position from lying down to sitting and from sitting to standing?	_____	_____

continues

Exhibit 11–6 continued

	Yes	No
61. Do you hold onto grab bars when you change position in the tub or shower?	_____	_____
62. Do you keep yourself in good condition with moderate exercise, good diet, adequate rest, and regular medical checkups?	_____	_____
63. If you wear glasses, is your prescription up to date?	_____	_____
64. Do you know how to reduce injury in a fall?	_____	_____
65. If you live alone, do you have daily contact with a friend or neighbor?	_____	_____

Once safety hazards have been identified and necessary changes have been listed and explained to the client, the GCM has to make sure that changes will be made by addressing hazards as problems in the care plan and writing an intervention for their solution. Often older persons are unable or unwilling to make changes. Suggested changes should be addressed with the older person, and every attempt should be made to get the person to agree and plan for the prompt implementation needed. If the older person resists, family or other support persons should be notified of the risk to the older person in remaining in the unchanged environment. These persons can often influence the older person and assist with the practical matters of implementation of changes.

Psychosocial Assessment

The purpose of the psychosocial assessment is to determine the client's ability to function and the level of functioning in a particular social environment. The social worker GCM is best suited by education and training to perform the assessment, although an RN GCM can also do the assessment.

The GCM assessing the older person should know the most common psychosocial problems faced by older persons and their families and be familiar with some of the potential life-enhancing methods of managing those problems. Care planning following the assessment often includes creative and individualized interventions since identified problems can be the result of more than one psychosocial deficit or maladaptive coping mechanism. In order to be useful, the planned interventions must meet the needs of the older person and be accepted by the client and family.

The psychosocial assessment includes a number of factors and is complicated by the various changes in the aging person and the complexity of the need for constant adjustment to change and loss. Components of the assessment should include coping skills, self-care ability, social support systems, values, finances, and legal planning. Some of these factors have a combined effect on the need for assistance and/or changes in the lifestyle of the older person as aging occurs.

The emotional needs and wishes of the client must be included in the assessment and the care planning that follows. The client may have accommodated to and accepted situations and conditions that in the GCM's opinion need to be altered. In ongoing research about life satisfaction, Campbell and Converse identified self-esteem and a feeling of control as critical components of life satisfaction and state that in any situation, it is impossible to predict whether it will be enhanced or will decline.[39] They theorize that perceived satisfaction increases as one becomes increasingly accommodated to a situation, even though the situation remains the same.

Life satisfaction in older persons has been widely researched, with low income, poor health, and lack of social interaction shown to be related to lower perceived quality of life.[40–42] The client's goals and concerns must be addressed and he or she must be included in planning decisions whenever possible. Client input and a plan tailored to the emotional, social, spiritual, and physical needs of the client will make necessary changes easier for the client to accept and will motivate the client to cooperate with necessary interventions, thus increasing the likelihood that the care plan will succeed and the client will be satisfied.

Coping skills are affected by physiological problems and cognitive deficits. As stated earlier, depression is common in older persons, and it is sometimes difficult for the GCM to sort out whether the underlying cause is a physical condition, medication interaction, cognitive decline, substance abuse, long-standing psychiatric illness, or simply the many life changes occurring as the older person ages and copes with multiple losses. Cognitive screening, when combined with a complete history, will help the GCM sort out whether the use of a maladaptive coping style has been a lifelong pattern of the client or is based on a change in judgment or inability to understand the issues of the current situation and the ramifications of the decisions the client is making.

It has been recommended that long-term care professionals do a systematic assessment of their clients' values and preferences as part of a comprehensive assessment.[43] This assessment can probably be done most effectively by a social worker. The assessment will assist both the client and the GCM to determine which aspects of life and care are most important to the client. The care plan must consider the goals of autonomy, informed consent, and quality of life. A values history can be conducted with the client. As one example, the client could be asked "is it more important to you to have the freedom to come and go as you please, or to be safe and accept some restrictions on your life?" Feelings and preferences regarding end-of-life issues must be explored with the client. Older persons may need time and assistance to clarify their thinking and determine who will carry out their wishes if they are unable to do so. GCMs are sometimes hesitant to ask questions about preferences for fear the client's preferences will be unrealistic. Clients may have a difficult time an-

swering certain questions due to lack of experience with some issues. In those cases in which the client's preferences cannot be included in the care plan, it is very important for the GCM to be aware as early as possible that the client will need education and assistance in adjusting to the reality of his or her care needs. Early knowledge will allow the GCM the opportunity to address those issues and prepare the client for necessary changes.

Some older persons are reluctant to discuss personal information with someone they have just met. If clients are willing to discuss the presenting problem, the interview should be started with that. Gentle probing will assist the GCM in determining the older person's awareness of the problem and comfort level in discussing it. If the client is reluctant to be forthcoming, the GCM can begin by gathering information from the client regarding lifestyle and residence. Much information can be obtained while the client is gaining a comfort level with the interview process and the interviewer. The discussion will have the tone of a friendly conversation. As the discussion proceeds and the client's comfort level grows, the client may reveal sensitive information that he or she would not volunteer to an interviewer asking questions from a questionnaire. Since many older clients fear that they will be relocated if they admit outside agencies or parties into their lives, it is important for the GCM to stress at the beginning that he or she is just gathering information and that the client will be involved in planning any changes. Conversations about lifestyle often include information about major life changes, social and family supports or the absence of these, demands of daily living, and coping skills. Ability to converse and access short-term and long-term memories will also be revealed to the GCM. Clients may indicate some of their perceptions about their current situation and their ability to deal with reality and exercise judgment. The client's perception of his or her health status should be determined. If the client is asked "How do you rate your overall health—excellent, good, fair, or poor?" responses may give the GCM insight into the individual's self-concept, need for knowledge, and motivation for change. If a client perceives that his or her health is good but actually has multiple chronic illnesses, the client may have excellent coping skills, including a positive attitude; may be in denial; or may fear being honest with the GCM.

If the client lives alone and has obvious care needs, the GCM should ask about assistance being provided by family, friends, or social or health agencies. Information will be obtained about adequacy of assistance, the client's willingness to accept help, family relationships, and the presence or absence of social support.

Vague responses may indicate either that the client is not connected to support systems or that cognitive impairment may be present. The client may mention persons whom the GCM should interview to gather additional information. Since it is frequently the perception (or desire) of older persons that family and friends will be available to provide as much assistance as is needed, any information from the client that adequate assistance is available should be verified with those family and friends named.

The client's lifetime coping patterns and methods of handling stress must be determined. This will provide information regarding support systems, healthy versus unhealthy ways of handling stress, the importance of religious or spiritual practices to the client, control issues, and psychological problems or mental illnesses. Information obtained will help the GCM in planning the intervention strategies of the care plan.

It is important to determine during the screening whether the older person or caregivers are impacted by problems prevalent among older persons, such as depression, substance abuse, and elder abuse. Geriatric depression is discussed in Chapter 13. Family caregiver depression is quite common and can affect the quality of care that the older person receives. Substance abuse can be related to depression or be an independent risk factor that, if ignored, can negate the success of the most well-thought-out care plan. Red flags for the GCM to investigate include frequent falls; multiple fractures; multiple bruises; isolating behaviors; reports of excess sleeping or insomnia; the presence of multiple

pain control or mood-altering drugs or alcohol in the home; and increased tolerance to drugs or alcohol. The GCM should also be aware that few substance abusers will be honest in their answers involving use. Family members and caregivers should be interviewed separately regarding the older person's usage, if at all possible. The home safety inspection can be useful in determining whether alcohol is present in the home, but it must still be determined whether the older person is actively drinking.

The GCM must have the opportunity to meet with the client alone when asking questions about elder abuse. The older person being cared for by family or others and being abused will not usually admit to the abuse for fear of caregiver abandonment or retaliation. The most common types of abuse or maltreatment are physical abuse, neglect, psychological abuse, violation of rights, and financial exploitation. The GCM should observe family interactions closely when in the home. Red flags include multiple bruises or burns, weight loss or dehydration, crying or agitation, poor hygiene, isolation of the older person, and lack of necessary items of daily living despite adequate income.

Financial assessment is a necessary category of assessment and a critical precursor to care planning. Finances are a determining factor in many decisions the older person and the family need to make. The disclosure of financial information is very difficult for many older persons, and GCMs may have difficulty approaching the issue. It is never appropriate for the GCM to use unverified observations and assumptions concerning the client's financial status to determine the care planning for that client. When loss of independence occurs and care must be obtained, financial capabilities must be taken into account.

Failure of the GCM to assess finances may result in expenditure of much or all of a client's resources prematurely or unnecessary conservation of adequate resources that could have been used to provide the client with a better quality of life. If the older person is cognizant, he or she must be included in planning for care that costs money and agree to any plan that requires expenditure of his or her assets. If the client is reluctant to spend money, he or she will feel in greater control if the plan reflects his or her goals and values. Family members can sometimes provide assistance by telling the older person that it is necessary to reveal assets during the assessment and by assuring the client that this is the time to spend some of those assets.

Whenever possible, the client's family members should be interviewed concerning their perceptions of the client's situation and their role in the client's life, the family structure, and family patterns of functioning. This will assist the GCM in determining whether there will be family support or obstacles in the implementation of the care plan. The ongoing involvement of and coaching and support from family members and other caregivers help ensure the success of the care plan. If the GCM and the client's family feel like members of the same team, the likelihood of success is enhanced.

WRITING THE ASSESSMENT FINDINGS AND DESIGNING THE CARE PLAN

Once all the information is gathered, it must be analyzed in a systematic, logical manner. Written assessment questionnaires assist in the categorization of data. Data can be classified according to a number of different parameters, including identified problems, functional deficits, chronic or acute illnesses, and coping mechanisms and deficits. The sorting and classification of data lead to the identification of areas of intervention.

Intervention strategies must be individualized. The report always begins with a statement of the presenting problem. In the case of Lena, this could be stated as "Problem: Older woman with multiple disabilities, at high risk for falls, living alone in unsafe environment." Sometimes the GCM will not consider the presenting problem to be the client's most urgent problem. Often there are several problems and the GCM can propose separate interventions. Frequently, priority must be given to life- or safety-threatening conditions or immediate concerns of the client and family. In some very urgent situations, these interventions may need to be initiated prior to the completion of the plan. Some data will be

obtained in the assessment that will be useful in the identification of more than one problem or the intervention strategy that will be most effective or most acceptable to the client.

The care plan can be divided into a number of categories, depending upon the requirements of funding sources who will be reimbursing for care, the educational and licensing status of those designing the plan and carrying out the care, and the policies and paperwork of any given agency or facility. There has been little research done on how GCMs make care plan decisions. The limited research available has shown some inconsistency from GCM to GCM when GCMs are given the same case study and asked to design a care plan. The researchers felt that professional judgment was one explanation for variations in care plans. Medicare and other government funding sources now require that standardized assessment tools (e.g., the OASIS) with multiple choice forced answers be used. This requirement should result in the development of more objective assessments and care plans with measurable outcomes.

The care plan always includes a list of problems, diagnoses, or functional variations from the normal. Each identified problem should be addressed individually with an intervention and a clear plan of how that intervention is to be operationalized. Language used must be as straightforward and objective as possible so that it is subject to the least amount of variation in interpretation by those carrying out the plan. If the plan is to be carried out by family, unskilled caregivers, or anyone outside the discipline of the writer, the use of terminology commonly used within that discipline but not necessarily understood by others should be avoided if possible.

The plan may include a timeline stating either frequency of intervention of the GCM, or number of interventions to be expected before the outcome point should be achieved. Additionally, the plan may include a measurable outcome or goal for each intervention. More than one intervention may contribute to a single goal. In the care plan for Lena (Table 11–1), the goal of the first two interventions could be listed as safety.

Since clients are older persons and many of their conditions are chronic, the goal usually involves improved safety or functional status, not complete absence of disease or return to normal functional status. All who use the plan must understand that it is subject to change as the client's condition changes and must be reviewed on a regular basis by the GCM and if possible the team to ascertain if the plan is still the most effective plan for that client.

The people who hire the GCM will not necessarily be happy with the findings and outcomes of the assessment. It is not uncommon for many more problems to be found than the family is aware of or is motivated to discuss or address. The solutions to identified problems may include the need for greater involvement of the family, greater expenditure of finances, more psychological intervention through social work contact, or major changes for the client that had not been anticipated. The GCM must provide detailed evidence in the report to back findings and recommendations. The greater the number of family members, fiduciary and legal represen-

tatives, physicians, and others whose cooperation will need to be obtained to carry out the plan, the more comprehensive and detailed the explanations and justifications for the interventions of the plan need to be.

Brief Example of Assessment and Care Planning Based on Case Study

Lena, the 83-year-old woman introduced earlier in the chapter, lives alone in a home that has not been modified for her disabilities. She has been assessed by the GCM as having four health and functional disabilities: her diagnoses of arthritis and heart disease, significant weight loss in the past year, hearing impairment, and pain in her hip and difficulty walking. Since Lena's expressed desire is to remain in her own home, safety issues must take priority.

Due to Lena's physical disabilities and the fact that she is at high risk for falling, and due to her arthritis and gait limitations, Lena needs

Table 11–1 Care Plan

Problem	Intervention
Lack of support/care providers	Implement care provision in home, including aide to assist with ADLs (bathing, medication reminders, light housekeeping).
Impaired home maintenance/safety issues	Arrange for handyperson to relocate client's bedroom to ground level, install grab bars in bathroom, and perform other household modifications and repairs as indicated. Arrange for aide to perform light housekeeping.
Pain and difficulty walking	Arrange physician appointment for health status update and medication review. Request physical therapy consult.
Isolation	Arrange for aide to provide stimulation, conversation, and company on outings. Arrange for hearing evaluation.
Weight loss	Arrange for aide to perform grocery shopping. Arrange for aide to prepare nutritious meals and record foods eaten and amounts for each meal. Check weight during each GCM visit.
Impaired financial management	Refer to bill manager to maintain finances. Refer to financial planner.

some assistance with ADLs if she is to remain at home safely. An aide should assist her with bathing, meal preparation, and housework. Lena should be evaluated by a physician and a physical therapist to determine if any of her pain and disability can be treated. The bedroom should be relocated to the downstairs portion of the house so that Lena can avoid climbing stairs and can rest well at night. An alternative for Lena to consider is a move to an assisted living facility where her physical needs could be met. Lena's hearing loss should be evaluated and the use of a hearing aide begun, if recommended. Inability to hear is resulting in decreased socialization and feelings of being out of control and isolated. Having assistance in the home will also provide her with socialization opportunities, both from spending time with the aide and from going out to activities with the aide's assistance. A bill manager should be hired to take over bill paying, and Lena should be encouraged to hire an attorney or estate planner to assist with asset management and estate planning. Lena should decide upon her advance directives and complete the necessary paperwork. Table 11–1 contains a care plan for Lena.

CONCLUSION

Once the assessment is completed and has been discussed with all concerned parties, the job of the GCM may be over, or just begun, depending upon whether he or she is asked to carry out the care plan. At times, the client or family may resist the changes recommended in the plan and decide that their connection with the GCM is finished. If and when a crisis arises in the life of the client, the GCM may be called upon to become reinvolved, adjust the plan to fit the needs of the current situation, and implement and manage the care plan. If this occurs, since the GCM has already acquired so much information about the client, the GCM is usually able to provide relatively quick assistance. In either case, the GCM has provided the client and family with a comprehensive blueprint of how to proceed and hopefully assisted them in seeing the value of using professionals for consultation and assistance.

NOTES

1. National Institutes of Health. "Consensus Conference on Geriatric Assessment Methods for Clinical Decision-Making." http://www.nlm.nih.gov (19 October 1987). Accessed April 4, 1999.

2. American Geriatrics Society. "Comprehensive Geriatric Assessment Position Statement." http://www.american geriatrics.org (October 1996). Accessed March 15, 1999.

3. National Institutes of Health. "Geriatric Assessment Methods for Clinical Decisionmaking: National Institute of Health Consensus Statement." http://www.nlm.nih.gov (19 October 1987). Accessed April 4, 1999.

4. Andresen E, Rothenberg B, Zimmer J. *Assessing the Health Status of Older Adults.* New York: Springer Publishers; 1997.

5. Matteson M, McConnell E. *Gerontological Nursing.* Philadelphia: Saunders; 1988.

6. Evans L, Forciea, M, Yurkow J, Sochalski, J. The geriatric day hospital. In: Katz P et al, eds. *Emerging Systems in Long-Term Care.* New York: Springer Publishers; 1999:67–87.

7. Naylor N, Prior P. Transitions between acute and long-term care. In: Katz P, Kane R, Mezey M, eds. *Emerging Systems in Long-Term Care.* New York: Springer Publishers; 1999:1–22.

8. Newcomer R, Harrington C, Kane R. Implications of managed care for older persons. In: Katz P, Kane R, Mezey M, eds. *Emerging Systems in Long-Term Care.* New York: Springer Publishers; 1999:118–148.

9. American Geriatrics Society. "Comprehensive Geriatric Assessment Position Statement." http://www.american geriatrics.org (October 1996). Accessed March 15, 1999.

10. Gallo J. *Handbook of Geriatric Assessment.* 3rd ed. Gaithersberg, MD: Aspen Publishers; 1999.

11. Fretwell M. Comprehensive functional assessment. In: Abrams W, Berkow R, eds. *The Merck Manual of Geriatrics.* Rathway, NJ: Merck & Co.; 1990:170–174.

12. VanSweringen J, Paschal K, Bomono P, Yang J. The modified Gait Abnormality Rating Scale for recognizing the risk of recurrent falls in community-dwelling elderly adults. *Phys Ther.* 1996;76:994–1002.

13. Soja M, Kippenbrock T, Hendrich A, Nyhuis A. A risk model for patient fall prevention. In: Funk S, Tornquist M, Champagne M, Weise, R, eds. *Key Aspects of Elder Care.* New York: Springer Publishers; 1992:65–70.

14. Harper M. An overview of mental health and older adults. In: Hogstel M, ed. *Geropsychiatric Nursing.* St. Louis, MO: Mosby; 1995:1–20.

15. Resnick N, Wells T. Maintaining and restoring continence. In: Funk S, Tornquist M, Champagne M, Weise, R, eds. *Key Aspects of Elder Care.* New York: Springer Publishers; 1992:135–154.

16. Semb S. Geriatric nutrition. In: *Continuing Education for California Nurses.* Sacramento, CA: CME Resource; 1998:1–14.

17. Gross P, Knutsen K. Integrating physical and psychosocial assessment. Presented at Geriatric Care Managers Conference; October 22–25, 1998; Chicago.

18. Pinholt E, Kroenke K, Hauley J, Kussman M, Carpenter J, Twyman P. Functional assessment of the elderly: a comparison of standard instruments with clinical judgement. *Arch Int Med.* 1987;147:484–488.

19. Morris J, Harues C, Murphy K. Designing the National Resident Assessment Instrument for Nursing Homes. *Gerontologist.* 1990;30:293–307.

20. Katz S, Downs T, Cash H. Progress in the development of the index of ADL. *Gerontologist.* 1970;10:20–30.

21. Mahoney F, Barthel D. Functional evaluation: the Barthel Index. *Md State Med J.* 1965;14:61–65.

22. Fillenbaum G, Smyer M. The development, validity and reliability of the OARS multidimensional functional assessment questionnaire. *J Gerontol.* 1981;36:428–434.

23. Moskowitz E, McCann C. Classification of disability in the chronically ill and aging. *J Chronic Dis.* 1957;5:342–346.

24. Heeren T, Lagaay A, vonBeck W, Rooymans H, Hijman W. Reference values for the Mini Mental State Examination in octo- and nonagenarians. *J Am Geriatr Soc.* 1990;38:1093–1096.

25. Tinetti M. Performance oriented assessment of mobility: problems in elderly patients. *J Am Geriatr Soc.* 1986;34:119–126.

26. Mathias S, Nayak U, Issacs B. Balance in elderly patients: the Get Up and Go Test. *Arch Phys Med Rehab.* 1986;67:387–389.

27. Lawton M, Brody E. Assessment of older people: self-maintaining and instrumental activities of daily living. *Gerontologist.* 1969;9:179–186.

28. Folstein M, Folstein S, McHugh P. Mini-Mental State: a practical method for grading the cognitive state of patients for the clinician. *J Psychiatr Res.* 1975;12:189–198.

29. Pederson N, Reynolds C, Gatz M. Sources of covariation among Mini Mental State Exam scores, education, and cognitive abilities. *J Gerontol.* 1996;51B:55–63.

30. Pfeiffer E. A Short Portable Mental Status Questionnaire for the assessment of organic brain deficit in elderly patients. *J Am Geriatr Soc.* 1975;23:433–441.

31. Smyer S, Hofland B, Jonas E. Validity study of the Short Portable Mental Status Questionnaire for the elderly. *J Am Geriatr Soc.* 1979;27:263–269.

32. Shulman K, Shedletsky R, Silver I. The challenge of time: clock drawing and cognitive function in the elderly. *Int J Geriatr Psychol.* 1986:135–140.

33. Mendez M, Ala T, Underwood K. Development of scoring criteria for the clock drawing task in Alzheimer's disease. *J Am Geriatr Soc.* 1992;40:1095–1099.

34. Tuokko H, Hadjistavropoulous T, Miller J, Beattie B. The Clocktest: a sensitive measure to differentiate normal elderly from those with Alzheimer's disease. *J Am Ger Soc.* 1992;40:922–935.

35. Administration on Aging. "Aging into the 21st Century." http://www.aoa.dhhs (September 1995). Accessed April 11, 1999.

36. National Safety Council and American Association of Retired Persons. *Falling—The Unexpected Trip.* Chicago; 1982.

37. Campbell A, Converse P. *Quality of Life in America.* New York: Russell Sage; 1976.

38. Kozma A, Stones M. Research issues and findings in the study of psychological well-being of the aged. *Can Psychol Rev.* 1978;19:241–249.

39. Larson R. Thirty years of research on the subjective well-being of older Americans. *J Gerontol.* 1978;3:109–125.

40. Spreitzer E, Snyder E. Correlates of life satisfaction among the aged. *J Gerontol.* 1974;29:454–458.

41. Kane R, Degenholtz H. Assessing values and preferences: should we, can we? *Generations.* 1997;21:19–24.

42. Hogstel M. *Geropsychiatric Nursing.* St. Louis, MO: Mosby Publishers; 1995.

43. Alcook D, Edwards N, Morris H. Home care case management. *J Case Manag.* 1998;7:167–173.

CHAPTER 12

Dementia and the Older Adult: The Role of the Geriatric Care Manager

Karen Knutson

Geriatric care managers (GCMs) devote significant time and energy to caring for clients experiencing dementia. Often GCMs are the first to identify unreported functional deficits and may provide services over many years, bringing continuity to clients and families by working across all care settings. As the population continues to age, GCMs will take on a more significant role. The challenge is to better understand the process of dementia; how clients, family members and caregivers experience this passage; and how families make decisions so GCMs can best help them. This chapter will provide an overview of the definition and diagnosis of dementia, explore the client and family caregiver's experience, and describe the GCM role in dementia care and work with other professionals. Finally, a model of care is described for training family members and paid caregivers who provide care to individuals with dementia. The model offers new insights into the ever-changing culture of dementia care. This chapter is organized in a way that best helps the new GCM understand dementia and the older adult. Causes of dementia and experiences by client and family caregivers are described first, enhancing the new GCM's understanding of what is important in comprehensive assessment, described later in the chapter.

INTRODUCTION

As the prevalence of older adults with dementia continues to increase, a majority remain undiagnosed until later stages of the disease, when the client's self-report is more difficult to obtain. Delays in detection result in untreated reversible types of dementia, further functional decline, increased difficulty managing complex health problems, and increased safety risks. Undetected dementia also results in lack of support for family members and caregivers when they are experiencing crises, are overwhelmed, and not prepared to take action. Up to 50% of primary family caregivers develop significant psychological distress.[1] Unmet needs have a profound effect on the client, family member, and caregiver.

Most dementia begins later in life, and it often occurs with chronic illnesses. At age 60 the incidence of dementia is about 1%, more than doubling every 5 years after the age of 60, up to 50% or more by age 85.[1,2] Common characteristics of dementia include the long period of functional dependency and the need for care in the last years of life.[3] More than one in five caregivers (22.4%) in the United States care for someone with dementia. This translates into an estimated 5,020,000 caregiving households nationwide that provide dementia care.[4] Alzheimer's disease alone accounts for about 70% of the many conditions that cause dementia, and the prevalence is projected to reach 14 million in the United States by the year 2050. Seventy percent of the 4 million Americans currently diagnosed with Alzheimer's disease are cared for at home. The annual cost of care is estimated at $100 billion, with families bearing the largest portion of that cost.[1] Although the majority of caregiving is provided by family members, the use of paid care is on the rise, and paid care will be increasingly needed in the future at a time when there will be fewer care workers available.

Perceptions of the person with dementia are undergoing significant change. Twenty years ago, losing the ability to remember, then called senility, was considered a normal part of aging. Care was provided by either family or institutional caregivers. Currently, it is recognized that decline in memory and other cognitive functions severe enough to interfere with activities of daily living (ADLs) is not normal aging. Experts have identified many types of dementia, some reversible, and noted that symptoms affect clients differently. Awareness of the need for screening, assessing, referring, determining the level of care needs, and selecting appropriate options has been heightened by the increase in dementia-specific strategies, home- and community-based services, and new research and treatment options. It is hoped that the future will involve greater acceptance of the client-/family-centered approach currently advocated by GCMs and which focuses on the whole person, integrating biopsychosocial aspects of care, and enhances quality of life for clients, family members, and caregivers.

DEFINING AND DIAGNOSING DEMENTIA

What Is Dementia?

Dementia is defined in many different ways. A clinical definition that is useful for GCMs describes dementia as the new onset of cognitive and comportmental alterations. Dementia features vary depending on the cause. The onset of dementia is usually insidious, which means that people cannot tell when it starts. *Cognitive deficits* are losses of memory, language, executive function, and visuospatial ability. *Comportmental changes* are alterations in personality, judgment, and insight. *Comportmental functions* help a person behave appropriately in social settings; make reasonable decisions; and plan, organize, and follow a logical sequence of steps to reach goals.[5] Most forms of dementia progressively worsen over time. These changes eventually impair ADLs skills: toileting, feeding, dressing, grooming, ambulation, and bathing. The changes also impair instrumental activities of daily living (IADLs): telephone use, shopping, food preparation, housekeeping, laundering, use of transportation, ability to take medications, and ability to manage finances. In addition to the decline in brain function, there may be changes in the social psychological environment and in patterns of relationship and interaction.[6]

Criteria for Dementia

In 1984, a work group sponsored by the National Institute on Aging, the Institute for Neurologic Diseases and Stroke, and the Alzheimer's Disease and Related Disorders Association developed criteria for the dementia syndrome (Exhibit 12–1). According to the work group, the syndrome consists of a decline in cognitive functions and is confirmed by clinical examination and neuropsychological tests. Consciousness is intact in dementia. The syndrome is based on behavior whereas specific causes of dementia are identified by diagnostic tests.[7] Dementia in itself is not a diagnosis.

The work group also developed criteria for diagnosing "probable Alzheimer's disease" for research protocols and clinical purposes. The onset of Alzheimer's disease is between 40 and 90 years of age and most often after age 65. Diag-

---

Exhibit 12–1 Criteria for Determining Dementia Syndrome

- decline in cognitive functions in comparison with client's previous level of function
- decline severe enough to interfere with social and occupational functioning
- decline confirmed by clinical examination and neuropsychological tests
- no disturbance of consciousness
- diagnosis based on behavior

nosis is determined by clinical examination and documented by the Mini Mental State Examination, the Blessed Dementia Scale, or a similar examination and confirmed by neuropsychological tests. Dementia is more likely present if there are deficits in two or more areas of cognition, including progressive worsening of memory and at least one other cognitive dysfunction. Alzheimer's disease cannot be diagnosed when there is a disturbance of consciousness (e.g., lethargy, drowsiness). The client must be alert for a diagnosis to be made (i.e., not affected by anesthesia, drug interactions, dehydration, and other problems). Ruling out any other possible diseases or disorders causing brain dysfunction is necessary.[7] If the client meets all of these criteria, the diagnosis of probable Alzheimer's disease can be made. If the criteria are applied clinically, the probability of an accurate diagnosis of Alzheimer's disease may increase to 90%.

There is a need to refine the criteria because there are other forms of dementia besides Alzheimer's disease. Nevertheless, the criteria provide a meaningful framework for the GCM when assessing clients (Exhibit 12–2). Assessing and documenting these criteria help a GCM screen for risk factors and undetected deficits, develop a plan of care, and refer clients to appropriate health care professionals for further evaluation. Referring for a dementia workup and neuropsychological tests to rule out other diseases or disorders impacting cognitive functions will be discussed later in the chapter.

Exhibit 12–2   Criteria Documented by GCM

- Mini Mental State Examination, Blessed Dementia Scale, or similar screening
- deficits in two or more areas of cognition
- progressive worsening of cognitive functions
- no disturbance of consciousness
- onset between 40 and 90, most often after age 65

Types of Dementia

In the field of dementia research, there is considerable debate around the issue of organic versus mental health disorder and wide variation in research findings on different types of dementia, related symptoms, and diagnostic progression. The *International Statistical Classification of Diseases and Related Health Problems* (ICD–10) lists dementia under organic disorders classified into 9 categories with 40 subcategories ranging from multi-infarct dementia to the more rare Creutzfeldt-Jakob disease (CJD).[8] The fourth edition of the *Diagnostic and Statistical Manual of Mental Disorders* (DSM–IV) divides dementia into 12 categories.[9] Both the ICD–10 and DSM–IV classifications agree in tracking the diagnostic progression through mild, moderate, and severe stages.[10] Readers who wish to extend their knowledge on the specific types of dementia are advised to consult the ICD–10 and DSM–IV manuals. This chapter will focus solely on the early symptoms of dementia for the purpose of earlier recognition, intervention, and treatment. Symptoms will vary depending on the part of the brain that has been involved. According to Kitwood, it is not always possible to clearly distinguish between neurological and psychological changes.[6] As the experts grapple to find common ground, practicing GCMs can develop their client/family approach to dementia care by viewing the biological, psychological, and social changes as equally important.

The most common types of degenerative diseases that cause dementia are Alzheimer's disease (including the Lewy-body variant), vascular dementia, dementia of the frontal lobe type, Pick's disease, dementia with Parkinsonism, and hydrocephalus.[11] Less common dementias include tertiary syphilis, Huntington's disease, nutritional deficiencies, and Wilson's disease. Acquired immune deficiency syndrome (AIDS) dementia and alcohol dementia are increasingly recognized. CJD, a rare viral disease causing dementia, has had increased public attention as a new variant of CJD emerged, transmitted by mad cow disease in British cattle, in 1996.[12]

The cognitive and behavioral symptoms of the most common dementias are highlighted in Exhibit 12–3 and are further described in the case studies.

Laboratory and Diagnostic Tests

After developing criteria for dementia in the 1980s, the American Academy of Neurology developed recommendations for laboratory evaluation.[13] Currently there are no specific diagnostic laboratory tests for Alzheimer's disease, but some tests can help identify other causes of the dementia syndrome. A blood-chemistry panel, complete blood count (CBC), tests of thyroid function, measurement of vitamin B12 levels, and screening for inflammatory and infectious disease are recommended. Computed tomography (CT) or magnetic resonance imaging (MRI) of the brain can rule out structural lesions (e.g., infarction, neoplasm, extracerebral fluid collection and hydrocephalus) that may contribute to dementia.[13] If indicated, lumbar puncture to rule out central nervous system infection or heavy metal screening may be performed. The blood tests and neuroimaging studies in Table 12–1 are important in the differential diagnosis to rule out metabolic and structural causes.

Causes of Dementia

The many causes of dementia are usefully divided into two categories: reversible and irreversible.

Reversible Causes

Reversible causes are generally not associated with permanent brain changes. The brain is normal but temporarily prevented from working properly. Usual factors include acute or subacute toxic agents such as alcohol or medications, cardiovascular or pulmonary diseases reducing the amount of oxygen to the brain, metabolic disorders such as hyper- or hypothyroidism, vitamin deficiencies, and sensory deprivation. These factors change the external environment in which the brain functions.[5]

Irreversible Causes

In irreversible dementia some brain tissue is affected and can no longer function normally. Depending on the intrinsic brain disease, there are many causes. The most common is degeneration or progressive death of nerve cells. Many mechanisms can cause brain cells to die. Alzheimer's disease accounts for about 70% of all cases of dementia. The typical course in Alzheimer's disease is one of progressive decline.[11] Strokes can also cause degeneration. Strokes close off blood vessels that support the brain, and tissues are impaired or without nutrients and oxygen. Trauma to the skull causing bruising of the brain can also cause dementia. Tumors can elicit symptoms of dementia. Sometimes seizures in the brain develop.[5]

Differentiating Dementia and Acute Confusion

The terms *acute confusion* and *dementia* are often used interchangeably. The former is more common in the nursing literature and the latter in the medical literature. Acute confusion is a disturbance in information processing and attention characterized by disordered cognition as well as disturbances in perception, thinking and memory, attention, and wakefulness.[14] Like dementia, acute confusion is characterized by global cognitive impairment. However, it is distinguished by acute onset, marked fluctuations in cognitive impairment over the course of a day, disruptions in consciousness and attention, and alterations in the sleep cycle. Hallucinations and delusions are common. Infection or drug toxicity typically cause acute confusion.

Dementia is a risk factor for acute confusion. Acute confusion and dementia often coexist, particularly in hospital settings, and are underdiagnosed and undertreated. Because acute confusion may vary in severity, it is important to identify mild confusion early enough to provide interventions that can prevent the development of more severe confusion. A referral for a dementia evaluation is essential when the acute confusion clears but the cognitive impairment persists.[14]

Exhibit 12–3 Early Symptoms of Dementia

Neurological/cognitive	Behavioral/psychosocial
Alzheimer's disease	
• slow, widespread, progressive symptoms	• slow, widespread, progressive symptoms
1. short-term memory impairment	1. personality changes (passivity to hostility)
2. inability to focus attention and recall events	2. decreased emotional expression
3. progressive disorientation (time and place)	3. diminished initiative
4. difficulty in word finding and impaired naming	4. depression and anxiety
5. impaired language comprehension and calculation	5. greater suspiciousness
6. visual and spatial deficits	6. visual hallucinations
	7. delusions (accusations of theft, infidelity, persecution)
	8. wandering
Vascular dementia	
• acute unilateral motor or sensory dysfunction	• sudden affective changes
• urinary dysfunction	• depression
• gait disturbance	• delusions
• masklike facial expression and rigidity	• psychotic symptoms
• aphasia	
Dementia of the frontal lobe type and Pick's disease	
• apathy	• prominent alterations in emotion, affect, and behavior
• language impairments (unfocused speech, spontaneous/compulsive repetition of words and phrases)	• disordered executive function (initiation, goal setting, planning)
• normal short-term memory	• little awareness of changes (denies any problems)
• normal or minimally affected cognitive testing	• disinhibited behavior
• normal visual and special abilities	• personality changes
	• withdrawal
Dementia with Parkinsonism	
• rigidity and postural instability	• disordered executive function
• general slowing of thought and action	• delusions
	• hallucinations
Hydrocephalus	
• gait disorder	• irritability
• urinary incontinence	• change in behavior
• cognitive decline (psychomotor slowing, impaired ability to concentrate, and mild memory difficulties)	

DEMENTIA EXPERIENCED

The Client's Experience

Often overlooked in the dementia process is the client's experience. When client losses take place as the result of dementia, grief reactions commonly occur. The denial, anger, fear, depression, acceptance, and reconstruction sequence found in other grief reactions is often experienced in dementia. Thus, grieving often goes unrecognized. The cognitive deficits of dementia can complicate the grief process. Client expe-

Table 12–1 Dementia Workup

Test	Rationale
Urinalysis	Rule out kidney dysfunction, toxic encephalopathy
CBC, sedimentation rate, electrolytes	Rule out anemia, electrolyte imbalance
Blood Urea Nitrogen (BUN)/creatinine, liver function tests	Rule out liver dysfunction
Thyroid function	Rule out thyroid dysfunction
Serum B12	Rule out vitamin deficiency
Syphilis serology	Rule out syphilis
HIV test	Rule out AIDS dementia
Neuroimaging studies: CT or MRI	Rule out tumor, subdural hematomas, abcess, stroke, or hydrocephalus

riences vary. At one extreme are clients who because of organic changes display very little insight. Others have an awareness of what is happening to them.[6] Accounts have been written by people with dementia when their cognitive functioning was still relatively intact. These accounts highlight issues such as the fear of being out of control, the fear of being seen by others as out of control, the feeling of being lost and of slipping away, the concern about being a burden and the desire to be useful, the anger with dementia itself, and the resentment that life has been marred by dementia. Some persons express acceptance of their disabilities and some their gratitude for the good things in their past. Many with dementia feel reassured by the company and support of other persons.[6,10]

The first interview below features a client experiencing early Alzheimer's disease and who has awareness of her memory loss. Her mother, a source of her inspiration, also experienced dementia during the last several years of her life. The ability of the client with Alzheimer's disease to discern impairment and have awareness is greatest when the disease is in its earliest stage.

Virginia P (Widowed Wife, Mother, Grandmother, and Great-Grandmother, Age 87)

I don't want to be a burden on my family. I don't want to intrude on their lives. I have to be brave. Time marches on and I have to make the best of it. I have days where I think it's not worth it but I just go on. Fortunately I have an upbeat nature. My memory is not that dependable. It makes me irritable. I don't know what I can do about that except try harder. I'd like to have my family back with me like the old days, but I can't turn back the clock. Sure, I'm lonesome a lot of the time. I enjoy people. The evenings get rather long and quiet. But a few hours with my family picks me up for several days. They are so wonderful to me and I'm so happy when they come to see me. I don't feel that one setback is the end of everything. My mother, who lived to be 101, is such an inspiration to me. I say to myself when I feel like giving up, my mother wouldn't do that. And that gives me the courage to go on.

The next interview describes a client with frontal lobe dementia. Even in the earliest stage of the disease, the client is unaware and has little insight. The client's early experience with frontal lobe dementia resulted in significant family stress, especially for her daughter. The client was living at home with her daughter, did not meet the court's definition of incapacity, had devised an escape plan, and was threatening to leave. The neuropsychologist who evaluated the client wrote her a letter indicating she had a mild dementia of the frontal lobe type, that the problem would not be obvious to her, and that her daughter should be helping more than the client believed.

Eva M and Susan (Mother and Daughter, Ages 78 and 59)

> My doctor says I have frontal lobe dementia but I don't think there is anything wrong with me. The only thing I've noticed is it's hard for me to concentrate when I read. My daughter has been influenced by my doctor. I don't want my daughter's help because she is trying to prove there is something wrong with me and I know there isn't. I refuse to see my doctor again. I will prove that they are wrong about this.

Eva M had good short-term memory but impaired executive skills, the hallmark and earliest finding of frontal lobe dementia. Executive skills consist of more complex higher-order functions directed by the frontal lobes of the brain and include organizing skills, planning, abstraction, social judgment, problem solving, insight, initiation or inhibition of behavior, reasoning, and sequencing.[15]

The Family Member's and Caregiver's Experience

Family members report satisfaction from caring for older adults with dementia, including the satisfaction of helping a loved one, doing something worthy, making a difference, and sharing precious time together. Families also experience substantial burden. This burden manifests itself in declines in the caregiver's own physical and mental health and lost wages. Moreover, family caregivers report three times as many stress symptoms as the general population, take more prescription drugs to treat depression and stress, and participate in fewer social and recreational activities.[16]

While much has been written about family caregivers of older adults with dementia, less has been written about the family caregiver's experience between the onset of symptoms and the pursuit of a formal evaluation and diagnosis. Current literature indicates that family caregivers wait an average of 2 to 3 years from the onset of symptoms before seeking an evaluation. Difficulties in defining and diagnosing dementia and lack of caregiver support are significant factors that lead to a delay in early intervention and care. An understanding of the family caregiver's experience can help GCMs to better assist clients and families in this difficult and complex transition.

Family members describe starting their journey as caregivers before recognizing the early symptoms of dementia. They describe the difficulty in distinguishing dementia from normal aging due to the gradual onset and intermittent nature of the symptoms. Signs and symptoms affect the older relative with dementia differently. Not all signs and symptoms are experienced with equal intensity. Some older relatives have different responses with different symptoms and responses, causing more distress than others. For example, some clients become emotionally agitated in addition to experiencing cognitive impairment. This behavior is very difficult for family members to deal with unless they have had some training. Time and experience are necessary to understand and comprehend symptoms. Some family members ascribe symptoms to their relative's personality, while others attribute them to depression. Family caregivers of those with short-term memory loss describe seeing their older relatives compensate for this loss by talking about the past, evading questions, or making up what they do not remember. Some caregivers minimize the impairment of short-term memory loss, unable to differentiate short- and long-term memory. The compensating behavior by the older adult with dementia adds to the family caregiver's difficulty in defining the disease. Memory-impaired older adults often maintain that their memory loss is normal for their age. Others who are aware do not want anyone to know and ask the family to keep the impairment hidden. Family members mention the difficulty in talking about the impairment and their reluctance to counter their relatives' wishes. Thus, the relative's experience affects the family member's experience, and the family caregiver's response is often to protect the relative with dementia.[17]

While there are differences in family caregiver attitudes and awareness, there are common significant themes. Family caregivers are afraid to know their relative has dementia. At the same time they are very anxious to learn all they can about the specific type of dementia. Family caregivers express a desire for more knowledge and emotional preparation. Different significant events lead family members to contact GCMs. Most family members describe waiting until they have reached a point of significant distress and are feeling overwhelmed.[17]

Laura R and Jane (Mother and Daughter, Ages 79 and 56)

During the first year or so, my mother just had a little bit of confusion now and then. It would disappear and she would be real clear for a while. This is what confused us. Looking back on old times, it is amazing to me what she could remember from years ago. That made me feel she was OK. We had a Fourth of July family reunion and spent the whole time talking about the good old days. My mother had a wonderful time. She could talk about the past better than I could. Then later, I thought my mother was depressed and just wasn't paying attention. She wasn't interacting with us very much anymore. I didn't know that depression and Alzheimer's Disease can have some of the same symptoms. She started following my father around the house. She would get very agitated and frightened when she was left alone. She said she was scared she wouldn't be here when we got back.

She just became more and more scared. I also thought it was her personality. This was just my mother. I thought she was getting older and just wanted my attention. It's hard to know what's personality and what's something else. She didn't want anyone to know. She would say to me, "If anybody asks, please don't tell them. I don't want to see them when I can't remember." She was so ashamed. That will always stick with me. She was so ashamed because she had this memory loss and didn't want anyone outside of the family to know. I felt protective of her. I went along with her trying to deny it to everybody else. I did what I thought was right, out of love, and did shelter her. But of course, you get to the time when you can't shelter anymore. I needed to talk to someone. Someone who would listen, and let me express my feelings and sort out some answers. I was feeling totally isolated and helpless. I just didn't know what to do.[17]

Caregivers often report a lack of support and understanding available to them during the diagnostic testing and treatment of their relative's dementia. Some family caregivers report that their relative's primary care physician assumed that the described symptoms were a normal part of aging and did not pursue an evaluation. This led to a further delay in intervention and care. Other family caregivers have difficulty believing the diagnosis. They often feel excluded from the confidential patient/physician relationship. Some family caregivers find their own families to be supportive. Others, however, experience a significant lack of support. They report that family and friends have a difficult time understanding dementia. Some family caregivers do not have other family members to turn to for support. Family caregivers describe contending with the negative changes in others' relationships with their dementia-impaired relative, as well as their own changing relationship with the relative. Family caregivers often delay getting help from formal services. Some family caregivers report difficulty getting help because of feeling overwhelmed, needing to deal with things one day at a time, and not knowing where to start. Others delay getting help because of the lack of time to learn about services and the difficulty in anticipating future losses.[17]

Bill and Sarah H (Husband and Wife, Ages 85 and 83)

I took her to her doctor. When the doctor came in, he asked her, "How are you doing?" She said, "I am just doing fine." We were all in denial for a long time. Finally he did some blood work and all of the follow-ups with the brain scan. Our doctor told us, "Alzheimer's disease is not black or white. You rule out what it isn't." I'm confident he knows what the disease is not, but not what it is. What confuses me is the diagnosis. It is important to make sure the diagnosis is right. Yet I understand that you can't really know, except by autopsy. I tried getting some support from my church. They have a friendly visitor who comes by. But the visitor told me there was no give and take in the conversation, so she wasn't coming back. I see that with our family too. Because they don't get back, they don't put energy into it. I worry about my own health. It's hard to worry about her and deal with the family at the same time. If something happens to me, I don't know what we'll do.[17]

One of the greatest difficulties for family caregivers is dealing with the dementia-impaired relative's resistance to help. This resistance is due at least in part to the increasing intolerance of change of all types. Resistance is often associated with a range of behavioral disturbances that the family caregiver does not understand. Family caregivers report that their relative's resistance makes it more difficult for them to get help or know how or when to take action.

Lorena H and Betty (Mother and Daughter, Ages 84 and 62)

My mother was diagnosed with clinical depression and later developed dementia. First she lost her husband and then her dog. She just stopped living. She has this compensating pattern so I can't rely on what she says. She says she is doing fine when she really is not. I have to actually see what is going on to know what is happening to her. When I try to help her she resists me. It is like dealing with a two-year-old having temper tantrums. One day we went out for lunch and had a lovely time. When we got back to her house I came in and told her I was going to help her. She wanted me to go home. She said she didn't need my help. She didn't want any interference as to how to live her life. I told her she wasn't doing things like bathing and brushing her teeth regularly, or paying her bills on time. I just wanted to help her out. She started screaming that I was going to take her out of her home, sell her home, and take all of her money. She then called my sister and told her I was stealing things from her. I felt like I was having a nervous breakdown.

Family caregivers experience many barriers to caregiving. An overwhelming barrier to early dementia care for family caregivers is the lack of education and training about the illness. Family caregivers describe the process of dementia as initially responding to the natural course of events in aging and later lacking belief in the diagnostic process. Watching the deterioration of their dementia-impaired relative, experiencing a lack of support from others, and contending with the deterioration of others' relationships with the dementia-impaired relative (as well as their own changing relationships with the relative) create demands that often outweigh the family caregiver's resources. This results in unbearable stress and delayed action.[17] Training programs provided by GCMs can address these gaps in caregiver knowledge and barriers to caregiving. Training family and paid caregivers about dementia care will be discussed later in the chapter.

THE GCM ROLE IN DEMENTIA CARE

As experts in dementia and family care, GCMs are paving the way for new approaches to care. Understanding the nature of the client and family experiences and how they want care delivered is critical to the GCM process. Figure 12–1 highlights the comprehensive GCM process and will be referred to as GCM activities are described below.

Interviewing Family Members and Caregivers

Cognitive deficits often prevent the dementia-impaired older adult from seeking help early or accessing needed services. Typically, family members make the initial contact with the GCM. They are often looking for help with decision making and care planning (e.g., how to keep parents together and as independent as possible while conserving their resources). GCMs provide significant support and information during this stressful time, assisting family members with a variety of strategies, including how to cope, how to be an informed consumer, how to choose health care providers who are knowledgeable, how to bring their undiagnosed/untreated relatives into the health care system, and how to determine what services and care can best meet their relative's needs.[17]

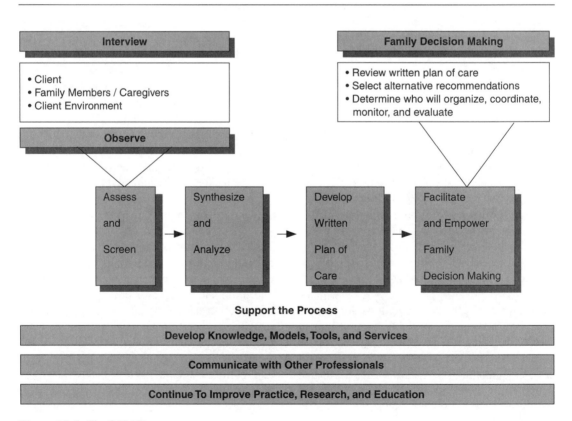

Figure 12–1 The GCM Process.

The GCM often talks on the phone or meets family members and caregivers in a separate location prior to being introduced to the client. Family members may want help with how to approach their dementia-impaired relative or how to influence their relative to get much-needed help. It can be difficult for family members and caregivers when clients do not recognize or deny loss of function or become suspicious, fearful, and angry. Poor short-term memory and the loss of ability to self-report what is currently happening are common with dementia. Interviewing family members ahead of time can help the GCM determine the best way to manage the client assessment. Communicating privately with family members also allows them to talk about what they are experiencing. The GCM can focus on the perspectives and needs of family members as well as acknowledge and reinforce their involvement. Family members often ask the GCM to contact other interested and concerned family members not present at the assessment. With the client's and/or authorized representative's permission, the GCM later contacts the various family members and assesses common objectives, trust, commitment to work together, and ability to communicate, all conditions necessary for collaborative family decision making.

The GCM assesses caregiver burden and stress to improve the quality of client/family relationships and to reduce caregiver burden and stress. The GCM screens for special problems faced by family members, such as not coping with the diagnosis, feeling loss and grief, dealing with anxiety and guilt, not setting limits, and feeling caregiver burnout. The GCM considers each family member's perspective as important in helping identify family issues and problems in communication. The caregiving needs of the client with dementia typically become the primary responsibility of one person. This can feel unfair to the person who has the primary responsibility or make others afraid of assuming any responsibility. The GCM evaluates how much assistance individual family members want to provide as well as realistically what they can provide. The level of family caregiver support helps the GCM to identify what additional needs for care exist.

Interviewing the Client

The client interview often begins with the family member and caregiver introducing the GCM to the client. During the interview the GCM focuses primarily on the client, as future recommendations will be based on the client's needs as much as possible. The client's degree of participation will depend on the progression of dementia, the GCM's approach, and the level of anxiety experienced by the client and family. At some point in the interview, the GCM speaks to the client privately and conducts the cognitive function and depression screens as well as ask the client to share any confidential information.

Communication Techniques

The GCM spends a significant amount of time at the beginning of the interview helping the client and family feel at ease. The GCM eliminates distractions in the client's environment that would interfere with the interview (TV, music, others talking) and attempts to maximize the client's ability to communicate (making sure the client is using glasses and hearing aids as appropriate, facing the client, sitting close enough to be heard). The GCM builds rapport with the client by establishing an atmosphere of trust and cooperation. The GCM is more likely to develop trust with the dementia client by looking at the world from the client's perspective. Establishing rapport with the client requires pacing or meeting the client on his or her level. The GCM observes the client's breathing, blinking, and vocal tone and tempo. Quantity of speech, spontaneity, hesitation, and perseveration in word use are observed. Attitude and reaction to the overall interview are observed. Is the client relaxed, tense, restless, or fatigued? Can he or she stay attentive? Does the client have insight into or attempt to cover up the disability? The GCM attends to all of the client's verbal and nonverbal messages. Understanding that the client responds more to what he or she sees than to what is said, the GCM makes eye contact and reassures the client with nonverbal gestures (e.g., a smile, a touch on the shoulder) in a nonthreatening, nonjudgmental manner. While open-ended questions are the hallmark of a good interview, the GCM recognizes that simpler, shorter, less complex questions decrease the demand on client memory and attention. When using functional assessment instruments, the GCM gives positive reinforcement to the client for responding to questions regardless of the answers.

Communication Difficulties

There can be many barriers to communication about dementia. Communication difficulties may occur between the GCM, client, and family as well as within the family itself. Clients with cognitive deficits may experience difficulty in comprehending questions and providing meaningful responses, making communication more challenging. Differences between people of different generations, genders, and ethnic backgrounds are also considerations when evaluating communication difficulties. For example, dementia-impaired clients who are ethnic minorities may live with several family members who share caregiving responsibilities. Family members/caregivers often have difficulty in identifying areas of cognitive deficits and accepting these changes. This contrasts with the family member living at a distance from an older relative living at home alone. Family members living with an older relative may have a greater opportunity to observe functioning, but may also experience greater conflict and communication difficulties between family members and between older relatives and family members.

Clients with progressive dementia have differences in self-awareness and may lack awareness of changes or loss of functioning. Anosognosia, or unawareness of deficit, is associated with higher levels of caregiver distress. Clients who lack awareness may engage in activities that might cause harm to themselves and others.[18] Anosognosia may interfere with the client accepting help. Often family members, caregivers, and professionals view unawareness as denial or deception on the part of the client. Unfortunately, this often leads to a lack of evaluation and treatment. Some-

times, even when clients are evaluated they are not told their diagnosis.

These problems are compounded by ageism, the assigning of more negative than positive traits to the client because of age. Preventing the negative effects of this type of stereotyping is challenging. The GCM needs to learn about the different symptoms of dementia and examine his or her feelings and biases about dementia and how they affect his or her ability to communicate.

Assessing and Screening the Client

Assessment is the key to maximizing the client's functioning and providing optimal care for clients and their families. The seasoned GCM thinks of all data being gathered as integrated and all GCM functions as closely related. For example, as soon as the assessment process begins, the experienced GCM looks for indications of cognitive deficits. The deficits influence the GCM's assessment of client functioning and in turn, the client's ability to maintain independence. Deficits affecting functioning and thereby independence are integrated over the course of the assessment. The new GCM, however, finds it helpful to focus on each assessment activity separately. This chapter describes the discrete activities of a GCM working with a dementia client and family.

Subjective and objective data are obtained. Subjective data includes experiences of the client from the client's perspective and the family member's perspective as well as demographic and financial information. Objective data include observations made by the GCM as well as data from functional assessment instruments conducted in the client's environment. The process is client/family directed, flexible in the order of information collected, and designed to support and protect the client's self-esteem. For example, the GCM may ask the client with poor short-term memory to first review his or her life history. The client may be able to describe where he or she was originally from and where else the family has lived but not provide current and recent information. Although certain information may be best obtained from the family member, the GCM is interested in interacting with the client in ways that include him or her in conversation and provide insights into his or her preferences and needs.

Subjective Data Collection: Integrating the Client's History

The GCM approaches assessment from a holistic perspective, integrating personal information that promote the client's values, beliefs, and preferences. The GCM gathers subjective information such as the time of onset of cognitive deficits, the progression of symptoms, and any family history of dementia. Then the GCM inquires about other past and current health (e.g., hypertension) and psychosocial (e.g., depression) conditions as well as changes in that health status, the client's and family's attitude toward dementia, and coping strategies used by the client and family. The following case study is an example of how the client's untreated Alzheimer's disease started and how the symptoms progressed, according to the client's son.

Sally B and Robert (Mother and Son, Ages 83 and 52)

The GCM spoke at length about Sally B's history of memory impairment with her son. The son described his mother's difficulty with memory as very gradual and intermittent over the past 5 years and accelerating over the past 2 years. It started with occasional inability to recall names. She also confused generations in the family. For example, at times she confused Robert, her son, with her grandson not only in name but in person. She also would not remember what she had done the day before. Robert said he would ask his mother how the visit with the grandson was yesterday and she could not remember a visit. About 3 years ago, Robert became concerned about leaving his mother alone. She

would leave the stove on. About 2 years ago, she began confusing her current home with her home of 60 years ago. He had not been able to talk about financial issues with her for the past couple of years.

Robert described an alarming event that really shocked him 2 years ago, although he did not express his dismay to his mother. They had been at the beach for a weekend visit, and it was getting to be evening. His mother was in the living room and he went in to tell her they were about to drive home. His mother was sitting on the sofa, and she had removed most of her clothes. She told him she was ready to go to bed. She calmly accepted his statement that they were driving back home. Once she was dressed and on the road she seemed to adapt to the new reality. She also confused mornings and evenings. For example, she remarked as the sun was setting that she "liked this time of the morning the best." Robert said that for the last year his mother had been living in the more distant past. She still had good long-term memory but asked few questions about the recent past. For example, she did not talk about her deceased husband who died 10 years ago, but she did talk about her early childhood and about her own mother. Robert stated that his mother was now making accusations and being suspicious of others. When the GCM asked him to explain this further, he said that his mother would converse pleasantly with him, then suddenly ask "Why are you taking all my money?" She accused paid caregivers of also stealing her money. Yet his mother retained many good social skills. "She's very friendly to people even when she doesn't have a clue as to who they are."

The client's education, work history, and past and current interests and hobbies are obtained. The client's history of medications, laboratory and diagnostic tests, and other treatments is documented. Medications are reviewed, including nonprescription medications, vitamins, and supplements, for frequency of use, dosage, and prescribing health care provider. Medications not being used but still in the home are also re-viewed. Lifestyle issues including sleeping hab-its and exercise are discussed. For example, if the client is sleeping during the day, difficulty sleeping at night may occur, affecting the client's and caregiver's needs. The names of past and current health care providers and avail-able medical records outlining past diagnoses and treatments are gathered. The GCM concen-trates on potential gaps in care such as the client's failure to make routine physician visits, lack of communication among multiple health providers, inability to take medication appropri-ately, and other difficulties in self-management of chronic health problems. Relevant health in-surance information, long-term care insurance information, and financial information are ob-tained. Information on income, expenses, and assets is also obtained. The GCM helps the client and family understand the costs of care, plan re-alistically, and identify funding sources. For ex-ample, family members frequently ask to pay for the GCM assessment and written report to deter-mine the plan of care, instead of clients them-selves paying.

Objective Data Collection: Integrating Observation and Functional Assessment Instruments

Objective data are collected through direct observation and utilization of functional assess-ment instruments. Direct observation of the cli-ent experiencing dementia is important for a number of reasons. Clients may not be able to assess their own functioning. Additionally, fam-ily members may not see the client often enough or know how to interpret their relative's func-tioning. Studies rating assessment of physical function have used nurses' ratings as the gold standard.[19,20] Nurses were more accurate than older adults, who rated their own function higher than the nurses, and family members, who rated it lower. Studies comparing older adults with in-tact cognition, family members, and physicians found that older adults were reasonably accurate in their self-assessments, family members were intermediate in accuracy, and physicians were the least accurate.[19,21]

Functional Assessment Instruments

Functional assessment instruments are impor-tant. They provide additional objective informa-tion in the overall assessment process. The GCM uses functional assessment instruments in a so-cial and nonthreatening way in the client's own environment. These instruments help the GCM determine the client's baseline function, screen for undetected problems and risk factors, and monitor improvement or decline in functioning. Because clients' abilities change in different ways over time, the functional assessment in-struments provide the GCM with more objective and practical information regarding individual deficits and strengths as well as insights into im-proving deficits and preventing further decline. Most often, a combination of such instruments is needed. Appendix 12–A at the end of the chapter evaluates some of the more commonly used functional assessment instruments and their use-fulness when assessing dementia. Being familiar with the strengths and weaknesses of the various functional assessment instruments will help the GCM select the most appropriate instruments for the individual client.

Comprehensive Functional Assessment

Chapter 12 describes comprehensive func-tional assessment primarily as it relates to de-mentia, as general GCM assessment is discussed in Chapter 11. Additional, more in-depth perfor-mance-based screening methods of key target areas are described in this chapter to help the GCM better differentiate the client's functional difficulties. For example, the difficulties com-monly associated with dementia, such as using the telephone and driving, are also commonly associated with vision and hearing impairments. The GCM conducts additional screening of vi-sion and hearing as well as mental status to dif-ferentiate the impact of each on the client's over-all functioning. Because the client with cognitive impairment and vision or hearing loss may not be able to report or discriminate be-tween these impairments, it is critical that the GCM screen for vision and hearing loss and to what extent the impairments affect cognitive functioning.

The functional assessment includes physical, cognitive, emotional, and social functioning as well as the physical and social environment.[22] The objective part of the assessment process is complete when the client and client environment have been assessed and the GCM can formulate a written report with care options. The target areas of functional assessment include vision, hearing, arm and leg function, bladder and bowel function, nutrition, mental status, emotional health, ADLs/IADLs, home environment, and social support.[23] These target areas have been identified from ADL and IADL instruments in the literature and allow for performance-based assessment in addition to self-report. Brief questions and easily observed tasks are used. The target areas are more realistic for the practicing GCM than previously published instruments that are lengthy, not performance based, too complex to score and administer in the home environment, and focused on a general rather than geriatric population. Appendix 12–B describes how impairments of the key target areas impact the dementia client's abilities.

Vision

The client and family are questioned about vision loss. The standard Jaeger card (Figure 12–2) is a brief test of functional vision. The client, wearing corrective glasses, if appropriate, is asked to

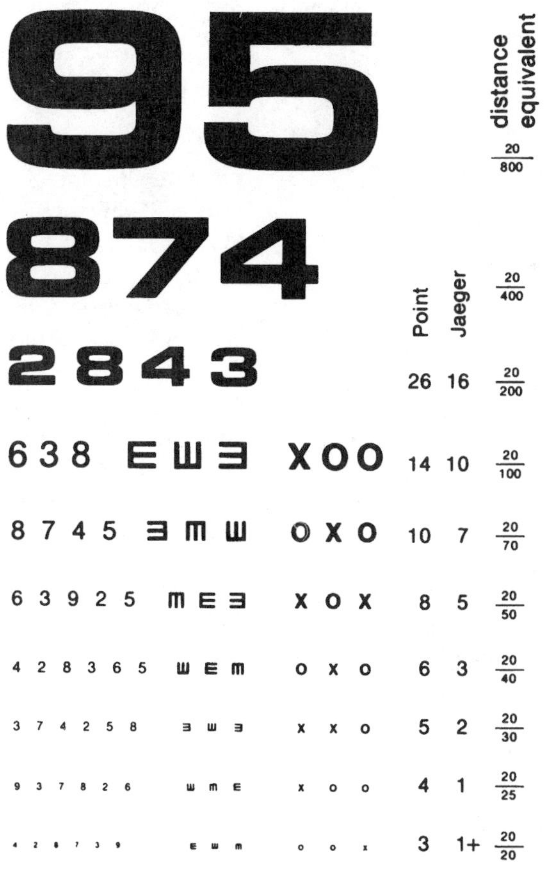

Figure 12–2 Jaeger Card.

read the card with one eye covered. The GCM holds the card 14 inches away from the client in good light. The procedure is repeated with the other eye. If the client cannot read the card at a level of 20/40 or better, a referral to an ophthalmologist is recommended.[23] Clients with cognitive impairment and vision loss may display improved cognitive ability with improved vision. Additional interventions specific to vision loss and risk of further decline are considered.

Hearing

The client and family are questioned about signs of hearing loss. During the interview, the GCM will find evidence of hearing loss by speaking in a normal voice and then observing how the client responds to questions. The whisper test is a simple test of hearing functioning and speech discrimination. The GCM stands about 18 inches from one of the client's ears and asks the client to cover the other ear. While making sure the client cannot see the GCM's mouth, the GCM whispers a few words. The client with normal hearing should be able to understand the whispered words in that ear. Clients found to have evidence of hearing loss should be referred to an audiologist or ear, nose, and throat (ENT) specialist. The GCM needs to consider what kind of support the client will need if hearing aids are recommended (e.g., helping with turning the device on and off, adjusting the hearing aid, and changing batteries). Clients with cognitive impairment and hearing loss may display improved cognitive ability with improved hearing.

Upper Extremity Function

Arm mobility is evaluated. The client is assessed for decreased muscle strength, limited range of motion, weakness, and pain. The GCM asks the client to touch the back of his or her head with both hands; with this exercise, the GCM can check for limitations of range of motion. The client is then asked to pick up a spoon. Inability to do the tasks should lead to a referral to the primary care provider and/or neurologist for a neurological and musculoskeletal evaluation.[23] Additional interventions to improve func-

tioning and decrease risk of further decline are considered.

Lower Extremity Function

Leg mobility is evaluated. The client is assessed for decreased muscle strength, balance problems, gait problems, limited range of motion, and pain. A functional mobility assessment that has been shown to be highly predictive of falls is to ask the client to rise from a straight chair, walk about 10 feet, turn around, and sit back down.[14] The GCM observes how the client walks. In observing this simple task, the GCM looks for possible factors that are causing risk. Clients with risk factors are then targeted for additional interventions. The GCM also tries to determine how individuals get from one place to another, inside and outside their living environment. Inability to do the functional mobility assessment should lead to a referral to the primary care provider and/or neurologist for a neurological and musculoskeletal evaluation.[23]

Bladder Function

The GCM asks the client, Do you ever lose urine and get wet? Are you aware of when your bladder is full?[23] If the client has incontinence, the frequency is noted. Is it mild, moderate, or severe? Is there a urinary tract infection? The client is then asked to direct the GCM to the bathroom. The GCM observes whether the bathroom is accessible to the client or has barriers. Clients with functional incontinence are then targeted for additional interventions, including adding bedside commodes and providing care that prompts or assists the client on a 2-hour toileting schedule. The client is assessed for acute confusion, which can occur when experiencing a urinary tract infection along with dementia. This sudden and temporary increase in confusion will occur until the urinary tract infection is resolved. A referral to the primary care provider or a urologist may be in order.

Nutrition

The GCM assesses the client's report of appetite, weight gained or lost, ability to swallow, and other items related to nutrition. The client's ability to obtain food and prepare meals is assessed. The GCM may ask the client to prepare a cup of tea or coffee or a snack. The GCM often will ask to inspect the refrigerator, especially if the client lives alone, to get a sense of the client's nutritional resources and need for nutritional support. Additional interventions to improve nutrition (e.g., in-home meals) are considered.

Mental Status

Cognitive processes assessed by the GCM include orientation, alertness, memory, attention, language, and visuospatial ability. The higher-order cognitive processes of problem solving, conceptualization, reasoning, and planning are assessed throughout the interview with the client. The Mini Mental State Examination (MMSE) (Exhibit 12–4, an adaptation of the exam in Exhibit 11–5 as given to Sally, a client introduced above) or Blessed Dementia Scale and additional cognitive function instruments such as the Clock Drawing Test are administered to the client privately in the client's environment.

MMSE administration and scoring, as originally delineated by Folstein and elaborated upon by Knutson and Gross, is described below.[24,25]

Orientation (10 Items). Orientation is assessed on the MMSE by asking the client questions about time (year, season, month, day of the month, and day of the week) and place (if the client's residence: state, county, town, home address, room; if a hospital: building, floor of the building, part of the city, city, state). The season should be correct within a day either way of the season change. One point is given for each correct response.[24,25] Sally is not fully oriented to her environment and may not always know what is going on around her; she scores 8 out of a possible 10 points.

Registration (3 Items). Registration is measured on the MMSE by asking the client to name three unrelated objects. The first attempt to say the three words is used in scoring. One point is given for each object. After completing the task, the client is asked to remember the objects and repeat them 5 minutes later.[24,25] Sally is able to

register current information, which means that she knows what happens to her as it happens; she scores a 3 out of 3. This is important in regard to her safety.

Attention and Calculation (5 Items). Attention refers to the ability to focus and concentrate on a particular task and is measured by asking the client to say digits or letters forward and backward, with backward repetition providing greater information about attention. Attention is assessed on the MMSE by asking the client to perform the Serial 7s, a test that also measures calculation ability. The GCM says, "I'd like you to count backward from 100 by 7. What is 100 take away 7?" The GCM does not give further reminders once the client has started. Then the GCM has the client spell "world" forward and then backward. For the latter count, the score is the number of letters that are in the correct order (DLOW = 4, DLDRW = 3, DLOLD = 2). The GCM uses the higher of the two scores (either the Serial 7s or the "world" backward score).[24,25] Sally is able to focus and concentrate as well as do the calculations; she scores a 5 out of 5.

Recall (3 Items). Recall is often impaired in dementia, and impaired recall is the most noticeable symptom in Alzheimer's disease. Memory is measured on the MMSE by asking the client to repeat the three objects that were said 5 minutes earlier during the Registration section of the test. The score is the number spontaneously recalled without a cue. One point is given for each correct answer.[24,25] Sally has poor short-term memory, meaning she not only has difficulty remembering recent events but also has difficulty making new memories. Her difficulties with ADLs (she needs prompting and standby assistance with personal care, including dressing and bathing) and IADLs (she has a hard time remembering appointments, managing medications, and managing bills and her estate) are due to her inability to recall experiences. She needs prompting by another person. Also, because of her memory impairment she has false ideas about things (e.g., that her son and paid caregivers are stealing her money) and an altered

Exhibit 12–4 Mini Mental State Examination

THE ANNOTATED MINI MENTAL STATE EXAMINATION (AMMSE)

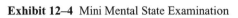MiniMental LLC

NAME OF SUBJECT _____ Age _____

NAME OF EXAMINER _____ Years of School Completed _____

Approach the patient with respect and encouragement.
Ask: Do you have any trouble with your memory? ☐ Yes ☐ No
May I ask you some questions about your memory? ☐ Yes ☐ No

Date of Examination _____

SCORE	ITEM
5 ( )	**TIME ORIENTATION**

Ask:

What is the year_____ (1), season_____ (1),

month of the year_____ (1), date_____ (1),

day of the week _____ (1) ?

5 ( )   **PLACE ORIENTATION**

Ask:

Where are we now? What is the state_____ (1), city_____ (1),

part of the city_____ (1), building_____ (1),

floor of the building_____ (1)?

3 ( )   **REGISTRATION OF THREE WORDS**

Say: Listen carefully. I am going to say three words. You say them back after I stop.

Ready? Here they are... PONY (wait 1 second), QUARTER (wait 1 second), ORANGE (wait one

second). What were those words?

_____ (1)

_____ (1)

_____ (1)

Give 1 point for each correct answer, then repeat them until the patient learns all three.

5 ( )   **SERIAL 7 s AS A TEST OF ATTENTION AND CALCULATION**

Ask: Subtract 7 from 100 and continue to subtract 7 from each subsequent remainder

until I tell you to stop. What is 100 take away 7 ? _____ (1)

Say:

Keep Going. _____ (1), _____ (1),

_____ (1), _____ (1),

3 ( )   **RECALL OF THREE WORDS**

Ask:

What were those three words I asked you to remember?

Give one point for each correct answer._____ (1),

_____ (1), _____ (1),

2 ( )   **NAMING**

Ask:

What is this? (show pencil) _____ (1). What is this? (show watch)_____ (1).

For more
information or
additional copies
of this exam,
call (617)587-4215

O   V   E   R

continues

Exhibit 12–4 continued

MiniMental LLC

1 ( )   REPETITION

Say:

Now I am going to ask you to repeat what I say. Ready? No ifs, ands, or buts.

Now you say that. _____ (1)

3 ( )   COMPREHENSION

Say:

Listen carefully because I am going to ask you to do something:

Take this paper in your left hand (1), fold it in half (1), and put it on the floor. (1)

1 ( )   READING

Say:

Please read the following and do what it says, but do not say it aloud.   (1)

Close your eyes

1 ( )   WRITING

Say:

Please write a sentence. If patient does not respond, say: Write about the weather. (1)

_____

_____

1 ( )   DRAWING

Say: Please copy this design.

TOTAL SCORE _____   Assess level of consciousness along a continuum

Alert	Drowsy	Stupor	Coma

	YES	NO
Cooperative:	☐	☐
Depressed:	☐	☐
Anxious:	☐	☐
Poor Vision:	☐	☐
Poor Hearing:	☐	☐
Native Language:		

	YES	NO
Deterioration from previous level of functioning:	☐	☐
Family History of Dementia:	☐	☐
Head Trauma:	☐	☐
Stroke:	☐	☐
Alcohol Abuse:	☐	☐
Thyroid Disease:	☐	☐

FUNCTION BY PROXY

Please record date when patient was last able to perform the following tasks.
Ask caregiver if patient independently handles:

	YES	NO	DATE
Money/Bills:	☐	☐	_____
Medication:	☐	☐	_____
Transportation:	☐	☐	_____
Telephone:	☐	☐	_____

perception of her environment (e.g., she confuses mornings and evenings). She scores 0 out of 3 on this section.

Language (9 Items). The Language section covers several key functions and includes assessing aphasia (difficulty expressing or comprehending language) and apraxia (difficulties where the client with intact motor and sensory pathways forgets motor skills [e.g., how to walk]). Language is measured on the MMSE by naming everyday objects, repeating, understanding a three-stage command, reading, writing, and copying. Naming is measured by holding up a watch and pencil one at a time and asking the client to name the objects. One point is given for each correct name. Repetition is measured by asking the client to repeat "No ifs, ands, or buts." One point is given for the completed repetition. The three-stage command is measured by asking the client to take the paper in his or her dominant hand, fold the paper in half, and throw the paper on the floor. One point is given for each command. (The three-stage command should not be repeated.) Reading is measured by asking the client to read "close your eyes" and to do what the phrase says. One point is given when the client performs that task, not when the client reads the phrase. Writing is measured by asking the client to write a spontaneous sentence. The sentence should be legible, but spelling and grammar errors should be ignored. One point is given when the client writes a sentence. Copying is measured by asking the client to copy intersecting pentagons so that they are about the same size as the first example drawn. The GCM should give the client a point if each pentagon has five clear sides, the overlapping angles form a diamondlike shape, and a complete side is not part of the overlap.[24,25] The GCM should ignore rotation or tremor. Sally has good language abilities (she scores 6 out of 9 points), which allow her to compensate well for her short-term memory loss, although she has trouble with the pentagon-copying task. She gives the impression that she is functioning at a higher level than she actually is. She compensates by "filling in the

blanks" of what she cannot remember, which is very common with dementia.

Scoring (Range 0–30). For college-educated individuals, scores of 25 or under are suspect.[25]

Visuospatial Ability

Visuospatial ability incorporates motor, perceptual, spatial, and memory processes and allows for navigation of the spatial environment, identification of visual information, and placement of objects into appropriate spatial relationships.[26] Some aspects of visuospatial ability are measured by drawing the intersecting pentagons on the MMSE and completing the Clock Drawing Test (Figure 12–3). In the clock drawing test, the client is asked to draw the numbers on a clock face. After the client completes the task, the client is asked to draw the clock hands at 2:45.

Sally has difficulty with visuospatial ability, as reflected in her difficulty drawing the pentagons and setting the clock at 2:45. This means that she is at high risk for future falls even though she currently walks without assistance. She is also at higher risk for accidents while climbing the stairs.

The GCM keeps in mind that the client does not lose all functions at the same time or the

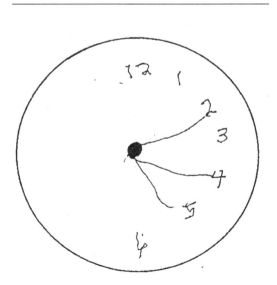

Figure 12–3 Clock Drawing.

same rate. For example, not all short-term memory is lost at once. In early dementia the client may have difficulty with retrieving information even though he or she can still recognize information. At a later stage the client may not be able to retrieve or recognize the information. Some clients may be able to copy but unable to write a sentence because the ideas do not flow. Identifying specific deficits becomes important later, when developing strategies to support the client. For example, arranging clothing by color and making sure the client's visual acuity is as good as possible are helpful for the client with visuospatial deficits.

Emotional Functioning

An example of the many screening tests for depression is the Yesavage Geriatric Depression Scale (Exhibit 12–5). A score greater than 10 suggests the client is experiencing depression.[27]

On the Geriatric Depression Scale, Sally scored 13 out of 30, which is suggestive of depression. One of the theories about depression is that it can occur, especially when a person is ex-

---

Exhibit 12–5 Geriatric Depression Scale

1.	Are you basically satisfied with your life?	yes	NO
2.	Have you dropped many of your activities and interests?	YES	no
3.	Do you feel that your life is empty?	YES	no
4.	Do you often get bored?	YES	no
5.	Are you hopeful about the future?	yes	NO
6.	Are you bothered by thoughts you can't get out of your head?	YES	no
7.	Are you in good spirits most of the time?	yes	NO
8.	Are you afraid that something bad is going to happen to you?	YES	no
9.	Do you feel happy most of the time?	yes	NO
10.	Do you often feel helpless?	YES	no
11.	Do you often get restless and fidgety?	YES	no
12.	Do you prefer to stay at home, rather than going out and doing new things?	YES	no
13.	Do you frequently worry about the future?	YES	no
14.	Do you feel you have more problems with memory than most?	YES	no
15.	Do you think it is wonderful to be alive now?	yes	NO
16.	Do you often feel downhearted and blue?	YES	no
17.	Do you feel pretty worthless the way you are now?	YES	no
18.	Do you worry a lot about the past?	YES	no
19.	Do you find life very exciting?	yes	NO
20.	Is it hard for you to get started on new projects?	YES	no
21.	Do you feel full of energy?	yes	NO
22.	Do you feel that your situation is hopeless?	YES	no
23.	Do you think that most people are better off than you are?	YES	no
24.	Do you frequently get upset over little things?	YES	no
25.	Do you frequently feel like crying?	YES	no
26.	Do you have trouble concentrating?	YES	no
27.	Do you enjoy getting up in the morning?	yes	NO
28.	Do you prefer to avoid social gatherings?	YES	no
29.	Is it easy for you to make decisions?	yes	NO
30.	Is your mind as clear as it used to be?	yes	NO

Scoring: Add the total number of capitalized responses. A score above 10 is suggestive of depression.

Total score: _____

periencing "learned helplessness," because of being in situations where the person has no control over negative events.[28] Sally has experienced some significant negative events, including the loss of her husband, her home, and some of her independence.

The GCM checks for changes in the client's behavior such as wandering, agitation, delusions, hallucinations, and acute confusion. These behaviors more commonly accompany the mid- to late stages of dementia and can be frightening to the client, family members, and caregivers. For example, poor short-term memory may interfere with the client's ability to keep a location in mind and lead to wandering. Pacing and other physical nonaggressive behaviors suggest unmet needs for socialization. The GCM also identifies behaviors that may be related to physical pain.[29]

The GCM checks for changes in personality such as irritability, temper outbursts, passivity, and greater dependence on caregivers. The GCM identifies passivity that could respond to specific interventions, as passivity may decrease a person's ability to carry out ADLs and IADLs. Is the client withdrawn and isolated? Is the client receiving sufficient stimulation? Is the client overstimulated? Are there side effects from medications (e.g., psychotropic drugs) that are causing the client to be passive?

The GCM asks the family about when certain behaviors or personality changes began, how often certain behaviors occur, and whether certain behaviors occur at particular times. The GCM also inquires about the presence of pain or fatigue. Understanding changes in behavior and personality helps a GCM individualize interventions for the client, coordinate the needed care, and refer the client for necessary treatment. GCMs can help family members by providing supportive counseling and referring them to support groups and/or psychological services as appropriate.

ADLs and IADLs

The GCM notes the client's overall dress, grooming, and personal hygiene, all indicators of self-care. Other important ADL and IADL activities cannot realistically be directly observed, and the GCM must rely on the client's and family members' reports. The GCM asks many questions. Can the client dress him- or herself, fastening buttons and tying shoes? Can the client retain enough memory to follow precautions in the home? The MMSE scores can give the GCM insight into the client's ability to perform ADLs and IADLs. For example, a score of 20–25 may be an indication that the client will have difficulty keeping appointments, using the telephone, obtaining meals, and traveling alone.[30]

Social Support

Social support in ADLs may be difficult for the GCM to directly observe. The GCM attempts to become familiar with the important friends and family members who provide support to the client. The GCM discusses with the client and family changes in or loss of roles (e.g., spouse, employee). Assessing for depression can give the GCM insight into social support and the loss of social roles, which can be a significant factor in depression. The GCM observes for loss of interest in relationships and activities, which could indicate the client is not receiving enough stimulation. The GCM helps the client find pleasant activities, perhaps activities the client has enjoyed in years past, that accommodate the client's current functioning. The GCM also encourages the family caregiver to engage in leisure and recreational activities to relieve the stress of caregiving.[31]

Physical and Social Environment

The GCM evaluates the environment for safety, including lighting, familiarity of the surroundings, security, barriers to accessibility and mobility, and effect on overall functioning. Clinical observations indicate that noise in the physical environment and high levels of activity in confined spaces (social environment) often increase wandering.[32] The GCM observes whether the client experiences loud noises or overstimulation in the environment. Specific environmental interventions include protecting the client from the stresses of overstimulation and maximizing environmental cues to maintain independence and prevent injury both inside and outside the home. Safety interventions may include the use of door locks to prevent wandering at night, participation in the Safe Return program through the Alzheimer's Association, and using medical alert bracelets.[1]

Synthesizing and Analyzing Assessment Data

GCMs synthesize and analyze the assessment data and identify problems/needs, deficits/strengths, preferences, resources, and informal support (Figure 12–1). GCMs need sophisticated interviewing and observational skills. They also need knowledge of aging and disability as well as family/caregiver dynamics. The GCM balances the client's perspective and the family members'/caregiver's perspective with what is observed in the assessment.

When assessing clients, the GCM differentiates normal age-related changes that affect sensory, motor, and cognitive functions and behaviors from indicators of dementia. For example, the slowed language processing of normal aging is differentiated from additional changes in language processing that occur with dementia. Likewise, the slower reaction time of normal aging is differentiated from the visuospatial and problem-solving impairments of dementia, impairments that significantly affect skills such as putting on clothes, walking down stairs, and driving a car. Hearing and vision may be impaired. Differentiating hearing difficulties from lack of comprehension may be accomplished by repeating questions in a louder voice and simplifying words used when repetition does not lead to understanding. Additionally, the functional assessment instruments provide objective data regarding the client's strengths and deficits. For example, asking the client to read and obey the statement "Close your eyes" on the MMSE helps differentiate between (1) vision loss, (2) lack of comprehension of the words, and (3) inability to do what the words say. Medications may need to be changed to help the client compensate for functional deficits: for example, diuretics in a client with gait imbalance may result in in-

creased risk for falls. Psychotropic medications with significant side effects can further impair functioning. Benzodiazepines (Xanax, Librium, Ativan) can lead to dizziness, which can produce falls, particularly in the client with dementia. Discussion with physicians about selecting medications to optimize the client's functioning is a priority.

Developing a Plan of Care

Developing a written plan of care involves defining the problems, developing goals from defined problems, and identifying alternative recommendations of ways to attain the goals (Figure 12–1). This means the GCM needs to know all of the activities involved in assessing clients as well as all of the community resources for alternative recommendations. Specific strengths and deficits in client functioning are discussed in the report, which forms the basis for future care and helps family members understand the level of support needed in client decision making. The report information is communicated by the GCM to the client and family to empower family decision making. The client's values and preferences help the GCM determine which alternatives to recommend for consideration. Recommendations include cost of services. In contrast to traditional home health services, GCM planning anticipates change rather than reacts to change and is individualized rather than standardized. For example, the dementia client at risk for falls due to changes in vision and cognitive functioning is assessed at home by the GCM and receives selected interventions to prevent falls and make the home safe. This is different from the traditional skilled home health services, which are available only after the fall and subsequent injury and provided only with a physician's order.

Special attention is given to keeping information simple for the client and communicating to the family that it may be necessary to do one thing at a time so as not to overwhelm the client. Recommendations include but are not limited to support for family caregivers, environmental changes, home care, day care, retirement communities, assisted living, and nursing homes. Specific recommendations that decrease family caregiver burden, increase caregiver effectiveness, and plan for the future are included.

The following case study is an example of how the GCM synthesizes and analyzes assessment data and develops the plan of care. The case study demonstrates how the combination of early dementia, significant hearing and vision loss, and clinical depression affects the client's current functional status. The GCM helps the client compensate for certain changes and behaviors (resistance to seeing her physician, resistance to help from her grandson) through a variety of problem-focused strategies. The GCM, in collaboration with appropriate health care providers, improves client functioning and arranges a caregiver to provide the assistance that is still needed. By identifying and addressing unreported functional impairments, the GCM improves the client's quality of life and decreases the frustration and time spent by the primary health care provider in managing the client's multiple chronic conditions. The GCM helps the grandson transition into the family caregiving role by providing education, counseling support, and alternatives that facilitate decision making.

Gladys P and Brian (Grandmother and Grandson, Ages 97 and 48)

Gladys P was referred to the GCM by her grandson Brian, who has power of attorney and lives many states away. According to Brian, his grandmother had misplaced her hearing aids and had been unable to talk to him on the phone for the past week. Usually, he talked to her every day. Gladys lived alone in a moderate-income senior apartment complex. She lost her husband when she was in her forties. Her only daughter, Brian's mother, had lived in the same city as Gladys until her death from cancer 3 years ago. Brian stressed, "While I'm her only family now, I'm standing behind her 100%, even though I'm at a distance." Brian described his relationship with his grandmother as good but fraught with anxiety. "I want to help her financially, but she

won't take any money from me. Yet she throws a lot of guilt my way."

While there was no family nearby, a woman from Gladys's church called and visited Gladys regularly as well as delivered meals occasionally. Brian was increasingly concerned because his grandmother had been getting more forgetful over the past several months. For the past 3 years he had tried to convince her to move to a retirement community or move closer to him, but she had refused. Brian asked the GCM to assess his grandmother and indicated that he wanted to fly in to visit her in 2 weeks and talk about options. A consent form was faxed to Brian with a request to return it as soon as possible, and an assessment was scheduled for the next day.

The GCM met with Gladys, who had found her hearing aids. When asked, Gladys told the GCM she was originally from Baltimore and moved to her current apartment in 1981. She had worked as a cashier in the food industry until she was 79. Unfortunately, the year she retired, the company cut the pension plan. As a result she was living off of her Social Security income and had $10,000 in the bank, which she was saving for her funeral expenses. When asked about her relationships, she described her daughter who died as her "pride and joy" and Brian as a "wonderful boy" who was very sympathetic to her. She didn't want Brian worrying about her. In her words, "I don't want him spending any money on me. I've lived a good long life. He has his own children and his own life to live." She then began crying and said, "I cry a lot. I miss my family," then added, "I never thought I would live this long." The GCM asked Gladys how she coped with her losses. She responded, "I pray every day. God is with me and I'm taking one day at a time. I used to read my Bible and go to mass every day, but I can't do that anymore."

The GCM assessed Gladys's functioning and found her to have severe hearing loss in both ears. The loss was more significant on the right, and her hearing aids were either broken or not working well. Gladys had severe vision loss in her right eye and moderate vision loss in her left eye. She also reported central vision loss and complained that the lines on the reading card were blurry and moved around. As she described it, "There is a big black hole in the middle." When asked further about her vision loss, Gladys responded that she thought she might be going blind. "I don't want to tell my grandson about this because he is out of town. So I just sit here and worry. I know if he were here, he would take me to the doctor right away." Gladys thought she had been wearing the same glasses for the past 5–6 years but wasn't sure. She did not remember when she last saw any physician but did know the names of her physicians. She said she had stopped taking her only medication, "a blood pressure pill," because she didn't think she needed it. She did not remember how long ago she had stopped her medication. Gladys received a score of 25 out of 30 on the MMSE and 16 out of 30 on the Geriatric Depression Scale. She was aware that her cognitive abilities were changing, and that embarrassed her.

During the functional assessment, Gladys used the walls and furniture to support her as she moved around the house, although she did not have significant problems with balance, coordination, or reaching. She washed at the sink because she was not able to get in and out of the bathtub by herself. She could fix her own meals, but the GCM observed decreased reserve capacity to do ordinary daily activities that required Gladys's maximum energy. She was able to go out of the apartment inside the building to get mail and do her laundry, but she did not drive, so she was dependent on her friend from church to buy groceries. She walked down the back stairway to use the coin-operated washer and dryer in the basement because the stairway was closer to her apartment than the elevator on the other side of the building.

The GCM used a holistic approach in synthesizing and analyzing the functional assessment information. Small decreases in Gladys's functioning included misplacing her hearing aid, not being able to talk to her grandson on the phone, not getting her vision evaluated, not having her hearing aid repaired, and not reordering her blood pressure medication. These factors made a significant difference in her functional independence. Her difficulty with ambulation appeared to be more from poor vision than an unsteady gait. Also, her inability to drive and get out of her apartment building barred her from getting the socialization and services she needed. And because of her cognitive impairment and depression, she was unable to set up and arrange transportation to appointments for the necessary evaluation of her health care needs.

A practical problem-solving approach was used to manage the client's resistance. The GCM asked Gladys what she wanted. Gladys said that she wanted to hear and see better and she didn't want anyone helping her do what she could do for herself. She also wanted to stay in her apartment but didn't want any strangers coming in. The GCM told Gladys she would help her, explaining what it would take for her to see and hear better. The GCM explained her role in arranging and following up on appointments. She asked Gladys to sign a consent form and left the apartment to call the grandson, who was anxiously awaiting her report of the assessment.

Family Decision Making

Problem-solving techniques can be used to make decisions among alternative recommendations. Once alternatives are selected, the GCM helps empower the client and family to determine who will organize, coordinate, monitor, and evaluate the ongoing care (Figure 12–1). Table 12–2 highlights the plan of care for Gladys as described in the written report, including problems, goals, and recommendations as conceptualized by the GCM. Additionally, the report noted that the recommended medical evaluations would be covered by the client's health insurance, but that new glasses and hearing aids, caregiver support, and bathroom supplies would be out-of-pocket costs.

Gladys was not able to report her functional impairments accurately. As a result of the GCM's assessment and written report, Brian became more knowledgeable about the problems his grandmother was experiencing. He also un-

Table 12–2 Plan of Care for Gladys P

Problems	Goals	Recommendations
Central vision loss	Improve vision and overall functioning	Ophthalmologist evaluation New glasses Large-print Bible and other books
Hearing loss	Improve hearing and overall communication	Audiologist evaluation ENT specialist evaluation New digital hearing aids
Cognitive impairment	Improve cognitive support	Primary care evaluation with dementia workup
Depression, lack of social stimulation and relationships	Increase social activities and level of communication, improve quality of life	Primary care provider evaluation Friendly visitor from the church Paid caregiver to assist with activities
No family nearby, stressed grandson living at a distance	Improve communication and decrease family caregiver burden and stress	Ongoing care management Counsel grandson on options for home care Educate grandson on coping skills and resources to relieve burden
Difficulty obtaining groceries, preparing meals, paying bills, taking medications, keeping appointments, using the telephone, doing laundry, and traveling alone	Improve nutrition and increase functional independence while providing support	Paid caregiver to assist with medication, bathing, shopping, and transportation In-home meals Daily money management service Assisted living options for future planning
Walking downstairs to do laundry	Decrease risk of falling Improve reserve capacity	Paid caregiver to assist client with laundry (using elevator and avoiding stairs) Raised toilet seat, portable bath bench Handheld shower hose

derstood that he needed to help her with decision making in a more significant way. By making additional phone calls, the GCM was able to obtain additional medical information for the written report. She reported that Gladys had been seeing the same primary care physician for the past 26 years, although she had not had a visit for the past year. Gladys did not have an ophthalmologist, and her ENT specialist had retired. According to her pharmacist, Gladys had not re-

filled her medication in the past 6 months. The GCM called the primary care provider after speaking to the pharmacist, and a medication refill was called in.

After reading and discussing the written report over the phone with his grandmother, Brian asked the GCM to work with his grandmother to implement all of the recommendations starting with the physician appointments. He wanted to support his grandmother in staying in her apartment with in-home assistance, starting out with 4 hours of care a day. He proposed a visit to a couple of the middle-income assisted living facilities and asked that the GCM arrange the appointments and accompany him and his grandmother on these visits. He further proposed an agenda for the day he would fly in: to review the implemented recommendations; to discuss Medicare and Medicaid issues, which he found very difficult to understand; and to discuss assisted living options as a backup plan. Because Brian wanted to help, he decided he would initially balance and maintain his grandmother's checkbook, be responsible for her monthly income and expense statements, and gradually transition into writing all of her checks. Gladys told her grandson she would not pay for new hearing aids, new glasses, or care in her apartment "because they were too expensive." Brian told the GCM he wanted to pay for those services initially.

The GCM scheduled appointments with a new ophthalmologist, a new audiologist, and a new ENT specialist followed by an evaluation with Gladys's primary care provider. The specialist appointments were scheduled for the same week as the GCM assessment, and the primary care physician appointment was scheduled for the following week. These evaluations resulted in diagnoses of early Alzheimer's disease, depression, macular degeneration more severe in her right eye, and hearing loss. New glasses and hearing aids were ordered. Gladys's primary care physician did not recommend an antidepressant for her, viewing her depression as more recent and associated with her isolation and inability to manage her activities. By arranging and taking Gladys to appointments with the health care providers and by communicating the client's functional status ahead of time, the GCM expedited the medical evaluations, saved time for health care providers, assisted the physicians in carrying out their medical plan of care, and helped relieve the grandson's burden and stress. The GCM screened and selected a paid caregiver, introducing the caregiver to Gladys at her appointment with her primary care provider, gaining the physician's support for the needed

care. After the visit the GCM wrote Gladys a letter indicating that her primary care physician wanted her to have 4 hours of caregiver care a day, providing information about her specific caregiver, and outlining the caregiver's responsibilities. The GCM later that week reintroduced the paid caregiver to Gladys at her apartment. While Gladys did not remember their first meeting, she had the letter, which reinforced that her physician, whom she had known for 26 years, wanted her to receive help from this specific person. The GCM also introduced the paid caregiver to the management staff of the apartment building. The GCM and paid caregiver then collaborated on organizing activities that matched Gladys's interests (e.g., going for drives, going to church).

Ongoing Care Management

Studies indicate a high level of chronic health conditions and medical complexity among functionally impaired clients receiving ongoing care management. The amount of care clients require is determined more by their functional deficits and strengths than by their medical diagnosis of dementia. The client's memory and organizational skills may be inadequate to manage daily routines or medical needs, as in the case of Gladys. The activities of service coordination and ongoing monitoring become critical in managing the unique needs and care of the client with dementia. To coordinate and manage the ongoing care, the GCM focuses on client functional status and self-determination over time. This approach differs from the episodic "acute care" perspective of the traditional health care system.

In the case of Gladys, the GCM made monthly visits and was on call 24 hours a day, 7 days a week. The paid caregiver made sure that Gladys wore her hearing aids and glasses and took her blood pressure medication every day. In-home meals started arriving. Gladys went grocery shopping with the paid companion once a week. She began going to mass daily and became reconnected with two longtime friends from her church. She began sleeping better since she was getting up at a regular time every day and having 4 hours of activities in the morning with her paid caregiver. According to the paid caregiver, Gladys was laughing more and seemed to be less depressed. She loved riding around with the caregiver, especially to church. As Gladys said, "My church is my strength, and I want to make sure it is still there every day." While Gladys's vision, hearing, and cognition were not restored to normal, her new hearing aids, glasses, and paid caregiver support resulted in improved functioning and quality of life. Once Gladys's depression improved and she stabilized at her new level of functioning, the GCM asked that the primary care provider evaluate Gladys for memory-enhancing medications. He agreed, and during his follow-up visit he started her on Aricept 5mg once a day, which resulted in an observable improvement in cognitive functioning. The major challenge for the GCM in this case study was to ensure the needed caregiver support for Gladys without decreasing her autonomy and self-sufficiency any more than necessary. This was most difficult, as is often the case with dementia clients, because Gladys needed more help than she recognized. Continued encouragement was required from the GCM, grandson, and primary care provider to keep the care in place.

One day, about 3 months after the initial assessment, the GCM was paged by the paid caregiver. The caregiver had noticed increased agitation in Gladys over the past few days. She also noticed increased confusion over Gladys's daily schedule. Gladys began yelling at the caregiver, saying she never took her anywhere and had not come for the past 3 days. On the day of the phone call, the caregiver told the GCM that Gladys had fired her and told her not to come back because she didn't need help. The GCM made a visit to the client's home that day. The GCM observed, in addition to increased agitation, that Gladys was going to the bathroom frequently, although she denied having urgency or frequency of urination. A call was made to the primary care provider, who worked Gladys into his schedule at the end of the day. The GCM took Gladys to the physician's office. A urinary tract infection was identified, an antibiotic was given, and Gladys's increased confusion and agitation resolved.

The effects of various medical treatments on function become an important consideration for clients with dementia. In this case, the memory-enhancing medication Aricept resulted in observable improvement of the client's cognitive function. Treating a urinary tract infection dramatically improved the client's increased confusion. Working collaboratively with other professionals, the GCM was able to optimize the client's functioning.

COMMUNICATING WITH OTHER PROFESSIONALS

GCMs communicate with other professionals while working with clients and their family members and caregivers. Communicating with other professionals supports the GCM process, improves care for the client with dementia, provides for more appropriate referrals, and improves the GCM's practice (Figure 12–1). The GCM understands that the client and his or her family experience relationships with professionals on a very personal level. The GCM supports the client's existing relationships with professionals, identifies the need for new relationships, and makes appropriate referrals with permission from the client and family. The GCM acts as the collaborative advocate for the client, ensuring that client goals are the focus of professional activities. As care coordinator, the GCM actively communicates with all professionals so they have timely and consistent information relevant to their roles and the roles of others. The GCM engages all professionals to integrate their care plans, achieving common goals for the client and family.

When family members live at a distance, the GCM is often the community contact, providing rapid response to crisis situations that may involve different professionals. In Gladys's case, the GCM's response to Gladys's sudden escalation of confusion facilitated the timely diagnosis and treatment of a urinary tract infection by the primary care physician and prevented the development of more severe confusion. The functional assessment of the GCM complemented the diagnostic evaluation and treatment provided by the primary care physician in this example, resulting in improved function and curing the infection.

Determinations of when consultation with a primary care provider, neuropsychologist, neurologist, or neuropsychiatrist is indicated depend on factors such as the client's history, the client's and family member's preference, the primary care provider's expertise in dementia care, and available resources. Most clients with dementia can be diagnosed and managed in primary care settings. Primary care providers may include physicians, nurse practitioners, and physician assistants. The GCM often communicates to the primary care provider through the provider's office or triage nurse. Because many primary care providers have limited time available to meet with and assess patients in today's managed care environment, the GCM needs to develop effective strategies in communicating client functioning to primary care providers and nurses.

Clients presenting with unusual symptoms and onset or atypical neurological findings are often referred to neurologists, geriatric psychiatrists, or geriatricians. Neurologists are particularly helpful for clients with Parkinson's disease, unusually rapid progression, or abnormal neuroimaging findings. Geriatric psychiatrists can provide behavioral management and monitoring of psychotropic medications. When the dementia is in the early stages or the diagnosis is unclear, neuropsychological testing may distinguish between normal aging and dementia as well as identify deficits that point to a specific diagnosis. The neuropsychologist may also aid in distinguishing depression from dementia or in determining competency for legal purposes.[1,13] Geriatric assessment units, if available in communities, are especially helpful when other medical problems are present. The GCM may refer directly to these geriatric specialists or may be instrumental in recommending to the primary care provider that a more comprehensive evaluation is needed based on the functional assessment conducted in the home. Appendix 12–C provides a referral checklist for the GCM to ensure that the necessary steps have been taken in working with health care providers.

Because clients with dementia may have other chronic illnesses or injuries, the GCM may work with a variety of professionals. Gladys's GCM worked with an ENT specialist, an audiologist, an ophthalmologist, and a pharmacist. GCMs also work with nurses, social workers, physical therapists, occupational therapists, and speech therapists. The relationship with these professionals varies depending on their setting: rehabilitation center, hospital, client home, or nursing home. For example, as part of an interdisciplinary team in a rehabilitation center, the nurse may screen for psychosocial and functional problems and work with an occupational therapist in deciding the client's equipment needs. The occupational therapist may focus on assessing ADL/IADL function as it relates to cooking and dressing. The physical therapist may focus on assessing ADL function as it relates to mobility and transfers. The social worker may facilitate the use of community resources and coordinate discharge planning.[26] In the hospital setting, the nurse case manager rather than the social worker may be responsible for coordinating discharge planning. In the client's home environment when the client qualifies for reimbursable home health care services, the physical therapist and the speech therapist may be the professionals in the home health care agency that assess ADL/IADL function. In the home environment when the client does not qualify for reimbursable home health care services, the GCM may be the only professional to provide functional assessment, decide equipment needs, and coordinate community- and home-based services. The GCM needs to understand how the professionals work in the setting providing services for the client. The GCM communicates with those professionals that come together for the client's needs at the time services are provided. The GCM adjusts his or her role to complement the professional services, looking at the client holistically, filling in the gaps as needed, but not duplicating reimbursable services. An important feature of the GCM's role is working with the client on an ongoing basis to ensure continuity. This arrangement promotes trust with the client and family members, but means working with different professionals in different settings over time. It also means following the client to whatever environment is needed.

Professionals in the mental health arena (e.g., social workers, gerontologists, psychologists) are important resources for the GCM. Ongoing counseling/therapy may be needed for family conflicts, family members not coping with the dementia diagnosis, loss and grief, depression, and feelings of anxiety or guilt. Family members may also need additional help dealing with caregiver burnout. Providing professional alternatives to addressing family conflicts and problems enables the client and/or family member to choose the most appropriate strategy.

GCMs work with professionals in organizations that provide dementia-specific services. The local and national Alzheimer's Association offers specific programs to educate family caregivers, including family support groups. Videotapes and caregiver books can also be borrowed or purchased through the local Alzheimer's Association. For example, the family member who wants to assist with bathing when that becomes necessary can read a booklet or see a training video on bathing and bed skills. Additionally, the Alzheimer's Association sponsors educational programs that benefit professionals. GCMs work with professionals in assisted living residences and long-term care facilities. For example, the GCM may work with an assisted living professional to find the right apartment or work with a nursing home professional to find a bed within a special dementia care unit. The GCM may meet with facility staff before the move, discussing specific needs of the client, and may after the move be retained by the family to provide oversight of services. When family members live at a distance, the professionals may keep the GCM informed about the client and work collaboratively to resolve problems.

GCMs work closely with elder-law attorneys, who provide legal planning. The GCM's functional assessment is often helpful in developing the legal plan. The GCM may suggest a consultation with an elder-law attorney for legal planning documents to let someone else make decisions when the client is no longer able. Families may need legal help when facing a Medicaid spenddown or when the client is being exploited by others. GCMs often work with elder-law attorneys when dementia and family relationships affect legal issues.

In summary, the GCM's role when working with other professionals is to break down barriers, share information, and use a collaborative approach to problem solving with an orientation toward advocacy for the client.

TRAINING FAMILY AND PAID CAREGIVERS ABOUT DEMENTIA CARE

Developing a Client/Family Framework

There are various models used to describe individuals and disability. The most common model is the medical model of disability, which responds to a person's medical condition. A second, the social model of disability, identifies the barriers present in society that truly disable people. In contrast to these models, a person-centered approach to dementia care developed by Kitwood describes the personal deterioration associated with dementia as resulting from not just the individual's neurological impairment but the social and environmental aspects as well. Kitwood's focus on personhood supports the notion that a person with dementia can be in a state of relative well-being by looking at the main problems that contribute to ill-being.[6] GCMs need to examine different models carefully when working with clients and families. The GCM may consider one model when working with other professionals on the diagnosis and treatment of dementia and another model when making recommendations to clients and families for physically safe care that also addresses issues of belonging and self-esteem. GCMs also need to use models to create programs to train family members and paid caregivers about dementia care.

I suggest the following model for a training program because it emphasizes quality of life issues and helps caregivers look for the "purpose" of behavior rather than search for its "cause." The model was also selected because it provides a new and innovative approach and adds to the literature about dementia care. The model focuses on goal-oriented behavior as being self-created rather than motivated by drives or causes. Dementia may diminish capacity, but behavior can be viewed as goal oriented and hopeful. While family and paid caregivers may not always understand the client's goals, they can provide valuable support when the goals are identified. Thus GCMs can help clients choose goals that encompass social interest, can be supported by others, and result in greater satisfaction and improved quality of life.[33]

Synergration: Integrating Self, Relations, and Work

This section describes a client/family framework for dementia care using a model of synergration created by David L. Hanson.[33] While fundamentally based on Adlerian psychology, synergistic psychology postulates three tasks of life critical to satisfaction: self, relations, and work. Each task has an independent psychological goal (Exhibit 12–6).

Synergration is a life task process that integrates self, relations, and work while striving toward the goals of significance, belonging, and usefulness. While tasks of self, relationships, and work are independent of each other, when balanced they create a higher quality of life.[33] This model will become clearer as the chapter looks at client, family, and paid caregiver relationships.

In a study of 20 interviews with dementia-impaired subjects, 60% indicated they did not see their current life as helpless or depressing, and 85% made positive statements regarding their

---

Exhibit 12–6 Three Tasks of Life

The goal of the **SELF** task is to be *significant* among others.
The goal of the **RELATIONS** task is to *belong* with others.
The goal of the **WORK** task is to be *useful* to others.

---

primary caregivers. The work ethic of the older generation was reflected in statements regarding the need to feel useful, as expressed by 60% of subjects.[34] According to Hanson, synergistic satisfaction is created in the synthesis of self, relations, and work.[33] Synergy means "working together," and the expansion of all three goals and three tasks results in an expansion of this satisfying synergy (Figure 12–4).

Synergistic deterioration occurs when there is deterioration of one or more tasks or goals. When clients with dementia lack the support of others, they often experience the regression in all three life tasks and goals, leading to extreme dissatisfaction (Figure 12–5).

According to Hanson, persons are born with innate responses to the environmental realities they encounter.[33] These responses to life originate from the following four situational realities: persons enter the world in motion, with needs not provided, as unique individuals, and as helpless infants. These four situational realities result in four basic feelings experienced by all humans from birth to death: feelings of inferiority, separateness, anxiety, and movement. While feelings generate compensatory responses, persons are free to make basic choices as they construct a world to help them feel secure. The purpose of behavior is to respond to these basic feelings by doing compensatory tasks to achieve desired goals. Persons compensate for feelings of inferiority by striving to develop the self, toward significance (connection). They compensate for feelings of separateness by developing relationships, to belong with others (cooperation). They compensate for feelings of anxiety through meaningful work, to be useful to others (contribution). And finally, they compensate for feelings of movement by engaging in activities, to create stability (community). While it is possible to sequence these four realities and their responses in different ways, it is helpful to think of these concepts as an encouraging sequence: persons move from connection, to cooperation, to contribution, and finally to community. In other words, persons first show up, then cooperate with others, then contribute to the greater good, and finally become part of the community. The model as-

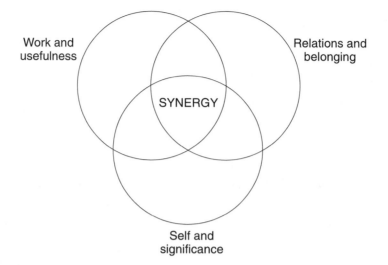

Synergy: satisfaction resulting from integration of the three life tasks and goals

Figure 12–4 Synergistic Satisfaction.

sumes that all behavior has a purpose and that persons increase the quality of their lives through developing activities, the self, relationships, and work (Exhibit 12–7).

Because of dementia-related changes, the client may not be able to adequately compensate for these basic feelings without support from others. As a result, the client may experience intensified feelings of inferiority, separateness, anxiety, and movement. An example is the extremely anxious client in constant motion, not knowing where he or she is going but unwilling

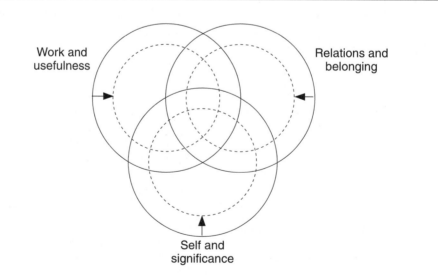

Deterioration: dissatisfaction resulting from regression in all three life tasks and goals

Figure 12–5 Synergistic Deterioration.

Exhibit 12–7 Feelings, Responses, and Goals (Tasks)

Basic feelings
Inferiority
Separateness
Anxiety
Movement

Basic responses
Self
Relations
Work
Activity

Basic goals
Significance (Connection)
Belonging (Cooperation)
Usefulness (Contribution)
Stability (Community)

or unable to rest. The following section discusses a person with dementia in this situation. A crisis (the death of the client's spouse) acts as a catalyst for the client's daughter to seek an evaluation.

Mary B and Cindy (Mother and Daughter, Ages 62 and 41)

Mary B was referred to the GCM by her neurologist, who had just told Mary that she had early onset Alzheimer's disease. The neurologist called the GCM and told her that Mary needed around-the-clock care and needed to stop driving because of her visuospatial and planning disabilities. The day after Mary got her diagnosis from her neurologist, the GCM met Mary and her daughter Cindy in the client's home after first talking to Cindy at length on the phone. Cindy lived in the next state and had taken a leave from work to stay with her mother after Cindy's father's death from cancer 2 weeks earlier. Having just learned of her diagnosis, Mary wanted to stay in her own home to "sort things out for herself." Cindy wanted her mother to move closer to her.

Cindy shared that her mother had been very active and sociable and loved traveling and

cooking. She was also very creative and had painted all of the pictures in the home. She loved gardening and made beautiful flower arrangements. Cindy's concern was that her mother had become withdrawn and isolated, probably because Mary had been caring for her husband before he died and did not have time to spend with family and friends. Now her mother was very fearful and anxious. To get her mother out of the house, Cindy had taken her shopping almost every day for the past 2 weeks. Cindy said the experience was extremely stressful. She described her mother as driven, unable to stop herself or unwilling to let Cindy stop her after being out more than 12 hours a day. She further described her mother as moody and irritable throughout the day, having difficulty getting dressed, putting on her makeup and jewelry in the morning, and counting out correct change in the store. Cindy said her mother refused to let Cindy do these things for her and got angry when Cindy corrected her. Cindy said that several things were misplaced daily and described instances of Mary losing her purse, misplacing jewelry, and even accusing Cindy of taking her mother's wedding ring, which was found later in her jewelry box. Cindy said her mother seemed especially distressed by these experiences of misplacing items. Cindy acknowledged that since she had been with her mother she had not had any time for herself and was not sleeping well. She wanted to help her mother but didn't know what to do. She also had to leave in a couple of days and go back to work.

During the interview, Mary privately confided to the GCM that she was very upset with her daughter. Cindy had moved things out of place and changed Mary's routine. According to Mary, that made things more confusing for her and made it harder to do things for herself. She described previously relying on her husband to help her. She said she also took care of him during his illness. "He was my memory, and I was his arms and legs. We could really work well together, as a team." Mary said when she lost her husband she felt like she lost herself as well. She started crying and said she was angry at Cindy but also didn't want to be a burden on her. She was worried about what this disease was going to do to her daughter. Mary said she didn't know how long she would be able to do the things she could do now and wanted to do as much as possible every day. The GCM gave Mary the opportunity to talk about her dementia and issues she was concerned about before proceeding with the functional assessment.

On assessment Mary had a high level of functioning during the early stage of her early onset Alzheimer's disease. Her MMSE score was 27 out of 30. She had good vision and hearing. She was misplacing things and having difficulty keeping up with appointments and medications without help. Because of her visuospatial problems, she perceived things correctly but had trouble judging spatial distances, requiring assistance with putting on jewelry and makeup and putting on her seatbelt. She could fix snacks or single dishes for herself, but because of her visuospatial problems she had difficulty using a knife to cut up vegetables and meats. She had no difficulty with ambulation and was not incontinent. Her home was all on one level and had no barriers that interfered with her functioning. Small changes, including her daughter moving the coffee pot and cleaning and rearranging other items in the house, made a significant difference in Mary's ability to function independently at home. Mary was unable to drive, manage her checkbook, or handle her estate. Overwhelmed by grief and struggling with a cognitive impairment, Mary was unable to make decisions without significant support from Cindy.

After the assessment, the GCM developed a plan that included live-in care at home, counseling for bereavement, attendance at an early onset Alzheimer's support group for Mary coordinated by a well-trained facilitator, a daily money management service, a family support group for Cindy, and a long-term goal of Mary moving to an assisted living facility near Cindy for people with dementia. Because Mary had walked 2 miles a day, the GCM recognized the client's need to walk and selected a paid caregiver to interview who also enjoyed daily walking, since letting Mary walk alone was risky. Working with Mary and Cindy to implement the plan, the GCM made weekly visits the first month to talk with Mary and determine her satisfaction with her paid caregivers. At Cindy's request, the GCM also set up a training program for family and paid caregivers providing verbal communication and written information. Additional services included supportive counseling for Cindy over the phone and being "on call" for crises such as when behavioral difficulties developed. At Mary and Cindy's request the GCM then made visits twice a month to monitor the plan of care after the first month.

Keady suggests that clients with dementia at this very early stage require distinct and separate services.[10] In particular, there is a role for an independent confidante who can act as a client advocate buffering the effects of dementia and the desire of the client to protect the family caregivers from the disease's effects. The GCM, partnering with the client, has the opportunity to take on this significant role. Dementia may be experienced, as described in the case study of Mary, as the loss of self, family, friends, and familiar places. There is no greater need than to help clients maintain a sense of self, a sense of purpose, and relationships with others in the face of their declining cognitive abilities. With clients' ability to compensate compromised, GCMs need to encourage their clients' abilities with meaningful activities and nurturing relationships. In the case of Mary, the GCM empowered the client and family to choose two paid caregivers from a number of screened caregivers so that the client and family could select caregivers who would provide the best companionship and want to participate in activities the client liked.

Family members and paid caregivers can help the client by responding to the client's feelings (inferiority, separateness, anxiety, movement), thus gaining a sense of what the client is experiencing, and then beginning to assist the client in the basic compensatory responses (self, relations, work, activity). By engaging in the tasks, clients with dementia can move closer to the basic goals of significance, belonging, usefulness, and stability. Family members and caregivers must learn to recognize and support the client's efforts in achieving these tasks. Exhibit 12–8 outlines strategies for Mary and her live-in caregivers and that were developed by the GCM working with Mary, Cindy, and the paid caregivers. It was possible for Mary to work through some of her fears and losses. According to Kitwood, individuals vary greatly in how they experience their neurological impairment.[6] Those who have lacked insight on various feelings are particularly vulnerable. Others may reach a point in their impairment where defenses collapse and raw emotions break through with agonizing intensity.[6] Yet others may be able to acknowledge losses, grieve, and let go. Efforts by the GCM, family members, and paid

---

Exhibit 12–8 Steps for Collaborative Dementia Care: A Plan for Mary's Caregivers

Step 1: Respond to client feelings
- Is the client experiencing feelings of excessive inferiority?
- Is the client experiencing feelings of excessive separateness?
- Is the client experiencing feelings of excessive anxiety?
- Is the client experiencing feelings of excessive movement?

Step 2: Help the client in the basic compensatory responses

- Assist in the development of the self task with the goal of significance
  1. Validate the client's feelings, providing reassurance and support
  2. Encourage the client to dress up and wear makeup, complimenting her on how she looks
  3. Communicate to the client that the assistance provided is to help her be independent
  4. Verbally cue her as needed, allowing her to do for herself, even when it takes longer
  5. Maintain the client's normal routine (eating, bathing, going to church, etc.)
  6. Working with client, prepare foods she likes, using her method of preparation
  7. Watch the client's TV programs, learn the characters, and talk about the programs
  8. When the client can no longer use silverware, prepare and eat finger foods with her

- Assist in the development of the relations task with the goal of belonging
  1. Provide companionship and encourage her relationships with supportive family and friends
  2. Keep open communication with family, initiating phone calls and visits
  3. Assist with family events and luncheons with friends in the client's home
  4. Maintain outside activities, attending art galleries, plays, and movies together

- Assist in the development of the work task with the goal of usefulness
  1. Continue planting, growing, and cultivating garden flowers and vegetables
  2. Include the client in preparing meals, value her opinion and make her feel a part of it
  3. Participate in expressive recreational therapies, including exercise and dance
  4. Take morning walks together and increase the number of pleasant events in the daily routine
  5. Participate in the early onset Alzheimer's disease support group at the local chapter of the Alzheimer's Association

- Assist in the development of an environment with less movement and more stability
  1. Develop a system to stimulate memory and orientation, including clocks, calendars, and to-do lists
  2. Put everything back in its place, every time, to decrease the client's confusion
  3. Modulate the environment, preventing too much or too little stimulation
  4. Structure schedule so client is home by 4:00 PM to minimize effects of "sundowning"
  5. Limit shopping to less than 3 hours to decrease sensory stimulation and disorientation

caregivers to maximize Mary's satisfaction and sense of significance, relationships, belonging, and work usefulness are important in Mary's plan of care.

With the goals of self-development and significance, the client can be empowered and encouraged to make independent choices that are not dependent on others or structured by the situation. For example, if Mary can still make her morning coffee without needing assistance, this encourages her sense of self even though she has diminished capacity.

Family caregivers find protective caregiving the most stressful part of providing home care.[10,35] Facing negative choices and not knowing what to do to help, family caregivers often withdraw into their own world. Paid caregivers can provide much-needed respite for family caregivers and offer protective caregiving to clients with dementia. Focused interviews of paid caregivers that I conducted indicated that protective caregiving (i.e., protecting the self-image of the client with dementia) was the most important part of providing dementia care. These paid caregivers also acknowledged that protective caregiving was difficult for family caregivers because of their desire to see their loved ones the way they had been in the past and the difficulty catching up to the "current picture" because of the continuous changes in the client with dementia. As described by one paid caregiver, "It's like trying to put a picture frame around a moving picture."

As the prevalence of long-term and chronic care services in the home and community (rather than in institutions) increases, there is a tremendous need for training, support, and supervision of paid caregivers. The rest of the chapter will focus on how GCMs can train paid caregivers in the process of care. It is critical that the paid caregiver enter the client's world, as uncomfortable as that may be, to encourage the client to achieve goals and perform tasks that will increase the quality of life. The client with dementia may express intense longings most of the time but communicate in ways that the caregiver may not understand. Examples include the client living at home who says "I want to go home" or the client who says "I want to see my mother"

although her mother died many years ago. Another example is the client, a retired plumber, who takes apart the plumbing in the bathroom and is unable to fix it. Clients respond to their own reality. This may be uncomfortable for the caregiver, who experiences a different reality. The paid caregiver may become impatient or frustrated, not understanding the client's experience or how to respond.

It helps if caregivers view clients with dementia as giving them the opportunity to practice service beyond self. If caregivers try to understand the fear of being alone at night, feeling lost, or not recognizing anyone they know, they can better identify strategies to help the client move toward self-significance, relationships, and usefulness. Caregivers focusing on the process of care will create responses and strategies based on the individual rather than using standard "one size fits all" strategies. The GCM can develop a training program to educate family members and caregivers in this process. The training involves more than encouraging kindness. It involves developing the sophisticated skills based on a holistic model that emphasizes quality of life and what individuals value. By encouraging caregivers to be more useful to clients, GCMs help caregivers improve their relationships with clients and client satisfaction.

Self above Service and Service beyond Self

Choosing the useful goal—service beyond self—leads to caregiver encouragement, while choosing the self-elevated goal—self above service—leads to caregiver discouragement.[33] A successful work effort requires that caregivers have or create a sense of self-significance, cooperate with others, and provide contributing service beyond their own self interests. Establishing a sense of self, cooperating with others, and contributing service that goes beyond the self results in a deep sense of having a purpose. In the case study of Mary, the paid caregiver listened to Mary's feelings, encouraged her, and gently helped her when she struggled to get dressed and put on her seat belt. Mary responded by continuing to participate in the activity and successfully completing it with help, which encouraged the caregiver, giving her the feeling that her role was meaningful. A satisfied caregiver recognizes, beyond his or her own self-care, the usefulness of service beyond self and experiences encouragement from the client and others. An encouraged caregiver is willing to contribute even more. Implementing the client's plan of care is always a group effort where the caregiver can become part of the larger team.

Putting the self above service leads to caregiver discouragement. Paid caregivers who seek to overcome feelings of inferiority by striving for superiority and put self above service meet with discouragement. For example, taking control when the client needs help and not giving the client an opportunity to participate because it is easier for the caregiver can result in behavioral difficulty, discouraging the caregiver. Discouraged caregivers often intensify their pursuit of self-elevation, leading to even more discouragement.[33] Instead of trying to control the client, the caregiver can look for the basic feelings experienced by the client and connect in a more meaningful way.

Three Goals of Collaborative Dementia Care

The three goals of collaborative dementia care are contribution, cooperation, and connection.

Contribution

A goal of contribution leads to the caregiver demonstrating interest in the client's family, the care plan, and the vocation and is persuasive, achievement seeking, and task centered. Striving for individual superiority is intimidating and self-centered and occurs at the expense of service to others and the plan of care (Exhibit 12–9).

By being familiar with the activities of contributing caregivers, the GCM can encourage the paid caregiver toward contribution and away from superiority.

Cooperation

The second goal in collaborative dementia care is cooperation. Cooperation involves being completely in harmony with others, working for the common good. Cooperation is equality seeking, encouraging, collaborative, affirming, and nurturing. In contrast, domination is power seeking, critical, manipulative, opposing, and revenge seeking. Domination leads to more discouragement, as others are intolerant of being placed in an inferior position and will ultimately reject the dominating person (Exhibit 12–10).[33]

By being familiar with the activities of cooperative caregivers, the GCM can encourage the paid caregiver toward cooperation and away from domination.

Connection

The third goal in collaborative dementia care is connection. The most basic form of encouragement and service beyond self is the willingness to be authentically present and also be in connection with others (Exhibit 12–11). Being

---

Exhibit 12–9 Qualities of Contributing Caregivers

Contributing caregivers tend to:	**Contributing caregivers do not:**
Recognize the importance of all individuals involved with the client	View themselves as all-knowing or all-powerful and rule over others
Make special efforts to invest in work beyond own self interest	Arrogantly brag about own accomplishments as being superior
Strive to respectfully persuade others	Dictate and intimidate others with a sense of presumed self importance
Strive to make unique contributions to the plan of care	Create special privileges for themselves and expect special treatment from others
Participate in activities that promote meaningful work	Place self-centered interests ahead of useful effort

Exhibit 12–10 Cooperative Caregivers

Cooperative caregivers tend to: Promote the attitude for treating others as equals Work toward helping others do better Guide others toward creating mutual work benefit Seek out ways to affirm others Understand the importance of nurturing others	**Cooperative caregivers do not:** Control others for the purpose of demonstrating power; or act stubborn Try to control others with the use of criticism Manipulate others or maneuver others for self-serving advantage Resist cooperation or intentionally work against others Become quick to retaliate in moody and crabby ways

in touch with oneself and having the courage to express oneself is the foundation for connection. The most discouraged movement resulting from the striving for self above service is withdrawal from others, as it moves against the human need to connect, cooperate, and contribute. Withdrawal puts self above service because withdrawal is an effort to overcome feelings of inferiority by escaping the anticipated negative judgment of others. Withdrawal includes self-indulgence, expressions of inadequacy, suppression of action, and interpersonal detachment.[33]

By being familiar with the activities of connected caregivers, the GCM can encourage the paid caregiver toward connection and away from withdrawal.

CONCLUSION

The increase in the population over age 85 also increases the need for dementia-specific care management services. The current literature on dementia care primarily discusses care for those with Alzheimer's disease because that is what researchers know about and understand. As they learn to better differentiate the many different types of dementia and the biopsychosocial changes that occur with each individual as dementia progresses, they will be more capable of understanding what education is needed for caregivers. Our interventions will then become more refined, with more emphasis on how dementia affects individuals differently, the differ-

Exhibit 12–11 Connected Caregivers

Connected caregivers tend to: Express positive energy toward task-related activities Initiate efforts in response to others Respond constructively and initiate action toward the tasks Assertively express ideas and thoughts Be friendly and initiate friendly interactions with others	**Connected caregivers do not:** Seem indifferent to task-related activities Act as if they cannot relate to others or seem insensitive to others Avoid using energy for ordinary work activity Hesitate to express thoughts and ideas or remain inexpressive Avoid interacting with others and become disconnected with others

ent types of coping strategies that can help in problem solving, and empowering the family. High-quality dementia care requires stable and secure relationships for the client. GCMs can demonstrate new ways of thinking about dementia, intervene early, support family and paid caregivers, and find ways to prevent premature institutionalization or disability associated with too little or no support.

This chapter has discussed the impact of dementia on the older adult and family caregiver, including the medical developments related to dementia, the client's and caregiver's experience of dementia, GCMs' work with people with dementia, and GCMs' work with other professionals on behalf of people with dementia. A model to train family members and caregivers is offered. The key to the model is maintaining social interest and stimulating creativity, thereby enhancing quality of life for clients, family members, and paid caregivers. The models and tools discussed in this chapter are important in developing the GCM's knowledge about dementia care. However, these models and tools are not intended to substitute for the benefits of supervised work with experienced GCMs. Each new GCM must develop insight and experience as to the models and tools' appropriate use and timely application on behalf of clients and families.

NOTES

1. Small G, Rabins P, Barry P, et al. Diagnosis and treatment of Alzheimer's disease and related disorders. *JAMA*. 1997;278:1363–1370.

2. Evans D, Funkenstein HH, Albert MS, et al. Prevalence of Alzheimer's disease in a community population of older persons: higher than previously reported. *JAMA*. 1989;262:2551–2556.

3. Meier D, Morrison R. Old age and care near the end of life. *Generations*. 1999;23:6–10.

4. National Alliance for Caregiving and American Association of Retired Persons. *Family Caregiving in the U.S.: Findings from a National Survey*. Bethesda, MD: 1997.

5. Weintraub S. Leading-edge research on Alzheimer's disease and dementia. Presented at National Association of Professional Geriatric Care Managers annual meeting; October 1998; Chicago.

6. Kitwood T. *Dementia Reconsidered*. Philadelphia: Open University Press; 1997.

7. McKhann G, Drachman D, Folstein M, Katzman R, Price D, Stadlan E. Clinical diagnosis of Alzheimer's disease: report of the NINCDS-ADRDA work group. *Neurol*. 1984;34:939–944.

8. World Health Organization. *The ICD-10 Classification of Mental and Behavioral Disorders: Diagnostic Criteria for Research*. Geneva, Switzerland: 1993.

9. American Psychiatric Association. *DSM-IV: Diagnostic and Statistical Manual of Mental Disorders*. 4th ed. Washington, DC: 1994.

10. Keady J. The experience of dementia: a review of the literature and implications for nursing practice. *J Clin Nurs*. 1996;5:275–288.

11. Geldmacher D, Whitehouse P. Evaluation of dementia. *New Engl J Med*. 1996;335:330–336.

12. Wallace M. Creutzfeldt-Jakob Disease. *J Gerontol Nurs*. 1999;25:17–23.

13. Corey-Bloom J, Thal L, Galasko D, et al. Diagnosis and evaluation of dementia. *Neurol*. 1995;45:211–218.

14. Funk S, Tornquist E, Champagne M, Wiese, R. *Key Aspects of Elder Care*. New York: Springer Publishing; 1992.

15. Moss M, Albert M, Kemper T. Neuropsychology of frontal lobe dementia. In: White, RF, ed. *Clinical Syndromes in Adult Neuropsychology: The Practitioner's Handbook*. Amsterdam, The Netherlands: Elsevier; 1992.

16. United Hospital Fund. *Families and Health Care Project*. New York: 1998.

17. Knutson K. Family caregiving and memory-impairment: why decision making is so difficult. *GCM J*. 1995;4:2–8.

18. Seltzer B, Vasterling J, Yoder J, Thompson K. Awareness of deficit in Alzheimer's disease: relation to caregiver burden. *Gerontologist*. 1997;37:20–24.

19. Applegate W, Blass J, Williams T. Instruments for the functional assessment of older patients. *New Engl J Med*. 1990;322:1207–1213.

20. Rubenstein L, Calkins D, Greenfield S. Systematic biases in functional status assessment of elderly adults: effects of different data sources. *J Gerontol*. 1984;39:686–691.

21. Elam J. Comparison of sources of functional report with observed functional ability of frail older persons. *Gerontologist*. 1989;29:308A.

22. Klein S. Case management. In: Klein S, ed. *A National Agenda for Geriatric Education: White Papers.* Rockville, MD: Health Resources and Services Administration; 1996:39–56.

23. Lachs M, Feinstein A, Cooney L, et al. A simple procedure for general screening for functional disability in elderly patients. *Ann Int Med.* 1990;112:609–706.

24. Folstein MF, Folstein S, McHugh, PR. Mini-Mental State, a practical method for grading the cognitive state of patients for the clinician. *J Psychiatr Res.* 1975;12:189–198.

25. Knutson K, Gross P. Advanced assessment: integrating the biopsychosocial needs of client and family. *GCM J.* 2000;10:4–13.

26. Carstensen L, Edelstein B, Dornbrand L. *The Practical Handbook of Clinical Gerontology.* Thousand Oaks, CA: Sage Publications; 1996.

27. Yesavage J, Brink TL, Rose T, et al. Development and validation of a geriatric depression screening scale: a preliminary report. *J Psychiatr Res.* 1983;17:37–49.

28. Selig M. *Learned Optimism.* New York: Knopf; 1991.

29. Cohen-Mansfield J. Measurement of inappropriate behavior associated with dementia. *J Gerontol Nurs.* 1999;25:42–51.

30. Galasko D, Bennett D, Sano M, et al. An inventory to assess activities of daily living for clinical trials in Alzheimer's disease. *Alzheimer Dis Associated Disord.* 1997;11:S33–S39.

31. Antonucci T, Sherman A, Vandewater E. Measures of social support and caregiver burden. *Generations.* 1997;Spring:48–51.

32. Kolanowsi A. An overview of the need-driven dementia-compromised behavioral model. *J Gerontol Nurs.* 1999;25(9):7–9.

33. Hanson D. *User's Guide to the Goal Evaluation and Matrix Analysis (Fourth Edition).* Charlotte, NC: Synergistic Psychology Associates; 1998.

34. Acton GJ, Mayhew PA, Hopkins BA, Yauk S. Communicating with individuals with dementia: the impaired person's perspective. *J Gerontol Nurs.* 1999;25:6–13.

35. Bowers B. Inter-generational caregiving: adult caregivers and their ageing parents. *Adv Nurs Sci.* 1987;9:20–31.

Evaluating Functional Assessment Instruments

ACTIVITIES OF DAILY LIVING AND INSTRUMENTAL ACTIVITIES OF DAILY LIVING INSTRUMENTS

Many of the activities of daily living (ADL) and instrumental activities of daily living (IADL) instruments came out of research studies and were designed as lengthy self-report questionnaires. While they can be given to family members, they cannot be successfully administered to clients with dementia and may not provide as much information about physical functioning as the geriatric care manager (GCM) requires. Performance-based assessment is preferred. In performance-based assessment, the GCM can observe the client doing certain tasks rather than having to ask whether the client can do the tasks. Although reliable and valid in discriminating those who can do the function from those who cannot, the ADL and IADL scales are not sensitive to changes in condition, especially in the highest-functioning clients.[1,2] GCMs using ADL and IADL scales will want to complement them with other measures of function that better establish a baseline and assess change from one visit to the next. The instruments listed below are commonly used in assessing basic activities of self care.

Katz ADL Scale

The Katz ADL scale assesses basic activities of self-care and is not sensitive to small changes. It is useful in rehabilitative settings.[1,3] The weak-

ness of the instrument is that it assesses a limited range of activities and the ratings are subjective.

Physical Self-Maintenance Scale (ADL)

The Physical Self-Maintenance Scale assesses self-care, mobility, and transfers.[1,3] It allows direct observation of a range of functions and is useful in a variety of settings. The weakness of the instrument is that it is time-consuming to administer and difficult to use with seriously ill or cognitively impaired older adults.

Scale for Instrumental Activities of Daily Living (IADL)

The Scale for Instrumental Activities of Daily Living assesses more complex activities, including food preparation, shopping, and housekeeping.[1,3] It has a higher range of performance than the Katz ADL scale but is not sensitive to small changes. The weakness of the instrument is that it is subjective and difficult to use in cognitively impaired older adults.

COGNITIVE FUNCTION INSTRUMENTS

While mental status instruments cannot establish that a person has dementia, they are important in identifying the client who needs further evaluation. Screening tests for mental status remain the cornerstone of documenting suspected cognitive impairment.[4,5] The client's age, education, ethnicity, and language have been shown to influence responses to mental status screening, all factors the GCM must consider in selecting the most appropriate instruments. Although there are several instruments for staging and following the progression of dementia, they have been used primarily in Alzheimer's disease, and their value in other dementias is less clear.[6] It is best to use the staging instruments after a formal dementia workup is completed and diagnosis of Alzheimer's disease is made. Cognitive function instruments can also be used to follow the progression of change in dementia. Another method for following the progression of change after a differential diagnosis of Alzheimer's disease is made is to combine the standard mental status tests with staging instruments. Future reassessments can then be compared to the baseline assessment to document changes in cognition. The instruments discussed below are commonly used in assessing cognitive function.

Folstein Mini Mental State Examination

The Folstein Mini Mental State Examination assesses a broader range of functions than the Short Portable Mental Status Questionnaire and is particularly useful in screening for moderate impairment.[1,7] It is a fairly quick and sensitive instrument and has been validated over time. The weakness of the instrument is that it will not detect mild cognitive impairment and is not designed to grade progression. Also, clients with primary expressive aphasia may appear more impaired because of difficulty with language.

Clock Drawing Test

The Clock Drawing Test assesses visuospatial difficulties and basic executive functions like planning and simple abstraction.[8] Studies have demonstrated that clients with normal mental status draw normal clocks and that clients with Alzheimer's disease draw abnormal clocks. Visuospatial skills may be the primary deficit in some clients in the early stages of Alzheimer's disease.

Global Deterioration Scale

The Global Deterioration Scale assesses seven stages in the course of dementia with well-specified observed criteria: mild Alzheimer's disease is stage 3 or 4; moderate is stage 5 or 6; and severe is stage 7.[6,9] The Global Deterioration Scale gives an overall picture of the disease process and assists the GCM in accurately placing the client at the appropriate stage of dementia. Language performance is not used to stage the dementia. The weakness of the instrument is that it has been used primarily in Alzheimer's disease and its value in other dementias is not clear. It provides information on the general progression of the disease and does not take into account individual variations.

Functional Assessment Staging Tool

The Functional Assessment Staging Tool (FAST) is for distribution to the family and provides specific information on the order in which various functions are lost.[9] FAST also provides the family members with an estimated time frame so they have an approximate idea of how long a given level of functioning will last. Along with the Global Deterioration Scale, FAST helps the GCM to understand each stage of Alzheimer's disease and make suggestions to clients and families regarding appropriate decision making (e.g., decision making about level of care and care needs). The weakness of the instrument is that it has been used primarily in Alzheimer's disease and its value in other dementias is not clear. It is an informational table about the general progression of the disease and does not take into account individual variations.

Short Portable Mental Status Questionnaire

The Short Portable Mental Status Questionnaire assesses a narrow range of basic mental functions including memory, attention, and orientation and is capable of detecting gross cognitive dysfunction only. The weakness of the instrument is that it is insensitive to small changes.[1,10]

Wechsler Memory Scale

The Wechsler Memory Scale assesses a broad range of memory functions and is sensitive to more subtle changes.[1,11] The weakness of the instrument is that it takes a long time to administer and has inadequate norms for the older adult population. The latest version, WMS–III, has norms to age 89.

DEPRESSION INSTRUMENTS

Functional assessment instruments for depression do not establish a diagnosis of depression but are important in identifying the client who needs further evaluation. Most of the depression scales are reasonably valid, reliable, and useful for screening and provide an assessment of the effects of therapy. Most of these scales have difficulty differentiating the effects of physical illness from those of depression since they include questions about physical symptoms such as fatigue and pain. Their usefulness may be limited in clients experiencing severe dementia.[1] The instruments discussed below are commonly used in screening for depression.

Geriatric Depression Scale

The Geriatric Depression Scale is designed for older adults, assesses symptoms of depression, and includes a broad range of questions about mood.[1,12] It is quick and reliable and avoids an excess of physical symptom questions. The weakness of the instrument is its limited usefulness in clients with severe dementia.

Beck Depression Inventory

The Beck Depression Inventory is a self-rating scale that assesses symptoms of depression and includes a broad range of questions.[1,13] It is validated in older adults and medical patients. The weakness of the instrument is that it relies too heavily on physical symptoms, making it less useful in older adults with physical impairments. It is also difficult for cognitively impaired clients to use.

Hamilton Depression Inventory

The Hamilton Depression Inventory assesses objective symptoms of depression and can estimate severity of depression.[1,14] The weakness of the instrument is that it relies on physical symptoms, thus making it less useful in older adults.

NOTES

1. Applegate W, Blass J, Williams T. Instruments for the functional assessment of older patients. *New Engl J Med.* 1990;322:1207–1213.

2. Johnson J, Mezey M. Functional status assessment: an approach to tertiary prevention. In: Lavizzo-Mourey, ed. *Practicing Prevention for the Elderly.* Philadelphia: Hanley & Belfus; 1989:141–152.

3. Guralnik J, Branch L, Cummings S, Curb J. Physical performance measures in aging research. *J Gerontol.* 1989;44:141–146.

4. Mercer B. Evaluating memory loss in older women. *Wom Health Primary Care.* 1998;1;785–797.

5. McKhann G, Drachman D, Folstein M, Katzman R, Price D, Stadlan E. Clinical diagnosis of Alzheimer's disease: report of the NINCDS-ADRDA work group. *Neurol.* 1984;34:939–944.

6. Corey-Bloom J, Thal L, Galasko D, et al. Diagnosis and evaluation of dementia. *Neurol.* 1995;45:211–218.

7. Folstein MF, Folstein S, McHugh PR, et al. Mini-Mental State, a practical method for grading the cognitive state of patients for the clinician. *J Psychiatr Res.* 1975;12:189–198.

8. Sunderland T, Hill J, Mellow A, Lawlor B, Newhouse P, Grafman J. Clock drawing in Alzheimer's disease: a novel measure of dementia severity. *J Am Geriatr Soc.* 1989;37:725–729.

9. Reisberg B, Ferris SH, deLeon MJ, Crook T. The Global Deterioration Scale for assessment of primary degenerative dementia. *Am J Psychiatry.* 1982;139:1136–1139.

10. Dalton JE, Pederson SL, Blom BE, Holmes NR. Diagnostic errors using the portable mental status questionnaire with a mixed population. *J Gerontol.* 1987;42:512–514.

11. Wechsler D. A standardized memory scale for clinical use. *J Psychol.* 1945;19:87–95.

12. Yesavage J. Development and validation of a geriatric depression scale: a preliminary report. *J Psychiatr Res.* 1983;17:37–49.

13. Beck A. *Beck Depression Inventory.* San Antonio, TX: The Psychological Corporation; 1987.

14. Hamilton M. Development of a rating scale for primary depressive illness. *Br J Soc Clin Psychol.* 1967;6:278–296.

Key Target Area Impairments: Impact on Dementia Clients' Abilities

VISION

A decrease in vision can decrease a client's ability to read, engage in hobbies, and recognize faces and objects.[1] Decreased vision can also affect taking medications, driving, housekeeping, and food preparation. These difficulties are also commonly associated with cognitive impairment. While vision loss is not life-threatening, decreased sensory input can be particularly disabling to clients experiencing baseline cognitive deficits. It can put the client at additional risk if stove dials or diabetic accucheck levels are not seen accurately, for example.

HEARING

Hearing loss is very common in older adults. Like vision loss, it may not be obvious and often goes unnoticed and undetected and remains misunderstood. Hearing loss can compromise the ability to perform activities such as using the telephone, communicating in groups, and driving. In addition to reduced sound, hearing loss can result in distortion of sound and difficulty understanding language. Difficulty understanding speech can lead to social withdrawal and depression. Additional characteristics associated with hearing loss include suspiciousness, sadness, withdrawal, irritability, and fatigue. These characteristics are also commonly associated with dementia.

UPPER EXTREMITY FUNCTION

A decrease in arm function can make it difficult for the client to perform motor skills with hands and arms and limits activities involved in pushing off from a sitting to a standing position, raising arms for bathing, grooming, getting dressed, cooking, and cleaning. Restriction of these activities can lead to dependency and the need for caregiver assistance. The experience of pain in addition to decreased activities can lead to depression. Difficulties commonly associated with decreased arm function are also commonly associated with dementia.

LOWER EXTREMITY FUNCTION

Lack of flexibility of the legs and feet, restricted knee or hip movement, pain, and degenerative changes including the spine and joints can lead to a fear of falling, restriction of activity, loss of confidence, decreased well-being, and increased risk of falls. Cognitive and emotional impairments contribute to the client's risk of falling. Additional factors include a variety of neurological deficits, vision impairment, gait disturbance, loss of muscle strength and coordination, side effects of specific medications (sedatives, hypnotics, tranquilizers, and antihypertensives), and environmental factors. Often multiple factors interact to cause falls.[2]

BLADDER FUNCTION

Urinary incontinence is often unreported, untreated, and mistakenly thought to be a normal part of aging. Incontinence can lead to social isolation, depression, anxiety, falls, skin breakdown, and institutionalization. Cognitive impairment can be a contributing factor in urinary incontinence. Clients with dementia are at highest risk for functional incontinence due to difficulty finding the toilet or recognizing bladder signals; limited mobility; and inability to unbutton, unzip, and undress independently. Environmental barriers such as the lack of a bathroom off of the bedroom can also contribute to functional incontinence.

NUTRITION

Good nutrition emphasizes eating to preserve health. Some of the sources of poor nutrition include medical problems such as chronic constipation, dental problems, social problems such as living alone, financial difficulties, decrease in appetite and physical activity, medications, and difficulty with shopping and cooking. Many clients with dementia, especially those that live alone, do not consume enough calories to have good nutrition. The client with dementia may be unable to drive, thus limiting grocery shopping, and be unable to cook because of difficulty connecting the steps into linked behaviors. As a result, many clients with dementia do not bother to put meals together. Malnutrition can cause physical and mental decline. Malnutrition and dehydration are common causes of memory loss, confusion, and delusions.

MENTAL STATUS

Cognitive function refers to mental and intellectual ability. A decrease in cognitive functioning results in a decrease in overall functioning and a decrease in the ability to perform activities of daily living. Many variables—including the type of dementia, the progression of the disease, and individual functioning—affect the individual client's abilities. For example, a client with early onset Alzheimer's disease may have higher functioning but may be more aware of and distressed by deficits, have higher depression scores, and need more help from caregivers than a client with late onset Alzheimer's disease. On the other hand, the client with early onset Alzheimer's disease may experience psychiatric symptoms of wandering, agitation, hallucinations, and delusions much later than the client with late onset Alzheimer's disease.[3] In this example, the geriatric care manager (GCM) would distinguish early onset Alzheimer's disease from an early stage of late onset Alzheimer's disease and develop a plan of care based on the unique needs of the client and family.

EMOTIONAL FUNCTIONING

Screening the client for depression is essential, as the client with undiagnosed depression will have greater difficulty making decisions. Clinical depression is treatable and not a normal part of aging. Depression coexists with dementia in 30% to 40% of the older population. When the client with dementia and depression is treated, depression and functioning improve.

Brain changes associated with dementia often result in behavior and personality changes. Changes in the client's behavior and personality can be very stressful for the client, indicate unmet needs or significant distress, and are significantly correlated with caregiver depression and burden.[4]

ACTIVITIES OF DAILY LIVING AND INSTRUMENTAL ACTIVITIES OF DAILY LIVING

The performance of activities of daily living (ADLs) and instrumental activities of daily living (IADLs) depends on factors such as sustained attention, motivation, and motor performance. It is difficult to predict from mental status screening instruments which ADLs and IADLs are likely to be affected.[5] In a study of community-dwelling people with Alzheimer's disease, ADLs such as walking, eating, toileting, traveling outside the home, and watching television were attempted by almost all people. Handling mail, writing, reading, discussing current events, and using household appliances were performed by most people with mild to moderate Alzheimer's disease but were attempted by fewer than 20% of severely demented people (Mini Mental State Examination < 10). Managing a checkbook was attempted by fewer than 10% of the people in the study.

SOCIAL SUPPORT

Social support is important in assisting the client with dementia in ADLs and IADLs. Emotional support from family members and friends is also critical. A related issue is caregiver burden. Social support and caregiver burden are multidimensional.[6] Caregiver stressors include the physical and psychological burden of caregiving as well as the indirect stressors of other family members, work strain, and financial distress. Opportunities to experience fun, leisure, and recreation can alleviate caregiver stress.

PHYSICAL AND SOCIAL ENVIRONMENT

The more frail the client, the more he or she depends on his or her environment for support.[7] The client is sensitive to cues in the environment, especially when there is memory impairment. The GCM conducts the assessment in the environment where the client resides. This is in contrast to the traditional health care assessment/evaluation, which is conducted in the health care provider's environment. The assessment in the client's environment provides a unique opportunity that does not exist anywhere else. In the client's environment, the GCM can see how the client lives and get a sense of the client's daily routine. The assessment provides a clearer picture of the relationship between the client's functional strengths and limitations and the environment. It also allows the client to demonstrate his or her best or usual functioning in his or her familiar environment.

NOTES

1. Kosnik W, Winslow L, Kline D, Rasinski K, Sekuler R. Visual changes in daily life throughout adulthood. *J Gerontol: Psychological Sci.* 1988;43:63–70.

2. Funk S, Tornquist E, Champagne M, Wiese R. *Key Aspects of Elder Care.* New York: Springer Publishing; 1992.

3. Gross P. Early-onset Alzheimer's disease: clinical, genetic, neuropathological, and treatment issues. *GCM J.* 2000;10:14–20.

4. Kinney J, Stephens M. Caregiving hassles scale: assessing the daily hassles of caring for a family member with dementia. *Gerontologist.* 1989;29:328–332.

5. Galasko D, Bennett D, Sano M, et al. An inventory to assess activities of daily living for clinical trials in Alzheimer's disease. *Alzheimer Dis Associated Disord.* 1997;11:S33–S39.

6. Antonucci T, Sherman A, Vandewater E, et al. Measures of social support and caregiver burden. *Generations.* 1997;Spring:48–51.

7. Hogue C. Injury in late life. *J Am Geriatr Soc.* 1982;30:276–280.

Referral Checklist

____ Is the primary care provider aware of the geriatric care manager's functional assessment?

____ Has a recent history and physical, including neurological exam, been conducted?

____ Have the necessary laboratory and diagnostic tests been ordered?

____ Has a differential diagnosis been made and communicated to the client and family?

____ Are there coexisting conditions such as adverse drug reactions, infection, or acute confusion?

____ Have current interventions (e.g., pharmacologic) requiring physician orders been initiated?

CHAPTER 13

Depression and the Older Adult: The Role of the Geriatric Care Manager

Miriam K. Aronson

Depression is not a normal part of aging, despite common misconceptions. Rather, it is a serious but very treatable illness. Depression remains underreported by older persons themselves, underrecognized by informal and formal caregivers, and undertreated by health professionals. This chapter will discuss the phenomenology of depressive illness in older persons and the role of the professional geriatric care manager (GCM) in its assessment and management.

Approximately 15% of Americans over the age of 65 report clinically significant depressive symptoms, but only approximately one-fifth of these individuals meet the criteria for major depression. The rest suffer from depression-related clinical and subclinical states. Prevalence rates are the highest among those in nursing homes and those in primary care settings and lowest (less than 3%) among healthy community-residing older people.[1,2]

Risk factors for depression in older persons are similar to those for younger populations; namely, it is more likely to affect women, persons who are unmarried, persons who are widowed, persons undergoing stress, and persons with poor social support systems. But *comorbid medical illness* is the hallmark of depression in older persons, the major difference between depression in older persons and depression in younger persons. In younger persons, the predominant comorbid disorders are personality disorders and substance abuse.

Symptoms of major depression, as defined by the fourth edition of the *Diagnostic and Statistical Manual* of the American Psychiatric Association, include a pervasive sad mood that lasts for more than 2 weeks or a markedly decreased interest or pleasure in all activities *plus* at least three or four of the following symptoms: sleep disturbance, decreased energy, poor concentration, appetite disturbance or problems, psychomotor retardation or agitation, feelings of worthlessness or guilt, and suicidal ideation.[3] Crying may be part of the depressive symptom complex. However, in and of itself, crying does not mean depression. It may be an involuntary poststroke phenomenon or a manipulative strategy. Expressions of guilt are less prevalent in older than in younger depressed individuals.[4] In older persons, there may be a range of physical complaints, as in the case of Mrs. W.

THE CASE OF MRS. W

Mrs. W was an 89-year-old widowed woman who had resided in an upscale assisted living facility for several years. She had a part-time private-duty aide to assist with bathing, grooming, and mobility. Mrs. W had been a controlling matriarch most of her life. She had a husband who was dominated by her, and she had three very devoted children. She had experienced episodic bouts of depression throughout her life and had exaggerated complaints of pain at various times. Her medical care was fragmented and resulted in polypharmacy. Most recently, a pain practitioner had prescribed strong drugs for osteoporosis-associated pain. The drugs were not taken as prescribed; in fact, Mrs. W developed a "stash" of pills that became a concern to her family and physicians and a tool for her to manipulate her family. She had alienated her primary care physician and was dissatisfied with her current medical care. Over the past few months, she had become increasingly unhappy. She withdrew from her accustomed activities and became more isolated. In addition, she had complaints of sleeplessness, fatigue, loss of appetite, inability to concentrate, pain, and loneliness. Despite treatment with pain medication and anxiolytic drugs (in addition to her blood pressure, heart, and osteoporosis medications), her depressive symptom complex did not abate. The more unhappy she was, the more demanding she became of her children, who were concerned about her but frustrated by her lack of response to all of the medications and physician visits, the beautiful environment in which she lived, and all of their efforts. They asked a GCM for a consultation.

Despite Mrs. W's being in an assisted living facility where there were opportunities for socialization, she was isolated and felt very alone. She had limited her activities to watching television, listening to music, and playing a very occasional bridge game. She did not attend any facility activities regularly and rarely ventured outside of the facility, despite her children's invitations and willingness to transport her.

The role of the GCM here was to assess Mrs. W in her facility and to develop a care plan. The GCM identified fragmentation of medical care, polypharmacy, and depression as areas of immediate concern in this cognitively intact woman. Additionally, her loneliness and social isolation were prominent. The GCM recommended that Mrs. W have a comprehensive medical evaluation by a geriatrician and that she engage the geriatrician to be her primary care physician. The geriatrician recommended an antidepressant and also set about addressing the pain and polypharmacy. The GCM also recommended emotional support for Mrs. W and her children, with a goal of improving her affect and also increasing her socialization and physical activity. Mrs. W was resistant to suggestions about nonpharmacologic interventions such as physical therapy, exercise, increased socialization, and a later bedtime.

The high comorbidity of medical illnesses and late life depression and the infinite combinations of medical and mood symptoms pose diagnostic and classification challenges to clinicians across all settings. Anxiety is associated with depression but also with other medical and psychiatric disorders. With depression and anxiety, older persons tend toward expressing their problems as somatic complaints, which they perceive as less stigmatizing than psychiatric illness.[5]

Because of the complex nature of late life depression and the multisystem involvement, there is a need for flexible and multidimensional approaches to treatment; thus, it has been proposed that late life depression be considered a geriatric syndrome rather than a single categorical disease.[6] This suggested classification may also be applied to other prevalent conditions, including cognitive impairment, incontinence, falls, and malnutrition.

Unexpected changes in life circumstances are common in the lives of older persons and are social and demographic risk factors for late life affective disorder. There are also losses of roles and losses of function. Feelings of grief over these losses are not uncommon. There are disease-related losses of physical function. Losses of friends and relatives are frequent, and the social support network inevitably shrinks. Changes in living arrangements may become necessary and these changes exacerbate feelings of loss and unhappiness. In fact, recently admitted nursing home residents are an at-risk population for depression (Exhibit 13–1).[7]

Bereavement is common for individuals of advanced ages. Grieving is a normal process and does not always require intervention; however, for some individuals, grief becomes pathological and requires psychological and pharmacologic intervention. Little information is available regarding when "normal grief" becomes "pathological grief," when treatment is required, and which interventions are most appropriate. Older adults are more likely than younger adults to develop a major depression following bereavement.[6]

Little is currently known about the relationship between depression and medical illness.

Exhibit 13–1 Sociodemographic Situations Associated with Depression

- Retirement
- Multiple role losses
- Bereavement
- Deaths of family members and friends
- Loneliness and isolation
- Responsibility for care for an older person with a disability
- Residence in a nursing home
- Elder abuse
- Neglect
- Substance abuse

Depressive disorders may themselves cause or contribute to medical illnesses. Conversely, medical illnesses may cause or contribute to depression (Exhibit 13–2).[8] Each condition complicates recovery from the other. Unfortunately, most clinical drug studies involving depressed older people have excluded persons with significant medical illness.[9]

Exhibit 13–2 Medical Conditions Associated with Late Life Depression

Cardiac and vascular conditions
  Myocardial infarction
  Cerebrovascular accident
Other medical conditions
  Acute pain
  Chronic pain
Neurological conditions
  Dementia
  Parkinson's disease
  Cancer
Physical disabilities
  Hip fracture
  Loss of mobility
  Trauma
Sensory impairments
  Vision problems
  Hearing decrements

Depression negatively impacts quality of life, functionality, physical health status, longevity, and family and other interpersonal relationships. Depression causes "excess disability," complicating the course of illnesses, slowing recovery, and compromising the impact of interventions such as rehabilitation. Depression is often a "silent partner" responsible for resistance to care, inconsistency of course, and negativity. It also causes excess pain and suffering. In addition to its social, psychological, and physical toll on affected individuals, depression is associated with significant costs to the health care system. Medical outcome studies have revealed that only serious heart disease had a greater negative influence on functional status and bed days than did depression and only arthritis had a greater association with pain.[10]

SUICIDE

Suicide is the extreme and life-threatening potential outcome of depression. Studies of depressed people have shown that their risk for death by suicide is approximately 30 times greater than for the general population.[10] Individuals with major affective disorder have been estimated to have a lifetime suicide mortality rate of 19%. Other research suggests that there is an increased risk of suicide in late life affective illness. Americans over age 65 have a suicide rate that is 50% higher than that of the general population. Older men have the highest suicide rate (38 per 100,000, but 50 per 100,000 near age 85).[11] While more women attempt suicide, more men succeed. The most significant risk factor for suicide is a previous suicide attempt. This and other risk factors are listed in Exhibit 13–3.

A study of primary care patients revealed that relatively few suicide completers had been treated by mental health professionals. In a study of suicide completers 75 or older, about three-quarters had seen a physician within 1 month and 35% within 1 week of death. Although a substantial number of these persons were determined, by psychological autopsy, to have substantial psychopathology, many were not treated at all. Among those whose psychopathology was

Exhibit 13–3 Risk Factors for Suicide in Later Life

- Previous suicide attempt
- Prior depression or other psychiatric diagnosis
- Advanced age
- Poor social support
- Delirium
- Advanced medical disease
- Lifelong alcohol abuse
- Substance abuse
- Poorly controlled pain
- High level of hopelessness

recognized by their physicians, treatment was inadequate.[9] Thus, suicide prevention is a very important role for the primary care physician.[12]

The GCM plays a very important role in the diagnosis and management of depression. He or she is on the front line and must recognize the presence of depression and initiate the diagnostic and treatment processes. In older persons, depressive symptoms may be present as physical complaints such as pain, fatigue, appetite changes, or sleep problems. A comprehensive psychosocial evaluation by the GCM will include obtaining information about severity of depressive symptoms, alcohol, or other substance abuse, suicidal ideation, plans for suicide, prior suicide attempts, impulsivity, and hopelessness.[13] Self-neglect may also be an indication that an older person is at risk for self-injurious behavior. It is often hidden and likely very much underreported. It is incumbent on the GCM to look for and report signs of self-neglect. These may include unexplained weight loss, poor hygiene, poor housekeeping, or lack of compliance with medical regimens.

SCREENING INSTRUMENTS

There are standardized screening tools that can be administered easily and at least "flag" depression as a possible problem. Some of the more commonly used screening tools are the Geriatric Depression Scale, the Zung Self-Rating Depression Scale, the Depression Inventory, and the Hamilton Depression Inventory. Some

of these instruments are described elsewhere, including Chapter 12 and an article by Aronson and Shiffman.[14] These instruments are not diagnostic, but abnormal scores indicate a need for medical or psychiatric evaluation and further follow-up. Which tool is selected is not as critical as the need for the GCM to include depression screening in the clinical assessment. This procedure will be 10 or 15 minutes very well spent. A history of other psychiatric conditions must be obtained as well.

Getting a depressed older person to agree to medical evaluation and treatment may be easier said than done. Resistance may manifest itself as denial, a struggle for power, nastiness, or fear. The GCM must always keep in mind that most older persons do not consult psychiatrists. Rather, they are treated for psychiatric symptoms by their primary care physicians, if at all. Thus, the GCM must establish rapport with the client, his or her family, and his or her primary care physician. It may take substantial time and effort to get the client to agree to an evaluation, let alone treatment. A substantial proportion of individuals may never agree to evaluation or treatment.

DIAGNOSING DEPRESSION

As noted above, depression is not a normal part of aging and can cause unnecessary discomfort and diminished quality of life. It is important that younger persons not impose their fears and stereotypes about old age on older persons.[15] Depressive illness covers a spectrum of conditions, including dysthymia, minor depression, situational depression, and major depression. Because of depressive illnesses' high comorbidity with medical illness in later life, a comprehensive assessment is recommended for differential diagnosis. Elements of a diagnostic workup are listed in Exhibit 13–4.

The GCM must work collaboratively with the physician to obtain a differential diagnosis and develop and implement a feasible care plan. The GCM can be an important resource for the physician, since he or she is able to offer insights into the client's living arrangement, family re-

Exhibit 13–4 Diagnostic Workup for Late Life Depression

- Psychosocial history
- Mental status (cognitive) screen
- Depression screen
- Assessment of activities of daily living and instrumental activities of daily living
- Assessment of sleep and activity patterns
- Assessment of severity of depressive symptoms
- Assessment of suicidal ideation and history of prior attempts
- Medical history
- Review of prescription and over-the-counter medications
- Physical examination
- Routine diagnostic tests (e.g., electrocardiogram), laboratory tests, or imaging (computed tomography scan or magnetic resonance imaging), if indicated to clarify diagnosis
- Psychiatric consultation, if needed for clarification
- Neuropsychological testing, if needed for clarification

lationships, social network, functional abilities, beliefs, compliance, coping style, and other factors that must be taken into account in determining appropriate treatment and management strategies.

DEPRESSION AND DEMENTIA

Symptoms of depression and dementia may overlap or occur as comorbidities with other medical conditions as well as with each other.[16] For example, vitamin deficiencies may present with depression as well as dementia. Hyperthyroidism may present with symptoms of decreased interest and energy, symptoms that are common to both depression and dementia. On close review, many symptoms are similar but not identical (Table 13–1).

For example, the sad affect of a depressed individual may often be confused with the blank affect of an individual with dementia. The lack of response to questions or slow responsiveness of the depressed individual due to poor concentration may superficially appear to be similar to the loss of memory of the individual with dementia. Poor hygiene and self-neglect may be common to both conditions. These similarities are confounded by the fact that depression occurs concurrently in about 35% of dementia cases.[17] The presence of depression often causes excess disability, worsening the dementia symptoms. Evaluation and treatment of both the dementia and the depression are warranted.[18]

The case of Mrs. C is illustrative of the fact that depression and dementia often coexist.

THE CASE OF MRS. C

Mrs. C presented to the GCM with early dementia after her husband and family had consulted with the GCM regarding care planning on several occasions. They were heartbroken by the diagnosis and fearful of the future. Mrs. C had been diagnosed with an "Alzheimer-type dementia" and was on no medication or other active treatment. She was an attractive, physically active, and extremely social woman in her early sixties. She verbalized anxiety about her condition and fear about her future. She described having "night terrors" with a recurrent dream about being in a coffin. She described crying spells. She also was unable to experience pleasure in her activities as much as she had previously. She had loved entertaining family and friends but had withdrawn from this activity. She had also started napping in the afternoon, which had never been part of her daily routine. The GCM believed that this individual had a comorbid clinical depression and guided the family into obtaining a psychiatric evaluation and active treatment for the depression. Additionally, the family was urged to seek the pharmacotherapies that were available for the cognitive impairment. The client's depression was brought under control and the overlay of "excess disability" was diminished. The family was advised to have her discontinue driving the car and to hire a companion, who would help Mrs. C participate in activities and would ensure mobility and socialization. These comprehensive interventions helped to stabilize her and en-

Table 13–1 Symptoms of Depression and Dementia

	Depression	Dementia
Affect/mood/demeanor	Pervasive sadness, dourness, negativity	Blank matter-of-fact expression Possible overlay of sadness
Memory	Poor concentration and temporary memory decrease	Progressive impairment of short-term memory, eventually long-term memory
Function	Functional ability diminished by lack of motivation	Functional ability (activities of daily living and instrumental activities of daily living) diminished by declining abilities
Organization	Impaired decision making	Impaired executive function (e.g., organization, prioritization)
Orientation	Intact or impaired orientation	Impaired orientation
Language	Slowed language	Trouble finding words and naming things
Motivation	Impaired motivation	Possible impaired motivation
Appetite/weight	Either decreased appetite and weight or increased appetite and weight	Trouble remembering to eat Decrease in weight with no obvious explanation
Sleep	Possible problems falling asleep, staying asleep, or waking up	Possible sleep problems or no sleep problems
Thinking/reasoning; Ability to learn	Slow thinking and reasoning Ability to learn is retained Inability to learn new things	Impairment
Danger	Possible suicide	Safety concerns because of impaired judgment
Somatic complaints/pain	Possible multiple or exaggerated somatic complaints Fatigue	Complaints that are underreported or perseverated upon Fatigue
Depression screening tool	Possible high scores	Possible high scores or low scores

able her to participate in a range of daily activities. Mrs. C remained on a plateau for at least a year but then experienced a gradual but noticeable deterioration. Her activities were adjusted and readjusted as her cognitive and functional abilities changed.

The overlay of depression in Mrs. C had eluded several physicians, including the primary care physician, who allegedly knew Mrs. C well. This is not uncommon.[19] The GCM was able to step in and facilitate the needed medical intervention. The treatment of the depression unquestionably improved the client's and family's quality of life. In the course of the GCM's work with this family, there had been care planning, entitlement counseling, advocacy, counseling about available programs and resources, and emotional support for the client, spouse and family. The spouse developed a clinical depression in response to the worsening of his wife's condition, which he had difficulty accepting and for which he resisted treatment.

In this case, the client was quite verbal and there were reliable historians to query, so needed historical information was available to the GCM to suggest that the client was depressed. Depression may be difficult to assess in individuals who live alone because they may be poor historians and there may be no one available to objectively report changes in socialization, motivation, sleep, anxiety, performance of activities of daily living, and nutritional status. In these situations, the GCM may have to locate an informant—a relative, friend, or neighbor who sees the client frequently and is familiar with his or her day-to-day life. Additionally, the GCM may have to make several observations over a period of weeks or months to ascertain the existence and persistence of depressive symptoms.

In the course of determining a differential diagnosis, there is a third "D," delirium, that must be taken into account along with depression and dementia.[20] Delirium is a state of acute confusion to which older persons with dementia are more vulnerable than older persons without dementia. Depression, dementia, and delirium are compared in Table 13–2.

The GCM, who follows clients regularly and knows their behaviors and routines, may be the first to identify a precipitous change in condition such as the development of a delirium. If a delirium is suspected, it is important that medical intervention be obtained immediately, as delirium may be a life-threatening condition.

DEPRESSION AND CAREGIVERS

Approximately 80% of the care of older persons is provided by family caregivers; spouses, who may be older and frail themselves; or adult children, most commonly daughters and daughters-in-law. Caregiving is a demanding job that often becomes overwhelming. For this reason, depression is quite prevalent among caregivers. Studies of caregivers of individuals with dementia indicate that the prevalence of depression is approximately 35%. The GCM must be sensitive to this possibility and must consider it in the assessment and care planning process. The depression of the caregiver impacts both caregiver and client. Research has indicated that depressed persons were less likely to recover when their caregivers reported more psychiatric symptoms, more difficulties in providing care, and poorer physical health themselves.[21] Unfortunately, caregivers resist seeing themselves as people who themselves need interventions, which have been shown to be effective.[22]

THE CASE OF MS. A

Ms. A, a 55-year-old widow and only child, had been the primary caregiver to her 84-year-old mother for 15 years. For most of this time, she also held a responsible full-time job. When she was forced to retire because of corporate reorganization, she became a full-time caregiver. As hard as Ms. A worked as a caregiver, her mother's dementia progressed, the incontinence worsened, and so, too, did her mother's propensity to fall. After about a year of full-time caregiving, Ms. A was considering placing her mother in a nursing home because the physical and emotional demands of caregiving had become overwhelming. As she deliberated over the decision to place, she herself began to cry frequently, had difficulty making decisions, had sleep problems, and had other classic signs of clinical depression. She became increasingly isolated and lonely. She became immobilized in the face of the need to make a decision and was unable to make the placement. With much encouragement from a GCM, she joined a caregiver support group and was advised to seek psychiatric evaluation and treatment for her depression. With group, individual, and psychopharmacologic interventions, she was able to make the placement successfully. This enabled her to mobilize herself to reenter the work force,

Table 13–2 The Three Ds: Depression, Dementia, and Delirium

	Depression	Dementia	Delirium
Onset	Usually within a period of weeks	Slow, insidious, over a period of months/years	Abrupt, may be within hours or days
Symptoms	Pervasive sadness or loss of pleasure, plus vegetative signs	Gradual decline in functioning, including recent memory loss	Fluctuation in consciousness and attention Possible hallucinations, delusions
Course	Episodic, treatable, resolvable	Progressive, manageable	Treatable, usually resolvable
Consequences	May complicate course of other illnesses May lead to decrease in self-care May lead to suicide and various safety problems	Results in decrease in ability to perform activities of daily living, poor judgment, and decreased ability to learn	May be harbinger of medical illness Can flag life-threatening emergency Requires prompt medical intervention
Phenomenology	Can coexist with other Ds, causing "excess disability," and may complicate course of other illnesses	May make depression and delirium harder to recognize	Is more prevalent in persons with dementia and hospitalized patients
Treatment	Multiple simultaneous interventions	Multiple simultaneous interventions	Medical intervention first, to address underlying illness

to rebuild her personal life, and to decrease her isolation and loneliness. In this case, the caregiver's immobility and inability to make the placement decision caused her pain and suffering and also denied her mother the level of care she truly needed. Once the caregiver responded to the interventions she required, the placement of the parent with dementia was able to occur.

The tasks of the GCM in this case were to assess both client and caregiver and to develop a care plan—in this case, placement of the older person with dementia and intervention for the overwhelmed caregiver. The GCM had to work with the caregiver, institution, and physician to facilitate the placement. She also had to recommend and support appropriate treatment for the

caregiver's depression and provide emotional support. It is incumbent on the GCM to educate and advise family caregivers about available resources for themselves as well as for the person for whom they are caring. In this case, the GCM was instrumental in supporting Ms. A through the process of rebuilding her life and her career and was able to witness the resilience of this caregiver.

Caregivers may themselves be resistant to following an appropriate care plan. This is especially true when it comes to making tough decisions such as taking over the finances or placing a loved one in a nursing home. Deciding to place a loved one is one of the hardest decisions a caregiver may ever have to make. The case of

Ms. A illustrates the painfulness of the placement decision and how caregivers can get stuck in a vicious cycle of depression, guilt, martyrdom, and self-neglect.

THE CASE OF MS. H

Ms. H, a 60-year-old widow, cares for her ailing father, who lives with her in a housing arrangement that is unsuited to her father's mobility limitations. Her father has severe cardiovascular disease with a history of stroke and a mixed (vascular and Alzheimer's) dementia. Access to their apartment involves a steep flight of stairs that her father is physically incapable of navigating. Ms. H holds a full-time job and uses a combination of part-time in-home caregivers and day care to get through the days. Both the client and the caregiver have limited incomes and assets.

While her father can be very pleasant at times, he is generally difficult to manage and resistive to personal care. He has intermittent sleep disturbance, which leaves Ms. H perpetually tired, frustrated, and angry. When she yells at him, she feels guilty; yet she cannot contain her anger.

Ms. H is an only child and is estranged from her children. She had a difficult upbringing, and so did her children. The family issues remain unresolved. She gets no help from her children, only criticism when she sees them occasionally. Ms. H cries easily, is anxiety ridden, and is frustrated. Physically, the caregiving is getting more difficult, and she is "maxed out" on the amount of help she can afford to hire to supplement what is supplied under the benefits entitlement system.

While her own health was deteriorating, with potentially serious conditions she tried to ignore, she was struggling with the idea of placing her father in a nursing home. Her ambivalence prevented her from acting. She felt guilty even thinking about placement, although she was overwhelmed and her father was not getting as much care as he needed. Although placement would allow her to break the vicious cycle she was in and become free enough to begin rebuilding her own life, she remained overwhelmed and immobilized. It took more than a year before she

was able to accomplish the placement. She became clinically depressed after placement and refused to visit her father for several weeks.

The GCM worked with Ms. H and supported her emotionally through this difficult time. The GCM also urged Ms. H to seek medical evaluation for pharmacotherapy to treat her depression so she could begin to cope with the placement and begin the process of rebuilding her own life. Placing an older person in an institutional setting is often traumatic and increases emotional distress, which may require crisis intervention.

Depression is generally underreported by older people themselves and underrecognized and undertreated by their health care providers, whether in primary care settings or specialized settings such as the rehabilitation hospital or the nursing home. Older people are underrepresented on the rosters of psychiatrists and other mental health professionals. If they choose to report their depressive problems at all, their therapist of choice is their primary care physician. There are definitely gaps in the treatment of depression in older people, and those gaps are related to transfer of knowledge, practice patterns, and therapeutic nihilism on the part of both depressed people and health practitioners.

Treatment for depression is available in outpatient settings, inpatient settings, and with increasing frequency, in day hospital programs—also called partial hospitalization or intensive outpatient programs. While hospitalization is necessary in severe cases, it is not always the best setting for frail older persons. Unfortunately, Medicare reimbursement favors inpatient hospitalization. For inpatient services, Medicare reimburses treatment for psychiatric illness as it would medical illness. For outpatient treatment, however, there are financial disincentives, including a large copayment (50%) and an annual limit for physician reimbursement. Furthermore, Medicare does not provide reimbursement for outpatient prescription drugs, which can be quite expensive.

Pharmacologic and nonpharmacologic interventions have been shown to be effective in treating depression.[23–26] When pharmacotherapy is utilized, doses must be therapeutic and clients must be closely followed. Pharmacotherapies may not be sufficient in and of themselves, but may make depressed individuals more amenable to other interventions. Supportive therapy is often effective in helping those older persons with adjustment disorders or difficulties in adaptation to losses or other stressors. Problem-solving therapies have been reported to be a suitable modality. Group or individual sessions may be utilized.[27] There is no evidence that any one therapeutic modality is better than another, and an eclectic approach may be warranted. Social and family support is integral to recovery, so it is incumbent on the GCM and other involved clinicians to mobilize, educate, and support the members of the afflicted individual's family and social network. While loss and infirmity are common, depression must be seen as an illness, separate from sadness over illness or loss. Therapeutic goals must be realistic. Older persons need to be treated so they can find meaning in their lives, despite their limitations.

There is a dearth of well-designed outcome studies on treatment of depression in older persons in general and frail older persons in particular. Most of the existing studies have been done on inpatient populations, which are not necessarily a representative sample of older depressed individuals. The data suggest that there is a higher degree of recidivism than for younger depressed persons. Clinical trials of pharmacologic agents have intentionally included subjects without significant comorbidities. Often, they have had an upper age limit as well. Thus, little is known about outcomes of treatment of frail older persons.

Hospitalization is indicated in severe or clinically complex cases or for those persons with no available at-home caregiver. However, for many older persons, hospitalization disrupts the routine of life and can be disorienting. Intensive outpatient treatments such as day hospitals and day treatment programs are good alternatives to hospitalization since they enable depressed persons to maintain their familiar surroundings and social ties.

Severely depressed individuals are always at risk for suicide and should not be left alone. Where supervision cannot be provided by family or paid caregivers, movement to a sheltered setting is indicated. Monitoring the person and making the house safer are important when dealing with a depressed person at home or even a treated person who returns to the community from the hospital. The GCM can be instrumental in this process. The family should be instructed to remove the following items from the home: weapons such as guns and knives and potential weapons such as axes, hammers, razors, and scissors. Poisonous household products such as cleaning solutions and solvents should be removed or locked up. Matches should be kept out of reach. Unused medications must be discarded, and available medications should be kept only in small quantities that are not lethal.

DEPRESSION AND THE ROLE OF THE GCM

The GCM should serve as the linchpin in the process of recognition, diagnosis, and management of depression, not only by working directly with the client, family, and physician but also by working with other health providers and formal and informal caregivers, providing emotional support and training.

Recognizing depression in older persons can be a challenge to professionals and laypersons alike. Professionals are not necessarily immune from ageism and therapeutic nihilism and all too often hold negative sterotypes that delay prompt diagnosis and treatment of depressive symptoms in older persons. This is confounded by the fact that older persons may not tell their health providers or their families directly about their feelings or physical symptoms because of a fear of being labeled "mental" or otherwise stigmatized. Rather, older persons with depression may look, act, or express themselves differently or may demonstrate a generalized "failure to thrive."[28] These changes may be quite apparent to those who know the older persons well but vague or inconclusive to others, including health providers. Thus, it may take time and patience for the health provider to identify the symptoms. Many health providers do not spend this time. In some situations, there may be economic disincentives toward spending the time needed to obtain an adequate history, do a comprehensive assessment, and provide carefully monitored and effective treatment. Thus, there is an ongoing search for a quick fix—perhaps a "magic pill."

THE ROLE OF THE GCM IN TRAINING

How can the GCM promote recognition of depression in frail older persons? Informal and formal caregivers must be taught to observe and assess the usual behavior patterns and activity level of the frail older person, so that they will be able to recognize physical, mental, and emotional changes if they occur. Changes can occur quickly and may have significant consequences. The GCM must make older persons themselves and their caregivers aware that they must not merely accept unexplained changes in mood and function, ascribing them to aging, illness, or loss; rather, they must report these changes to their health providers. It must be emphasized that depression is an illness in and of itself and occurs in addition to social losses and physical infirmities. It is a treatable and manageable illness, with the potential outcome of treatment being an improvement in quality of life for the individual and those around him or her. All depressed individuals, including frail older persons, deserve competent assessment and appropriate treatment.

The GCM must present basic strategies for identifying and managing depression. The starting point in identifying depression or other mood changes is to determine how the client feels and how he or she functions. The GCM will use a combination of techniques to assess the client. Basic assessment techniques include observation and listening. The assessor must listen carefully to what the client says and must get a good history from a reliable informant, if necessary.

As an individual becomes clinically depressed, his or her appearance changes and the assessor must look for these changes. While the changes may be subtle at the beginning and difficult for an individual who sees the client daily to detect, they will probably be apparent to the

Exhibit 13–5 Changes in Appearance

- Newly stooped posture
- Slowing of movement
- Slowing of thought processes
- Unexplained weight loss or weight gain
- Clothing that does not fit
- Poor grooming
- Poor maintenance of clothing
- Poor hygiene
- Diminished energy level
- Unexplained fatigue
- Sad affect

trained eye of the GCM. Possible changes are listed in Exhibit 13–5.

As a clinical depression develops, there will also be changes in behavior and activity level. The GCM must gather this information as well. Some more common behavior and activity level changes are described in Exhibit 13–6.

The affected individual may make statements indicative of hopelessness or self-deprecating comments during the assessment or these types of statements may be reported by the caregiver. Exhibit 13–7 contains some of these statements.

Exhibit 13–6 Changes in Behavior and Activity Level

- Decrease in social participation
- Increase in isolation and social withdrawal
- Decreased interest in things
- Difficulty with decision making
- Difficulty concentrating
- Unusual negativism
- Hopelessness
- Inconsistency
- Newly poor hygiene
- Unexplained anger
- Increased anxiety level
- Increased complaints of pain
- Complaints of sleep difficulties
- Changes in appetite or eating habits
- Noncompliance with medications

Exhibit 13–7 Statements That May Be Indicative of Depression

- I'm not the person I used to be.
- I can't manage to get anything done.
- I'm awake all night and then get to sleep in the morning.
- Nobody can do anything for me.
- I don't care if I die.
- Things are hopeless.
- I don't want to be a burden to anyone.
- I've heard that medicines have too many side effects, so I don't want any.
- I may be nervous, but I'm not mental.
- Who's to care?
- Nobody wants me.
- I'm too poor to afford that.

Exhibit 13–8 Strategies for Communication with and Outreach to a Depressed Person

- Listen.
- Recognize *changes*—trust your eyes, ears, sense of smell, and general intuition.
- Remain calm—do not panic.
- Acknowledge the person's feelings. Do not try to talk the person out of the feelings.
- If the person expresses suicidal ideas, refer the person for immediate psychiatric evaluation and treatment.
- Be reassuring. The person is ill, and things will get better.
- Don't be judgmental. Depression is an illness and not something the person has chosen.
- Provide positive reinforcement, as appropriate.
- Acknowledge positive steps toward recovery.

In working with depressed individuals, caregivers need to use various strategies for interaction and communication. The GCM can serve as a role model in this regard. Suggestions are contained in Exhibit 13–8.

CONCLUSION

Depression is a prevalent and perplexing problem in the geriatric population. It is underacknowledged, underreported, and undertreated at this time. Given the baby boomers' greater knowledge about health issues and psychiatry, tomorrow's older persons will be more likely to seek diagnosis and treatment than today's older generation. The projected explosion of the older population and their increasing longevity make it necessary to address the gaps in information and training regarding depression in older persons and the anticipated shortages of mental health professionals.

NOTES

1. Unitzer J, Simon G, Belin TR, Dott M, Kayton W, Patrick D. Care for depression in HMO patients aged 65 and older. *J Am Geriatr Soc.* 2000:48:871–878.

2. Hughes CM, Lapane KL, Mor V, et al. The impact of legislation on psychotropic drug use in nursing homes: a crossnational perspective. *J Am Geriatr Soc.* 2000;48: 931–937.

3. American Psychiatric Association. *Diagnostic and Statistical Manual of Mental Disorders.* 4th ed. Washington, DC: American Psychiatric Press, 1994.

4. US Department of Health and Human Services. *Depression in Primary Care.* Vol 1. AHCPR Clinical Practice Guideline Number 5. 1993.

5. Smith SL, Sherrill KS, Colenda CC. Assessing and treating anxiety in older persons. *Psychiatr Serv.* 1995;46(1):36–42.

6. Kennedy GJ. The geriatric syndrome of late-life depression. *Psychiatr Serv.* 1995;46:43–48.

7. Hagans E, Hanscom J. Assessment of depression in a population at risk: newly admitted nursing home residents. *J Gerontol Nurs.* 1998;24:21–29.

8. Lyness JM, Bruce ML, Koenig HG, Parmelee PA, Schulz R, Lawton MP, Reynolds CF. Depression and medical illness in late-life: report of a symposium. *J Am Geriatr Soc.* 1996;44:198–203.

9. Caine ED, Lyness JM, Conwell Y. Diagnosis of late-life depression: preliminary studies in primary care settings. *Am J Geriatr Psychiatry.* 1996;4:S45–50.

10. Conwell Y. Outcomes of depression. *Am J Geriatr Psychiatry.* 1996;4:S34–44.

11. Conwell Y, Lyness JM, Duberstein P, et al. Completed

suicide among elder patients in primary care practices. *J Am Geriatr Soc.* 2000;48:23–29.

12. Wittenberg JS. Interventions for older suicidal patients. *Geriatr Consultant.* 1993;12:24–27.

13. Szanto K, Reynolds CF, Conwell Y, Begley AE, Houck P. High levels of hopelessness persist in geriatric patients with remitted depression and a history of attempted suicide. *J Am Geriatr Soc.* 1998;46:1401–1406.

14. Aronson M, Shiffman JK. Clinical assessment in home care. *J Gerontol Soc Work.* 1995;24:213–231.

15. Rimer S. Gaps seen in treating depression in the elderly. *New York Times,* September 5, 1999, 1.

16. Merriam A, Aronson, MK, Gaston P, Wey S, Katz I. The psychiatric symptoms of Alzheimer's disease. *J Am Geriatr Soc.* 1988;36:7–12.

17. Katz I, Aronson MK, Lipkowitz R. Depression secondary to dementia presents an ongoing dilemma. *Generations.* 1982;7:24.

18. Aronson MK, Gaston P, Merriam A. Depression associated with dementia. *Generations.* 1984;9:49–51.

19. Katz IR. What should we do about undertreatment of late life psychiatric disorders in primary care? *J Am Geriatr Soc.* 1998;46:1573–1575.

20. Breitner JCS, Welsh KA. Diagnosis and management of memory loss and cognitive disorders among elderly persons. *Psychiatr Serv.* 1995;46(1):29–35.

21. Hinrichson GA, Zweig R. Family issues in late-life depression. *J Long-Term Home Health Care.* 1994;13:4–15.

22. Mittelman MS, Ferris SH, Shulman E, et al. A comprehensive support program: effect of depression on spouse-caregivers of AD patients. *Gerontologist.* 1995;35(6):792–802.

23. Schneider LS. Pharmacologic considerations in the treatment of late-life depression. *Am J Geriatr Psychiatry.* 1996;4(1):S51–S65.

24. Zistook S. Depression in late-life: special considerations in treatment. *Postgrad Med.* 1996;100(4):161–167.

25. Zarit SH, Knight BG. *A Guide to Psychotherapy and Aging.* Washington, DC; 1996.

26. Duffy M, ed. *Handbook of Counseling and Psychotherapy with Older Adults.* New York: John Wiley & Sons, 1999.

27. Clark WG, Vorst VR. Group therapy with chronically depressed geriatric patients. *J Psychosoc Nurs Mental Health Serv.* 1994;32:9–13.

28. Katz IR, Beaston-Wimmer P, Parmelee P, Friedman E, Lawton MP. Failure to thrive in the elderly: exploration of the concept and delineation of psychiatric components. *J of Geriatr Psychiatry Neurol.* 1993;6:161–169.

CHAPTER 14

Incorporating a Spiritual Perspective into Geriatric Care Management

Leonie Nowitz

In the last decade there has been a growing interest in spirituality in American society and an increasing appreciation for spirituality's valuable contribution to health and well-being.[1] In the health care literature there is evidence that prayer and a belief in a higher power contribute to healing and a general sense of well-being. There is also growing interest in the search and creation of meaning in the second half of life as conferences, courses, and books address these issues under the title of "conscious aging."

The search for meaning and purpose in life often begins at times of illness, crisis, and suffering. A geriatric care manager (GCM) helps older persons and their families, friends, and paid caregivers find meaning and strength in coping with changes in function, increased caregiving, and reduced resources. A spiritual perspective offers the GCM an opportunity to broaden his or her vision of meaning and values and to be open to clients' viewpoints, struggles, and ways of finding meaning in life.

In 1975 the National Interfaith Coalition on Aging defined spiritual well-being as "The affirmation of life in a relationship with God, self, community and environment that nurtures and celebrates wholeness."[2] It is that which unites all aspects of ourselves and brings together concurrent paths of spiritual and psychological well-being. If GCMs can view more positively the frailty and finiteness of life, they can help older persons and their families find meaning and value in their situations, helping them care for each other, accept life's realities, and transmit the value of caring to future generations.

A spiritual view challenges the negative attitudes about aging in a society that celebrates youth, achievement, financial success, and power. This perspective enables GCMs to help their clients find meaning when productivity fails and they become dependent on others.

This chapter will address the meaning of spirituality for older persons and their families and consider the purpose and spiritual tasks of life's last stages. Assessment and intervention tools for the practitioner will be offered. Qualities with which GCMs need to address clients' struggles will also be discussed. The final section discusses the facilitation of spiritual connections with persons who have dementia and their families.

THE PURPOSE OF LIFE'S LAST STAGES

According to Carl Jung, "We cannot live the afternoon of life according to the program of life's morning, for what was great in the morning will be little in the evening and what in the morning was true will in the evening have become a lie."[3] To help clients evaluate their lives, GCMs need to ask several questions. What is the purpose of life after 65? What are clients' values, wishes, and dreams? How can clients stay true to their values and accomplish their dreams?

After age 65, there may be a transition from professional work to volunteer work and from ability to disability. Social networks may diminish as friends move away or die, which leads to an increased focus on family. Changes in family roles may ensue due to changes in health and dwindling resources. Everyone in the family needs to make a shift. As some members increasingly need care, others may need to assume caregiving responsibilities in addition to their current work and family roles. Though painful, transition and loss provide the opportunity to re-evaluate one's life goals. Who am I without my work role, when I am disabled and need to depend on others? Why am I here? What is it I still want to do and be? These important questions were inspired by the work of Schachter-Shalomi and Miller.[4]

By reflecting on these questions and attending to clients' thoughts and values, GCMs can help clients redefine themselves. GCMs can help their clients find meaning in loss by offering a loving presence and allowing a trusting relationship to develop. This process may involve listening to clients mourn and find meaning in their losses as they reflect on their lives, struggles, and strengths, and acknowledging the gifts clients have given and continue to give to others. The GCM needs to transcend the dominant culture's status- and youth-driven values and respect each client's feelings regardless of age, function, and status. When the GCM takes this approach, it can help clients shake off the culture's focus on autonomy and independence and instead see themselves as who they are based on a lifetime of experience.

It is important that GCMs acknowledge and respect a client's values. If a GCM notices a client's kindness, wisdom, dignity, depth, joy, integrity, wholeness, confidence, or peacefulness, the GCM should tell the client. This respect will help clients reestablish a connection within themselves, with other people, and with God, if they so choose.

Kenyon notes that:

> advanced human aging may also be a time for the possibility of a transition from having to being. Something new may now be taking place that goes beyond loss. Inner activity may increase.

Silence provides an opportunity for simply being with oneself which can be peaceful or anxiety provoking through confrontation with new aspects of ourselves. The experience of inner silence and being can result in an increased ability to be present to others, involving the ability to be more open to others and less preoccupied with self.[5(pp4–5)]

To provide a broader framework, it is helpful to consider traditions that offer another perspective. The Hindu tradition embraces loss as a natural part of the life cycle and thinks of the third stage of life as one in which one frees oneself from daily roles and moves to the performing of rituals and the reciting of sacred texts with all energies directed toward union with Brahman, the divine ground of the universe. Losses are considered "modes of liberation contributing to spiritual growth."[6(pp17–21)]

The Western counterpart to the Hindu journey would look upon late life as a natural monastic period.

> The aging process often strips the person of the distracting pleasures of the world by shrinking both actual life space and even the physical ability to participate in the adventures of life. It's as if God offers a new kind of intimacy and says to the frail elderly person, "You have lived a long life enjoying the pleasures of my creation. Sometimes you have enjoyed creation more than you have ME, but I understand because creation is so wonderful. Now that you are housebound and can no longer enjoy the physical and mental pleasures of your past, we have an opportunity to really get to know one another before we meet face to face at your death!"[7(p9)]

Accepting brokenness in a positive light is a part of many spiritual traditions. Most religious traditions view frailty and loss as meaningful, valuable parts of life. The Jewish rabbinical traditions speak of the value of brokenness. The Kotsker rabbi recognizes that nothing is as whole as a broken heart and that the brokenness and deficits create an opening up to possibilities of humility and seeking union with God.[8] Rav Kook noted that a broken heart was beloved before God, and Reb Nachman said that in the brokenness itself is the yearning for God.[8] Similarly, Ralph Waldo Emerson said, "There is a crack in everything God has made."[9] It has been said that as we age, the cracks begin to show. Are they just about darkness and brokenness? Or are they also a place for the light of spirit to stream through?

Spirituality has many faces and takes many forms. It is important to recognize the unique essence of clients, their families, and caregivers and to be open and available to the form of spirituality favored by individual clients and the people around them. There are four ways persons commonly experience their spirituality:

1. as a connection to something beyond themselves that comforts and guides them
2. as a connection to all living things, earth, and the universe
3. as a part of a faith tradition or having a close personal relationship with God or both
4. as a process of finding answers to life's difficult questions

Some older persons tend to turn inward. Others move from the inward view toward more meaningful relationships with others. And others experience spiritual awareness through religious traditions that sustained them in the past.[10] Moberg describes "spiritual" as referring to the very essence of each human being that relates everything consciously or unconsciously and either positively or negatively to God and that makes everyone valuable.[11]

SPIRITUAL TASKS IN OLD AGE

Genevay and Richards question the nature of growth in old age. Is spiritual growth separate from psychological growth, or is there one concurrent path that leads to mental, emotional, and spiritual growth in the last stage of life?[12]

Many believe that there are spiritual tasks to be accomplished in late life. The following tasks were suggested by Father Richard Sweeney at the 1991 American Society on Aging Forum and church and mental health workers at the 1997 American Society on Aging annual meeting:

1. making a conscious effort to know oneself and clarify one's personal values
2. establishing a sense of self-worth apart from life's externals
3. letting go of dimensions of life where there is no longer ability
4. seeking and sharing wisdom and love
5. mentoring others
6. viewing life as imperfect and facing issues of death and the afterlife

Many writers have shared their viewpoints on making meaning. Victor Frankl, a concentration camp survivor, writes about the search for meaning and how one's attitude toward one's experience creates meaning.[13] His works focus on how to turn suffering into human triumph and the importance of self-discovery, responsibility, and self-transcendence. Zalman Schachter-Shalomi and R.S. Miller, in the book *From Age-ing to Sage-ing*, talk about the concept of generativity, harvesting gifts of a lifetime and giving them back to family, friends, and society: "The archetype of the Inner Elder is a divine image representing the wisdom of the ages. This image of the Inner Elder calls forth the wisdom of older people at a time when our culture desperately needs it."[4(p139)] Allan Chinen's work offers much richness in noting the tasks of the elder: "learning to heed the dictates of the soul, being generative in inspiring the younger generations with practical counsel and noble inspiration, seeking self-confrontation and transformation through painful insight and authentic reformation."[14]

Carter Catlett Williams talks about the wonderful opportunity for self-discovery in later years. Paying attention to one's inner life, a person can make later life a time for growth, self-reflection, rediscovery, and self-exploration.[15] Finding meaning through suffering is the focus of Polly Young-Eisendrath, a Jungian psychotherapist who shares stories of people who have sustained major losses to their health and of family members.[16] She describes how they transcended these losses to develop, through their pain, compassion for and understanding of others. Through this process, they learned to accept the impermanence of life and allowed the formation of a new identity.

If GCMs view frailty and brokenness as valuable, meaningful parts of life, they can witness and be present to the suffering of clients. Often GCMs will witness great wisdom, understanding, and courage of their clients and families.

WAYS TO FACILITATE THE SPIRITUAL PROCESS IN GERIATRIC CARE MANAGEMENT

Psychological and spiritual growth can be nurtured by introspection and a search for meaning in life. Some ways the GCM can foster spiritual connection and growth in clients are discussed below.

Life Review

In reviewing their lives with an empathetic listener, clients can find meaning. Clients can review the struggles and the wisdom gained, the values lived and acquired, the mistakes made, and the opportunities missed. Healing can come from the process of facing hurtful experiences and letting go. Telling one's story in the presence of an empathetic listener allows a reworking of it.

Chinen notes that "in remembering the past, older adults transform it. The reflective individual comes to terms with mistakes and opportunities missed, learning to forgive himself and others. The elder embraces the past, not to regress, but to illuminate all of life."[14]

This process can be facilitated by the GCM (who may be a social worker or a nurse), paid caregivers, and family members (to whom the shared stories can transmit history and legacy). GCMs can help get their clients involved in senior center and day care programs. Participating in storytelling and the creative arts can enrich older people's lives and cultivate a sense of community. "When elders hear others reveal dimensions of their lives, they notice similarities and differences with their own experiences. They can be empowered to claim and reclaim the wisdom of their own lives."[17]

The GCM needs to be sensitive to each client's willingness to engage in this process and should engage with clients at their own pace.

Ethical Wills

The tradition of bequeathing a spiritual legacy in a conventional will, a codicil, or a separate document has its roots in the Bible. The desire was to pass on an instructive account of ideas and values close to the older person's heart—an ethical will.[18]

An ethical will can be used to pass values and a sense of what is important in life to future generations. If clients have no family members, the GCM can listen to clients' account of their values, a process that will strengthen the connection between the GCM and the clients. If clients are unable to articulate their values, GCMs can tell clients what they know of them based on stories the GCMs have heard that reflect the clients' values and character. This process will help clients feel that they are being understood and valued. Additionally, it helps clients recall old memories and gives them an opportunity to receive positive feedback and be seen for their deeper values.

For instance, Mr. K, a 96-year-old widower with a moderate degree of dementia, was working with a GCM. The GCM acknowledged Mr. K's generosity to his family and political causes as well as the extensive care he gave to his wife before she died. While he did not initially remember some of these actions, he began to remember his wife, how he loved her, and how important it was for him to make her life comfortable when she was ill. As this example illustrates, when the GCM shares his or her view of the older person's values as exemplified by his or her life story, the older person is validated. This can stimulate memories in an environment of trust.

Prayer and Meditation

Prayer and meditation are common in all religious and spiritual traditions. Eighty-one percent of caregivers for people with Alzheimer's disease say they use prayer in coping with the demands of caregiving.[19] GCMs might consider praying with their clients. They might want to check with family members whether the older person has prayed in the past. GCMs would ask family members whether opportunities for prayer should be provided to the older person. If a GCM is uncomfortable praying with a client or comes from a tradition different from the client's, the GCM could find another professional on the care team (e.g., a nurse, a social worker) who is familiar with the client's religious tradition. Many home care workers are comfortable with prayer and are willing to read from the scriptures and pray with clients, which can give clients a sense of peace and well-being.

Sacred and Secular Rituals

Performing sacred and secular rituals can help clients experience familiar memories and reconnect them with their faith and communal traditions. The GCM can find out what traditions and practices are familiar to clients and help recreate them. For instance, a traditional Christmas or Passover meal could be made. The GCM can ask clients and caregivers to help with planning (e.g., what foods they would like, what readings they would like to have) and can be present at a Passover Seder or Christmas meal. In addition, the GCM can help clients attend services by contacting places of worship to find out about wheelchair accessibility. The GCM can arrange for a friend to accompany the client and/or a caregiver to create more of a feeling of family and community.

Grief Counseling

Grief counseling to resolve the current and multiple losses of a lifetime is important to help clients heal their pain in the presence of a caring and empathic listener. The GCM can provide this counseling or can refer the client to another professional.

Focusing

In focusing, a GCM helps a client clarify and resolve all kinds of issues (e.g., unresolved relationship issues) and make all kinds of decisions (e.g., decisions about health care).

For example, Ms. F's aunt was not able to swallow food after surgery. Her physicians felt that the insertion of a peg tube was necessary to ensure adequate nutrition and hydration. Ms. F was ambivalent about this procedure. She questioned the quality of life of her aunt, who had recently experienced the onset of a dementia. Ms. F thought her aunt would not tolerate being mentally and physically dependent. The GCM helped Ms. F explore her feelings about other relatives who had lived in a seriously vegetative state for several years. The GCM encouraged Ms. F to think about her aunt's life and what interests and people had sustained her. The GCM shared with the niece the possibility that the peg tube might not always be needed if her aunt's condition improved. She encouraged Ms. F to talk with other relatives and explore what Ms. F's aunt would want for herself. Her aunt had not expressed any negative feelings about being ill and dependent. After discussion with family members and review of her aunt's life and her own reactions to others who were disabled, the niece recognized that she needed to come to terms with her aunt's changed functioning. She also realized that her aunt was not as debilitated as her other relatives. The GCM listened to Ms. F's fears about the quality of her aunt's life and helped Ms. F clarify her decision regarding surgery. Ms. F's aunt got the peg tube and after several weeks regained her capacity to swallow.

Broadening Clients' View of Themselves To Include Deeper Values

Many older persons who have suffered losses of family and friends and changes in health tend to view themselves in a negative light. It is helpful to appreciate the deeper values that have sustained and enriched the client.

For example, Mrs. D, a widow who suffered from dementia, had no friends and only a distant relative. She reminisced with the GCM about her life with her husband, a famous physician, and how she enjoyed traveling. "Those were the good days, and they are no more," she said. She described her present existence as one in which God was punishing her by squeezing the life out of her little by little. She focused on her past life, talking about how she was valued for being the beautiful wife of a famous physician. "Then I was something; now I'm nothing," she said. The GCM said, "Mrs. D, I see how valuable your past was to you in terms of your beauty and your sense of adventure. But in addition, I see a woman who has an inner beauty, who loved her husband and took care of him. You were hospitable to his friends and later you volunteered at a hospital and brought much caring to sick people. You visited them and gave so much of yourself." Mrs. D listened but did not respond. The GCM repeated her viewpoint many times because Mrs. D continued to think negatively about herself. The GCM talked to her about the wholeness of life and that if persons defined themselves by only one time in their lives they were bound to feel unworthy at other times that were different. The GCM continued to listen compassionately to Mrs. D's pain and sadness about the losses in her life. She shared what she valued about Mrs. D: "I value your courage and ability to endure the pain of so many losses, your warmth, your kindness, and your wisdom and ability to laugh at life." By reflecting on Mrs. D's lifelong values, the GCM attempted to help Mrs. D appreciate her many positive attributes and acknowledge her inner resources. The GCM brought small problems to Mrs. D from time to time, and Mrs. D reveled in the opportunity to share her wisdom by providing practical solutions. Mrs. D continued to view herself in a diminished capacity but also showed more comfort in being valued and grew more trusting in her relationship with the GCM and her caregivers.

Hearing the Spirit beneath the Words

GCMs working with clients, especially those with dementia, need to listen to the meaning behind the spoken words. Older persons may not always be able to say precisely what they mean, but an attentive and sensitive listener will hear what an older person is really saying.

For example, Mrs. T was frightened of "men" in her bedroom. Her caregivers would check her room each evening to assure her it was empty. She was a religious woman and the GCM asked her pastor to visit her. On his visits he prayed with Mrs. T for God to protect her and keep her safe. He dealt with her feelings without specifically talking about the "men." By praying with her, the pastor acknowledged Mrs. T's fears and offered comfort and a sense of safety.[20]

Awareness of Countertransference

"Countertransference describes the personal feelings that a professional experiences in relation to a client that can affect his or her professional interventions."[21]

In facilitating the spiritual process, GCMs need to be aware of their own values. They can ask, "How can we facilitate resolution of past issues and letting go of emotional baggage that hinders at the end of life? Can we listen to older people and allow them to come to their own recognition of what they need?"[12(pp4–5)] To be effective, the GCM needs to be in touch with his or her own concerns and how he or she resolves them. The client may have a different perspective that needs to be respected, particularly when it conflicts with the GCM's view.

The next section discusses how GCMs can go about examining their own values, spiritual beliefs, and family history.

GCMs LOOK AT THEIR OWN VALUES, SPIRITUAL BELIEFS, AND FAMILY HISTORY

In helping clients deal with the multiple losses in their lives, GCMs are offered the opportunity to examine their own feelings about aging and dying and consider their own values. GCMs should ask themselves these questions: How do I view my own aging? What models of care do I embrace for myself? What makes me anxious and reactive to clients? With what family systems am I most comfortable and uncomfortable? GCMs need to consider values that are acquired from three sources:

1. their family
2. their culture
3. their professional training

GCMs need to be aware of the values they transmit to their clients and the impact of their values on their clients. The following exercise can help GCMs consider their own values at different stages of the life cycle and understand their clients' evolving values and beliefs. By answering the questions for themselves and considering how their clients might answer them, GCMs will broaden their perspective and learn to not impose their values on their clients. The questions were inspired by the work of Schachter-Shalomi and Miller.[4]

- How have you valued yourself at different times of your life?
- What were your beliefs about aging, interdependence, and family connections as a child, as an adolescent, as an adult, and as a person with an illness or a disability?
- Have your values been similar at different stages, or have they changed as you have aged?
- How has your belief system served you throughout your life?
- How does it serve you at a time of loss and diminishment?
- What is the meaning of your life now, despite losses that have taken place?

ASSESSMENT OF CLIENTS' VALUES AND SOURCES OF MEANING

In *Assessing Spiritual Needs: A Guide for Caregivers*, George Fitchett includes a spiritual assessment tool that can help GCMs evaluate their clients' spiritual life and struggles (Exhibit 14–1).[22] The tool contains a number of categories that GCMs need to consider.

This spiritual assessment is part of a holistic assessment that includes the medical, psychological, family systems, psychosocial, ethnic, racial, cultural, and social dimensions that affect

Exhibit 14–1 Spiritual Assessment Tool

1. beliefs of the client that give meaning and purpose to the client's life
2. vocation and obligation: beliefs that create a sense of duty or moral obligation
3. experience and emotion that may be related to the sacred, the divine, or the demonic
4. courage and growth
5. ritual and practice
6. community
7. authority and guidance

older persons. This tool provides a comprehensive picture of a client. The text below considers each of the seven dimensions listed in Exhibit 14–1 in turn, with illustrative cases discussed for each dimension.

Beliefs That Give Meaning and Purpose

GCMs should ask what beliefs a person has that give meaning and purpose to his or her life. These can be religious beliefs and practices of the past. There are also other sources from which persons derive meaning and purpose.

Mrs. N

Mrs. N, a 75-year-old African-American woman who was divorced and living alone and a very feisty and strong-spirited person, lost one of her daughters a few years ago. She had another daughter who lived out of town, as did several siblings. Diagnosed with Alzheimer's disease, she gradually accepted a few hours of home care over a long period of time and sporadically visited a day care center. A woman who was very autonomous, she found it difficult to receive help. During one visit the GCM asked her what gave her the strength to deal with her memory loss and life situation. She said she had been raised as a Catholic and went to church all her life. She talked about God in personal terms, "I feel God is close to me—whatever happens during the day I talk to him at night and he listens. I couldn't be this age and in the world without God. He gives me strength in difficult times." The GCM asked Mrs. N about the times things did not work out the way she had hoped. She said "I accept God's will. My mother died; she might have suffered more if she had lived. God does what is best." Mrs. N's faith and personal relationship with God gave her courage and strength to face her deteriorating health and the losses in her life. The GCM's interest in what gave Mrs. N strength encouraged Mrs. N to talk about her strong belief in and relationship with God.

Mrs. B

Mrs. B, who had a moderate dementia, talked about her very strong connection to nature by reflecting on the woods outside her apartment and how comforting it was to have the trees there. "I have always loved nature; my family found it a source of nourishment and strength," she said. Some of Mrs. B's frightening dreams found resolution in the woods. Mrs. B's source of healing and support was her lifetime connection with nature. Nature was a nurturing and reassuring presence in times of difficulty. The GCM acknowledged and helped Mrs. B remember her connection with and comfort in nature.

Mr. J

Mr. J was a 95-year-old widower with severe sensory losses who walked minimally and suffered from moderate to severe dementia. Prior to his illness, he was an engineer who traveled extensively with his wife. While his interests were wide-ranging prior to his illness, once he was ill Mr. J was confined to his apartment, where he watched ballgames and nature shows and enjoyed going to the nearby park to feed the squirrels and watch the boats sail by. These activities were the central focus of his day. Mr. J drew pleasure and a sense of connection from the park (he always loved nature) and from ballgames; these were activities he enjoyed in the past and could continue to enjoy. The GCM shared Mr. J's enthusiasm for ballgames. She also discussed with him the pleasure he got from feeding the squirrels and watching activities in the park.

Vocation and Obligation

It is important to consider the client's or their caregivers' beliefs and whether they create a sense of duty or moral obligation. Are clients or their caregivers able to fulfill these obligations, or are clients and caregivers frustrated and guilty about not being able to fulfill them? Both the older client's and the family member's sense of obligation may provide stress, but there may be positive experiences such as a strengthened relationship.

Mrs. C

Mrs. C's health was deteriorating rapidly due to her congestive heart failure and multiple health problems. Her daughter hired a GCM to assess her mother's situation and to provide counseling to her mother as her health declined. She also had the GCM arrange home care and access other resources. The daughter was very stressed but continued to coordinate her mother's medical care and call her daily. The GCM noted the stress the daughter experienced because of the time associated with Mrs. C's care and the emotional drain of her mother's illness and decline. The GCM listened to her concerns about her mother and the emotional drain of caregiving. The GCM offered to help her with some tasks, but the daughter refused, feeling obliged to continue her role as primary caregiver. In ongoing discussions, she talked about the stress and drain of caregiving. After several months of the daughter refusing to accept any help, the GCM asked the daughter why she continued to do as much as she did. She said it helped her feel connected to her mother. This helped the GCM understand the meaning of her sense of obligation and to continue to be respectful of her wishes. In time the daughter was able to let go of the daily coordination of care and continued her daily calls to her mother, which gave her that continued sense of connection.

It is important for a GCM to understand the meaning of the caregiver's caregiving experiences and to be respectful of the caregiver while acknowledging the stress of caregiving. The GCM needs to respect the caregiver's timetable and wait until he or she is willing to relinquish tasks to the GCM or to others in the system.

Experience and Emotion

The GCM needs to ask what direct contact with the sacred, divine, or demonic the older person has had. What emotions or moods are associated with these contacts and with the person's beliefs and sense of meaning in life? What past illnesses or crises in life were connected with spiritual experiences? How does spirituality affect the current situation? What sources or rituals provide comfort?

Mrs. G

Mrs. G was a 91-year-old widow, a musician who lived with her caregivers and who was visited by her two sons regularly. Her sons hired the GCM to oversee Mrs. G's care, as they were frequently out of town. Mrs. G had strong mood swings, which may have been due to a long-standing personality disorder or to dementia. A strong-willed women who was not able to walk, she viewed herself as capable and was often frustrated in her efforts to care for herself. Her sense of self fluctuated depending on her mood. During visits, the GCM listened to her fears and frustration and encouraged her to tell stories about herself and her accomplishments and to reminisce about things that came to mind. While Mrs. G's family was Jewish, they observed no rituals. Mrs. G told the GCM many times that she did not believe in God and did not like her caregivers reading the Bible or praying. In one of the conversations, she talked about preparing for death. "I keep wondering at night how I continue to survive. Perhaps with the help of the Lord."

"Do you believe in God?" the GCM asked.

Mrs. G answered, "I talk a lot to God when anything goes wrong. I blame God with great pleasure and affection, but then I think what a hell of a job he has." She went on to say that she felt God was somewhere around but that she had told him to go away. The GCM asked if Mrs. G was concerned about seeing God. She said she was. "If he comes close I will die." The GCM asked if Mrs. G believed God comes for persons when they die. Mrs. G said yes.

"So you're not ready to die now?" the GCM asked.

"Not at all; there is time." The GCM asked Mrs. G about whether she believed in connecting with God after death, as the soul rises to take its place with God—which is part of the Jewish tradition. Mrs. G thought that would be a great thing but thought God was too busy for her. After reflection, she said, "There is a mysterious thing that guides us. If I try to go too far I get lost. Something in us guides us; it's not a person, it's a mystery. We just have to follow it." The GCM asked her if she was talking about her soul or God. She said, "I would rather not put a finger on it." Mrs. G is not involved in any rituals or practice, but she has strong spiritual connections.

It is important for the GCM to be aware of spiritual resources that give clients meaning and strength and to be open to the conversation about such resources even if clients deny them. The GCM's interest and openness give the client the opportunity to share his or her beliefs and fears. The GCM should be guided by the client's expression and support the beliefs of the client. If the client's beliefs create fear, the GCM can listen to these fears and offer additional opportunities to resolve these fears by encouraging familiar clergy or family members to comfort the client.

Courage and Growth

Must new experiences, including problems, always be explained by a person's preexisting beliefs, or can a person let go of existing beliefs in order to allow new ones to emerge? When do persons' new life experiences challenge their existing beliefs in God? Do crises of faith or self-doubt result? It requires courage to enter the dark night of the soul, come to terms with a new set of circumstances, and accept changes in oneself. How can GCMs help their clients accept changes?

Ms. H

Ms. H was a 77-year-old single woman who had had a stroke, was able to walk with assistance, and had a moderate degree of dementia, which affected her memory and made it difficult for her to articulate her thoughts. Ms. H's sister, who lived several thousand miles away, was her only living relative. The sister hired a GCM to oversee Ms. H's care and be accountable to the sister.

Ms. H was initially an opera singer and later worked in an administrative capacity for a major corporation. She was very knowledgeable about music and art and went to many concerts and museums. Her sense of self was diminished by her strong negative attitude toward being old and a societally induced emphasis on youth and beauty. It was difficult for her to say anything positive about herself.

The GCM tried to expand Ms. H's sense of self, encouraging her to modify her lifelong beliefs about youth and beauty. She tried to help Ms. H value her experience, wisdom, and knowledge and the fact that she was witty, caring, and loving. At times Ms. H was able to take this in. The GCM encouraged the caregivers to acknowledge Ms. H's strengths, points of view, and kindness, and Ms. H was receptive at times. At other times she stuck to her old negative beliefs about herself. The challenge of the GCM's work with Ms. H and her caregivers was to acknowledge her losses and traumas and help her view herself in a positive framework by mirroring positive views of her, to stretch her beyond her old beliefs.

Many clients have negative beliefs about aging and disability. In order to help clients accept their situations, GCMs can help clients explore their feelings toward God, if they express any feelings toward God at all. If clients do not have a religious connection, helping clients like Ms. H view themselves in more affirming ways can help them let go of entrenched beliefs that cause them to suffer.

Ritual and Practice

It is important for the GCM to know what the client's rituals and practices are and what they were in the past. This would include traditional religious practices, services, prayers, and holiday celebrations. It would also include nonreligious rituals such as family gatherings for celebrations or birthdays. If the GCM's clients do not have family or do not participate in any rituals, the GCM needs to find out what events were celebrated in clients' lives that had meaning to them. The GCM might ask what the clients would like to do (e.g., go to church or synagogue, receive communion at home, or have their priest or rabbi visit). Would clients like to say prayers with caregivers or have scriptures or other spiritual material read aloud? What holi-

days would they like to celebrate and how? The GCM can work with caregivers to provide holiday foods and organize or participate in holiday celebrations. Providing a service for older persons in their homes generates a sense of community for clients and caregivers. When clients have forgotten rituals of their past, the GCM can find out about these rituals by trial and error, by saying a familiar prayer, lighting candles, or singing familiar songs or hymns from the person's religious tradition. These rituals can engender a sense of deep connection to clients' past and tradition. The GCM needs to respect clients' wishes and move in a sensitive manner.

Mr. G

Mr. G was Jewish but did not remember the rituals of his childhood in an orthodox home. During Chanukah, the GCM asked him if she could say a prayer when he lit the menorah candle. At first he declined and said he was agnostic. The GCM accepted his wishes, but he was curious and encouraged her to do so. She read the prayer slowly in Hebrew and English while Mr. G watched attentively. He later told her he appreciated her saying the prayer. Mr. G insisted on lighting the candles on all future Jewish holidays, including lighting the menorah on Passover.

Clients can be responsive to music from their tradition. Responses to the singing of melodies can range from joyful participation to the more subtle response of a smile or tapping finger. It is important to follow the older person's lead in this. It is helpful to involve pastoral connections and staff familiar with the rituals to say prayers and sing religious songs. In these ways, the GCM will help clients build a sense of connection to the past and create a sense of well-being.

Community

Is the person part of one or more formal or informal communities of shared beliefs, rituals, or practices? What is the person's participation in these communities? The GCM may ask what it means to the client to be part of the community and how active the client is in the community. The GCM should consider both spiritual and other communities of family, friends, organizations, neighbors, and caregivers. The GCM may have to educate the clergy or lay volunteer if the client has dementia or is aphasic as to how to respond appropriately to the client. It is important to stress to the spiritual leader how valuable his or her visit would be to the client, as would other types of connection with the community of faith.

Past versus Current Communities

Frail, homebound clients tend to have small communities. Families may live far away, and the clients may have lost touch with friends who have moved or are too ill to visit. Other friends and family members may have died. Because of illness, clients may not currently be connected to religious organizations. If a client is not part of any faith community, the GCM should assess past involvement in and current willingness to be part of a faith community. Would clients want to participate in services outside their home, or would they like the members of their former community to visit? It is important to talk with clients about their current community as well as their emotional connections to organizations or communities that had meaning to them in the past. The GCM can help access important people from the client's past by asking the client and his or her family for names. The GCM can encourage clients to contact whoever they were close to or offer to make the calls on behalf of clients. In addition, the GCM can arrange for new opportunities to widen clients' circles, such as attending day care programs or respite programs, having friendly visitor volunteers, and participating in activities the client likes.

Mr. R

Mr. R was a 95-year-old client who was a successful artist and was cognitively impaired. The GCM encouraged Mr. R's caregivers to take him to art shows where his work was represented. He was significantly affected by his dementia, but he loved to see familiar faces at these shows and receive acknowledgment for his work. The con-

nection to the art community affirmed his self-worth. It is important for a GCM to involve a client with those who have had meaning in the client's life (e.g., former associates, neighbors, friends).

Home Care Community

The community of home care providers often becomes the surrogate family, providing great meaning for and connection with the client. It is important to support the home care staff so that they maintain good relationships with clients and care for clients' wellbeing. Many home care workers are spiritual people and view their work as the work of God, so they take naturally to caring for and loving their clients.

Mr. H

Mr. H suffered from dementia and physical incapacity. He was often agitated. His care workers were religious and had a daily ritual of saying prayers at the morning shift. At times he told them to stop. At other times, he joined the workers in their prayers. GCMs need to be vigilant that the caregivers are not imposing their viewpoints on clients, making clients uncomfortable.

Authority and Guidance

The GCM should consider where clients look for guidance when faced with doubt, confusion, tragedy, or conflict. To what extent do clients look within or outside themselves for guidance?

Mrs. L

Mrs. L's family lived out of town and hired a GCM to oversee her care. Mrs. L was visually impaired and at home in bed after a fall in which her arm and leg were injured. She could hardly move. She talked to the GCM about the difficult hospital experience. She hated not being in control and was glad to be at home in her bed. "I'm just lying here wondering what purpose I have. I don't know, but I know I've been through a lot of difficult struggles. I'm a tough egg. I've gone through difficult times but met people who had substance—that's what made the difference."

"So you valued the connections with people?" the GCM asked.

"Yes, that is right—I really liked them a lot."

"Do you wonder about the meaning of your life now?" continued the GCM.

"Yes, I don't know what I'm needed for, but that's all right, I am here and observing."

"So instead of thinking of what to do, you're just living in the present moment."

"Yes, that is what I am doing," said Mrs. L. She was quiet for a few moments. "I love listening to the music and to the voice that is coming from you."

"I appreciate that," the GCM responded. "I know you have meaning to your family."

"For a time I didn't think so, but they seem interested in me now."

"How do you feel about that?" the GCM asked.

"Oh, I love them visiting and talking with them; I really enjoy that." The GCM asked Mrs. L about her grandson. "That's right, I am a grandmother," said Mrs. L. "I remember Steve's visits a long time ago." The GCM reassured her that the caregivers and the GCM cared and loved her and that she meant a lot to them. Mrs. L said she was glad to hear that. The GCM's goal was to follow up on Mrs. L's statement about the purpose of her life and encourage her to reflect on the meaning of her life. All GCMs need to listen to the thoughts and feelings that guide clients and to follow clients' lead as they reflect on their lives.

Mrs. N

A GCM worked with an adult daughter who had difficulty caring for her autocratic, independent mother, Mrs. N, who had a significant dementia, was visually impaired, smoked incessantly, and lived alone in a tiny apartment. Mrs. N, a refugee who worked and brought her family to the United States, where she fought for the rights of workers in a union, was a proud woman who was writing about her martyred father who was killed in Eastern Europe.

For 2 years, the GCM provided consultation to her daughter concerning providing care to her mother, who often refused it, and helped the daughter in her efforts to balance caring for her mother with caring for her own family. In the process the daughter discussed her unresolved relationship issues with her mother. She admired her mother but was saddened by her mother's limited emotional nurturing. The daughter found students to read to her mother and introduced home care in a sensitive manner, using the GCM's services intermittently when problems arose.

The daughter brought her mother to her home for holidays, despite the difficulty in providing care. Mrs. N had another stroke, and the daughter honored her wishes in not taking her to the hospital. Mrs. N's daughter moved into her mother's apartment and took care of her. The GCM talked with the daughter about her mother's condition. A hospice program began to provide care to her mother; the hospice program did not provide workers on a few shifts, but the daughter stoically filled in the gaps in physical and emotional care.

A week after the stroke took place, the daughter called to tell the GCM that her mother had died the previous night. The daughter said the experience had been perfect; it was beautiful to be alone with her mother. She had gone out with friends for dinner and came home relaxed. She sat on the floor and spoke to her mother.

> I told her gently that she was dying— that she had been sick since Monday and now it was Friday. I talked about all her accomplishments, how everyone admired her, including her home care workers. I told her I loved her and that I knew how much she loved me. It was an exquisite moment. I went on to say that I knew that she didn't believe in heaven but suggested that if it were possible that there is a heaven, then perhaps mother could meet and continue her discussions with Roger, [a family friend] in heaven.

Mrs. N was very deaf, very ill, and cognitively impaired and her daughter was not sure she had heard her. But Mrs. N smiled, took a few breaths, and then stopped breathing. The GCM said it was wonderful that the daughter could be so present to her mother. The daughter said that she did not feel guilty but perfectly at peace.

Initially, Mrs. N's daughter had great difficulty providing care for her mother because she resisted it. Over time, with the support and encouragement of the GCM, she was able to help her mother come to accept the help she needed, while the daughter did what she found possible. Despite her sadness at her mother's earlier emotional unavailability, the daughter was able to consistently care for her mother or use the GCM when she was not able to do so. She was able to help her mother die by being present to her both physically and emotionally, acknowledging her life's gifts and enabling her mother to leave her life with good feelings about herself and her daughter, and with hope for the future. The GCM's support, acknowledgment of the daughter's feelings throughout the difficult caretaking period, and help in providing the daughter with home care assistance and the GCM's presence when needed were all important to the daughter. The daughter was able to rise above her ambivalent feelings and provide care and nurturing to her mother in a loving manner. The GCM witnessed the daughter's inner resources and strength as her mother died and supported all the daughter did for her mother. By being present to their clients' struggles and providing emotional support and concrete assistance, GCMs can help people solidify their own authority to care for their parents.

Ways To Affirm Clients' Spiritual Needs

There are seven ways that GCMs can affirm clients' spiritual needs.

1. GCMs can develop a trusting relationship with clients and help them feel safe to express their suffering. Being present to their pain helps clients feel cared for, valued, and respected.
2. GCMs can be open to the meaning of illness and loss and to their clients' view of the world.
3. GCMs can help clients view themselves beyond just their roles (e.g., father, wife).

4. GCMs can talk with clients about clients' beliefs and what has brought meaning to their lives.
5. GCMs can appreciate clients' life stories and acknowledge their strengths, struggles, triumphs, and losses.
6. GCMs can respect clients' agenda, words, and ways of doing things.[23]
7. GCMs can be open to learning from clients and interactions with them, being open-minded and nonjudgmental.[23]

FACILITATING SPIRITUAL CONNECTIONS WITH PEOPLE WHO HAVE DEMENTIA AND THEIR FAMILIES

How do GCMs overcome society's negative attitudes toward people with dementia and treat impaired clients with dignity and value, maintaining a person-centered approach? One way is to empathize with the frustrations of clients, whose symptoms will vary over the course of the illness. They will experience changes in their ability to do everyday tasks and will have to abandon work and familiar activities. They may have difficulty communicating and expressing their wishes clearly, have changes in personality and mood, and lack initiative. All these changes can lead to feelings of anger, frustration, fearfulness, anxiety, and sadness. "Living with Alzheimers means living in a world of fragments. There is a lack of connection. How did I get here? What am I supposed to do next?"[24]

To preserve the humanity of persons who have lost what this culture considers the defining quality of human beings—the ability to think and reason—GCMs need to move to an ethos of care based upon the emotional and relational qualities of human life.[25] GCMs are able to experience the person with dementia without having the emotions of the family, who have witnessed the changes in functioning of the person. In addition to listening to caregivers discuss their difficulties, the GCM should find out what the person's past interests, activities, and roles were and what has changed. What are the person's remaining cognitive abilities, and what does he or she like to do now? Listen to music? Take walks? The caregivers and friends can provide information on the client's values, such as working hard or caring for family members, as well as his or her life story. This helps the GCM better understand the person and be sensitive to the client's values and traditions.

It is important to understand each client's needs and to help the client feel respected, appreciated, loved, known, and understood. Persons with dementia need a sense of belonging—to feel part of a community, to share and give love, and to be productive, helpful, and useful. Because those with dementia lose their ability to fulfill these needs, they may feel frustrated, confused, isolated, and embarrassed.[26]

GCMs need to help clients experience positive connections with caregivers and the GCM. It is important for the GCM to be patient, sensitive, responsive, caring, encouraging, enabling, and empowering in his or her work and to serve as a model for both family and professional caregivers.

Being loved, responded to empathetically, and cared for can help the person with dementia feel more whole and provides a sense of security and peace. Bell and Troxel elucidate a positive and interpersonal approach in working with people with dementia and their families.[26]

Improving Spiritual Connections

In helping persons with dementia experience spiritual connections, it is important to have an idea about their traditions and bring familiar rituals to them to broaden their connections and sense of well-being. For persons with Alzheimer's, familiar symbols of faith connect with the heart rather than the intellect. The emotional or sensory aspects of spirituality take on a greater significance. "Music, hymns, prayers, familiar bible passages and rituals learned early in childhood can reach people with dementia and become a way to express themselves and receive comfort."[27(p2)] GCMs should ask clients and families what these familiar aspects of spirituality might be. "Touch, pictures, poetry, music and faith symbols can be used to communicate in individual

contacts and in communal worship."[27(p2)] Clients may respond by joining in or showing nonverbal responses such as nodding, tapping a finger, or moving their body. Rituals of faith are usually learned early in life and can be part of a lifetime of religious practice. "Because they do not completely depend on the intellect they reach emotional levels and tap earlier memory which can connect the client to his past."[27(p2)]

If the client is religious, going to a church or synagogue or otherwise participating in a religious community can help the client feel God's presence as a reassuring haven of stability. It can also provide spiritual assurance that the client is worth more than just his or her cognitive capacity and offer hope to overcome fears about diminished capacity and the uncontrollable. For those without a specific faith tradition or belief system, spiritual needs may be addressed in other ways, such as sharing a sunset, listening to music, holding hands, praying together, or watching services on television.

Improving Family Connections

There are practical, emotional, and spiritual components to working with families whose relatives have dementia. In the following example, a GCM helps some adult children through the various stages of their father's illness and an adult daughter is able to experience her father in a holistic frame, beyond just his illness.

Mr. K

A GCM was contacted by the daughter of a 93-year-old man who had dementia, Mr. K. She lived out of town and needed assistance in providing care for her father. Her stepsister lived near her father. The GCM's relationship with the K family spanned 5 years. During this period, the GCM met regularly with the daughters on a schedule that fit into their visits with the father. She focused on understanding how the experience of dementia affected them and helped them listen to each other's perspectives. The GCM encouraged discussion about Mr. K's changed functioning, his forgetfulness, and his intermittent confusion. She encouraged them to reflect on the changes in his behavior, to share their feelings, to empathize with each other, and to work together. The GCM shared information about dementia with the daughters, acknowledging the changes they experienced and recommending books, tapes, and educational meetings to them. She encouraged the daughters to seek support from their partners and friends.

The GCM helped the daughters grieve over losses in their father's functioning while remaining receptive to Mr. K's remaining ability to share his love, his point of view, and his sense of humor. His daughters shared their good experiences in taking him to the ballet, watching him enjoy art shows, and helping with his care. They continued to share a warm and loving relationship with him.

The GCM engaged the daughters in discussions along the continuum of care from 8 hours a day to two 12-hour shifts of care. The daughters thought a day care program would be helpful for their father. The GCM helped Mr. K get accepted into a day care program that he enjoyed and that provided stimulation for him and oversight of his home attendants. The GCM helped the daughters plan in small steps care for the future, arranging visits to facilities and helping them decide to have the father remain in his home unless it was medically necessary to transfer him to a nursing home. The GCM visited Mr. K and his caregivers and oversaw his care. She provided feedback to his daughters on a regular basis.

Mr. K died peacefully in his home at the age of 98. The tribute that his daughter wrote to him after his death speaks of her love, care, and spiritual growth and the importance of her connection to her father. In this poem she recognizes the contribution her father made as an artist and as a communist: his struggle to make art accessible to the people and for a living wage for artists.

> Were you kidding around with me or
>   was this for real?
> I found this both disturbing and amus-
>   ing
> I struggled to make sense of what was
>   happening
> You didn't know who I was?

I began to feel like I was your memory
you were 93 years old, the main man
    in my life
we were kindred spirits, though we
    were separated by 59 years
and you were always there when I got
    home from school

Your loss of memory coincided with
    the collapse of the Soviet Union.
I was careful to protect you from
    knowing that your cherished system
    was crumbling

I wondered if you lost your cognitive
    memory to spare yourself the
pain of watching the capitalist class
    toot its triumphant horn
I remind myself that you were 23
    when the Russian revolution shook
the world up, and you with it.

Your loss of memory coming as it
    does in the middle of these celebra-
    tions
makes me feel like the context of my
    youth is slipping away
I rush to remember the historic mo-
    ments that became family mantras
the Spanish civil war, the state murder
    of Ethel and Julius Rosenberg
the FBI's witchhunt against commu-
    nists, gay people and labor unions

Have I now become a messenger of
    this history that you no longer re-
    member?

As you aged, body connection became
    our major communicator.
It was difficult to watch you lose your
    memory
one of my mirrors was gone
but like you I am learning to be in the
    moment
not lacking history but assuming it
At some point I stopped reminding
    you that I was your daughter
Our relationship had been transformed
    by your loss of memory

we just were
Because of you I now understand that
    memory is most importantly
about our bodies and our hearts.
without these we cannot do justice to
    our histories

Your memory of the struggle was em-
    bedded in your body and in your
    heart
but the details were gone

You had a physical and emotional
    memory of justice and fundamental
    truth
You had an emotional essence
You were an essence in your stillness
You are the essence of Harry. That's
    what I get:
little fleeting moments of the essence
    of Harry.
It is a different way of seeing the
    world and
I take it as a gift.[28]

This daughter's experience of her father throughout her life as a wonderful caregiver helped her value the positive connections between them that continued despite his dementia.

GCMs' work with families whose relatives have dementia challenges GCMs to help families go beyond grief to find the positive in the situation. The GCM can help the family shift their expectations of their relative, see their relative beyond the dementia, accept the situation, and live in the present. The family member can try to appreciate the relative's deeper values and the values of mutuality and caring throughout the life cycle. GCMs can encourage family members to draw on their inner strength and spiritual resources. Family members can think about how their parent cared for them or how they wish they were cared for. In being fully present to family members, GCMs can help them shift to being present to their relative, as they resolve their grief. Dementia offers persons the opportunity to treasure the moments they share together and live more fully in the present.

CONCLUSION

By incorporating a spiritual perspective, GCMs can be a resource in building compassionate communities of care. This perspective broadens the GCM's scope in working with chronically ill and elderly clients and their families in an attempt to help them find meaning and value in their lives.

By viewing the client's frailty as a potentially meaningful part of life, the GCM can share with the client the contributions he or she has made and continues to make. In reviewing his or her own values and spiritual beliefs, the CCM can discern the differences between personal values and client values and be open to and interested in the diverse ways clients find meaning in their lives.

As delineated in this chapter, the spiritual process can be facilitated in many different ways. It is important to enable family members and caregivers to experience the client's spirit beyond his or her illness, and encourage the client to share personal spiritual resources by valuing them, carrying out rituals, and being present to them. In this way, the client's sense of connection to himself or herself, the community, and God can be enhanced.

NOTES

1. Atchley B. Atchley on aging and spiritual growth. In: Seeber J, ed. *Aging and Spirituality*. 1998;10:6.

2. National Interfaith Coalition on Aging. Spiritual well being: a definition. Presented at National Interfaith Coalition on Aging; 1975; Athens, GA.

3. Jung C. *Modern Man in Search of Soul*. New York: Harcourt Brace; 1933.

4. Schachter-Shalomi Z, Miller R, eds. *From Age-ing to Sage-ing: A Profound New Vision of Growing Older*. New York: Time Warner; 1995.

5. Kenyon GM. Aging and possibilities for being. *Aging and the Human Spirit*. 1992;2:4–5.

6. Leder D. *Spiritual Passages: Embracing Life's Sacred Journey*. New York: Tarcher/Putnam; 1997.

7. Thibault JM. Review of *Spiritual Passages: Embracing Life's Sacred Journey. Aging Human Spirit.* 1997;7:9.

8. Magid S. Wrestling with despair: a Jewish response to worry and depression. Presented by the Drisha Institute and the National Center for Jewish Healing; June 14, 1998; New York.

9. Emerson RW. *Essays: First Series.* 1841.

10. Atchley RC. The continuity of the spiritual self. In: Kimble, MA, McFadden SH, Ellor JW, Seeber J, eds. *Aging, Spirituality and Religion.* Minneapolis: Fortress Press; 1995:68–73.

11. Moberg DO. Spiritual well-being defined. In: Ellor JW. *Aging and Spirituality.* 1997:2–3.

12. Genevay B, Richards M. Spiritual growth and psychological development: a concurrent path as we age. *Aging Spirituality.* 1997;9:4–5.

13. Frankl VD. *Man's Search for Meaning.* Boston: Beacon Press; 1959.

14. Chinen AB. *In the Ever After: Fairy Tales and the Second Half of Life.* Wilmette, IL: Chiron Publications; 1989.

15. Williams CC. Explorers without a map: charting a course to value and meaning. Presented at the American Society on Aging Annual Conference; 1998; San Francisco.

16. Young-Eisendrath P. *The Resilient Spirit: Transforming Suffering into Insight and Renewal.* Reading, MA: Addison Wesley Publishing Company; 1996.

17. Snorton TE. From struggles, dilemmas, and events in ages past. *Aging Spirituality;* 1995;7:3.

18. Riemer J. *So That Your Values Live On: Ethical Wills and How To Prepare Them.* Woodstock, VT: Jewish Lights Publishing; 1991.

19. Alzheimer's Association, National Alliance for Caregiving. *Who Cares? Families Caring for Persons with Alzheimer's Disease.* Washington, DC: 1999.

20. Personal communication with Marty Richards, 1999.

21. Genevay B, Katz RS. *Countertransference and Older Clients.* Newburg Park, CA: Sage Publications; 1990.

22. Fitchett G. *Assessing Spiritual Needs. A Guide for Caregivers.* Augsburg, MN; 1992.

23. Simon D. Healing and the spirit: tapping spiritual resources to facilitate a more positive experience of life's final stage. Presented at the American Society on Aging, Summer Series; July 1998; New York.

24. Gwyther L. Helping congregations maintain a connection to spirit in the Alzheimer's disease experience. Presented at the Annual Meeting of the American Society on Aging; March 1999; Orlando, FL.

25. Post SG. *The Moral Challenge of Alzheimer Disease.* Baltimore: Johns Hopkins University Press; 1995.

26. Bell V, Troxel D. *The Best Friends Approach to Alzheimer's Care.* Baltimore: Health Professionals Press; 1997.

27. Richards M. Meeting the spiritual needs of the cognitively impaired. *Aging and Spirituality.* 1994;7:2.

28. Gottlieb A. *In Living Memory* [videotape]. Toronto, Ontario: VTape; 1997.

PART V

The Future

CHAPTER 15

The Future of Geriatric Care Management

Merrily Orsini

When care managers started helping older persons and their families back in the early 1980s, care management was a unique service, and most practitioners were working alone. In the last 20 years, as the U.S. population has aged and as more and more women have begun working outside the home, geriatric care management has moved more into the mainstream. Future demographic changes, especially in the older population, will have a huge effect on the geriatric care management of the future.

Technology has also brought huge changes in the last 20 years. Fax machines were unheard of 20 years ago. Computers were still mainframes, and the personal computer was just being introduced, mostly for games. Rapidly changing technology will affect the geriatric care manager (GCM) of the future.

The range of professionals offering geriatric care management has expanded considerably in the last 2 decades. Care management began with professional persons within the health care system who were more and more frequently solving problems for older persons and their families. As was logical, the first care management professionals were usually nurses and social workers. As the industry has grown and become more mainstream, other professionals who interface with older persons and their families have begun offering care management services.

- Attorneys who specialize in estates are starting to offer care management.

- Accountants' entry into care management is fairly new but highly organized.
- Trust officers have been involved with care management for as long (or longer) than the profession has existed. The trust officer was often the one person who serviced the older adult who had no support system. In many locales, the trust officer is arranging care, ordering groceries, paying bills, and supervising the situation: the core of the care management business. Trust officers also began using GCMs in-house and as contractors very early on.
- Rehabilitation specialists and physician's office staff members are also entering care management.

One has only to look at the growth of Humana, first as a hospital chain, then as an insurance company, to see the effects of growth on an industry that understands the reimbursement rules. When Humana became the first for-profit hospital to accept insurance reimbursement, it set about learning how to maximize reimbursement for services. By looking at reimbursement in categories and studying profitability for each category, one can increase profitability by "selling" services in higher profit categories. This ability to target and grow more profitable reimbursement categories enables companies to have some control over their profits through targeting services based on their profitability. Thus manipulated and understood, third-party reimbursement can become the goose that laid the golden egg.

As America ages, insurance companies will have to rely on care management for their frail customers. Care managers understand the nuances of care needs and in which setting a patient can thrive. They understand the variety of costs associated with hospitalization, home care, and nursing home care, and the instances when it is cost effective to utilize home care rather than hospitals or nursing homes. Preventing rehospitalization and keeping persons out of nursing homes will be paramount in saving health care dollars. Deciding which customer needs care at home, can thrive in a congregate setting, needs Meals on Wheels, or needs other support will be of foremost importance as the number of older persons grows and begins using the long-term care policies that are so popular now. This understanding is not unlike the usage of categories for profitability in reimbursement. Because the care manager can save the insurance company money, third-party reimbursement to the care manager will be utilized.

MANAGING CARE AS A MAINSTREAM BUSINESS, NOT A BOUTIQUE BUSINESS

What is a boutique business, and what is a mainstream business? A mainstream business is one that is easily recognized by all, one with good name recognition. It is a place where people customarily would turn for help. For instance, if there is an emergency at home, everyone knows to dial 911 and expects to go to the emergency room. For eye problems, persons see optometrists or ophthalmologists. If women are pregnant, they go to obstetrician/gynecologists. The field of geriatric care management is still so relatively new that when a geriatric care management problem arises, persons in need do not know where to go. Geriatric care management is not a household word, and at this time the GCM is not someone who is turned to first when there is a geriatric care problem.

A boutique business is a small one- or two-person business that serves a relatively small number of people with limited services. The boutique geriatric care management business keeps its client numbers down so that each client gets personal attention. Weekly or daily visits are not uncommon. The care manager is the "surrogate family member" and responds to all the client's needs in a timely fashion. The boutique geriatric care management business will continue to be a model of business in the future, particularly in rural areas or ethnic areas of large cities. However, as U.S. demographics change, these boutique services will grow as the need for service grows.

To understand the drastic changes that this nation will experience in the need for GCMs, one has only to look at the statistics.

> Described by the Census Bureau as a 'human tidal wave,' the baby boom generation is technically defined as those born within the fertile periods between between 1946 and 1964. This cohort is 70% larger than the generation born during the prior 2 decades. Now in their most economically productive years (ages 36 to 54 in 2000), these 'boomers' currently comprise more than one-third of the U.S. population. As the baby boom generation ages, U.S. society will be transformed. While those over 65 years of age are now a relatively small part (12%) of the population, by 2030, this age group will constitute fully one-fifth of the population, a sizeable segment of all consumers, voters, homeowners, and patients. Increasingly, every social institution and sector will be required to accommodate the needs of older people. Resources will have to be mobilized to serve them.[1(p1)]

Over the 20-year period of 2010 to 2030, the older population will increase from 39.4 million to 69.4 million (13.3% to 20.1% of the total population) in what is projected to be the most rapid growth period for older persons of the 21st century. In other words, by 2030, as the last of the baby boom cohort reaches retirement age, one out of five persons will be at least 65 (Figures 15–1 and 15–2).[1] This growth in the older population and the changes that it brings will have the biggest impact on geriatric care management services for the future.

The knowledgeable geriatric care management business of the future will be in great demand given the projected infirmities of the aging population.

> As America ages the number of people with chronic conditions will increase. Approximately 88% of the elderly have at least one chronic condition. Such conditions limit the activities of nearly two-fifths of the elderly with one-third of these disabled elderly requiring help with either personal care or home management. Chronic diseases are, in fact, the primary cause of disability among the elderly. Having more than one chronic condition adds considerably to the health burden, increasing the likelihood of disability as well as the use of health care services. This risk of co-morbidity increases with age among persons diagnosed with at least one chronic condition. One in six children (17%), more than one-quarter of those aged 18 to 44, half of those aged 45 to 64 and 69% of those 65 years and older have multiple chronic conditions.[1(pp23–24)]

Given the care needs discussed above and the likelihood of more and more frail elderly persons having chronic conditions, the need for a GCM in the future seems to be certain. Looking at the other side of the equation, the availability of caregivers, that certainty seems even greater.

> As the baby boom generation retires and the need for caregiving increases, the supply of family caregivers is projected to decline. This decline can be traced to lower fertility rates in the caregiving generation and to family networks that are getting smaller. In 1980 there were 11 potential caregivers to every one older person. By 2010 this ratio will decline slightly to 10 to 1 and it will continue to decline as the size of the older population grows. By 2030, the ratio of potential caregivers to elders will be reduced to 6 to 1.[1(pp12–13)]

Currently, over 50% of the persons in nursing homes have a dementia.[2] However, the future projections for this population are uncertain.

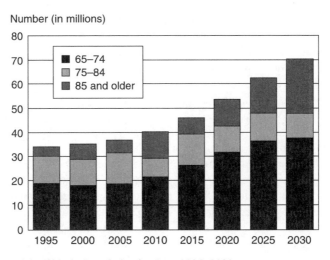

Figure 15–1 Projection of the Elderly Population by Age, 1995–2030.

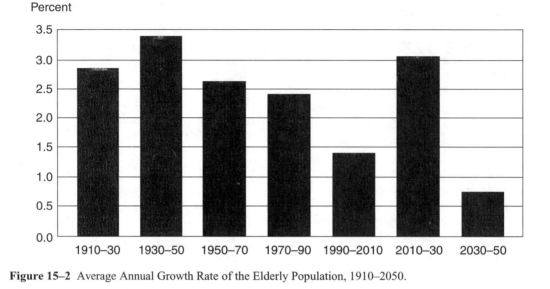

Figure 15–2 Average Annual Growth Rate of the Elderly Population, 1910–2050.

Dementia in the elderly population, most particularly Alzheimer's disease, may have tremendous long term care implications over the next 40 years. Drugs now in development may eventually reduce the rate of cognitive deterioration from these conditions and could thereby significantly reduce the number of persons who need supportive assistance in their activities of daily living. Currently, about half of those in nursing homes and 30% of those in residential care have some measurable cognitive deficits. The proportion of these persons who have no physical conditions that also necessitate supportive care is unknown. Will baby boomers be subject to rates of Alzheimer disease similar to those currently seen in their parents' generation? Will drug treatment cut the incidence in half? Or perhaps a higher level of independent functioning, such that many of those now in special care units can be transferred to home or assisted living settings? Dementia will be a powerful factor in shaping the

quality of life and the cost of health care in an aging America.[1(p49)]

America is aging. More Americans will be older than ever before. Americans are still likely to have families with two wage earners. Some professionals will need to oversee older persons' care, monitor their progress, coordinate services, and advocate for the frail elderly. It is possible that GCMs will fulfill this role in the future.

As the GCM solves problems, meets needs, and integrates into the elder care service network, geriatric care management will become a mainstream business.

DIVERSE PROFESSIONALS DELIVERING GCM SERVICES: THE LAWYER, THE ACCOUNTANT, THE TRUST DEPARTMENT

For the 75-year-old, "the future" is obviously the next 10 years. City planners, on the other hand, may have the next 50 years in mind. GCMs need to deliver services in the immediate future while keeping an eye on changes they will want to be ready to make during the first half of the 21st century. There are two distinct demographic strata for the future: conditions during 2000–2010 and conditions during 2010–2050. During the first period, older persons as a proportion of the total population will not increase,[1] giving GCMs time to assimilate current changes in their caregiving landscape. Diverse providers of services and technology hopefully will be in place then to adjust to the burgeoning senior population from 2010–2050. One can look at the projected need and the growing numbers in a variety of ways. Medicare managed care projections are just one visible measure of the impact the numbers will have on our systems. Figure 15–3 shows the projected growth in Medicare managed care enrollment between 1991 and 2007.

Looking at two groups of seniors, those aged 65–74 and those 75 and above, it is predicted that between 1990 and 2010 the first group will increase by 16.3% (to 21,075,000), while the older cadre will grow by 39.7% (to 18,352,000; Figure 15–4). From 1990 to 2010, seniors aged 65–69 will increase in number by 52.7%, those 70–74 by 19.8%, those 75–79 by 11.9%, those 80–84 by 41.3%, and those over 85 by 84.1%.[3]

As noted above, the increased number of persons potentially needing care is offset by a corresponding decrease in caregivers who are in the family or who are informally hired (Figure 15–5).[1]

'Support ratio' or "dependency ratio" is a measure used as a crude indicator of future care needs. Expressed in terms of the support ratio, the simplest comparison is of those at retirement age (presently age 65 and older) to those of working age (aged 18 to 64). It is projected that between 1995 and 2010, the support ratio will hold steady at 21 persons aged 65 and older for every 100 persons. That old age support ration, however, will rise 71% between 2010 and 2030, increasing from 21 to 36 older persons per 100 persons aged 18 to 64.

When one looks at the support ratio for persons 85 years and older per 100 persons aged 50 to 64 years there is even more cause for alarm for caregivers. The ratio of these adults over 85 in 1995 numbered 10 for every 100 persons aged 50–64 years. In 2010–2030 that ratio will increase to 15 adults over 85 for every 100 person aged 50–64. The chief result of this shift is that those persons in that 50–64 age group with grown children will possibly face the dilemma of caring

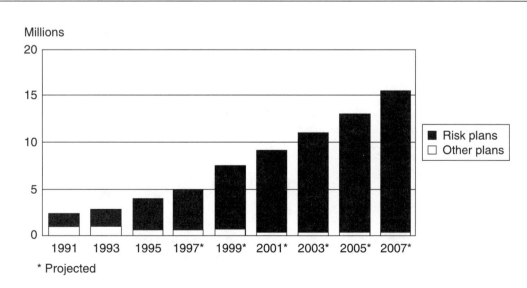

Figure 15–3 Medicare Managed Care Enrollment, 1991–2007.

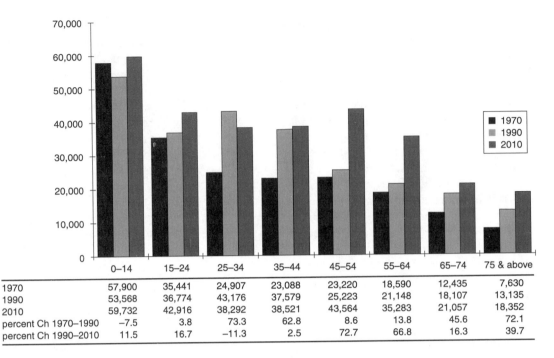

	0–14	15–24	25–34	35–44	45–54	55–64	65–74	75 & above
1970	57,900	35,441	24,907	23,088	23,220	18,590	12,435	7,630
1990	53,568	36,774	43,176	37,579	25,223	21,148	18,107	13,135
2010	59,732	42,916	38,292	38,521	43,564	35,283	21,057	18,352
percent Ch 1970–1990	−7.5	3.8	73.3	62.8	8.6	13.8	45.6	72.1
percent Ch 1990–2010	11.5	16.7	−11.3	2.5	72.7	66.8	16.3	39.7

Figure 15–4 Population of the United States (000), 1970–2010.

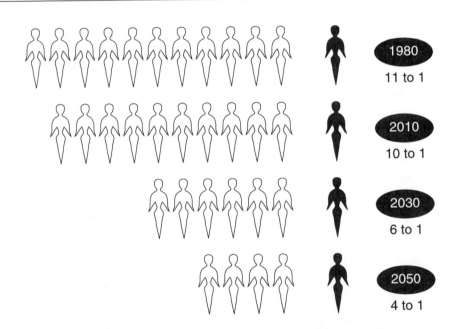

Note: In 1990, the ratio of the population in the average caregiving age range, ages 50 to 64, to the population aged 85 and older was 11 to 1. By 2050, there will be only four potential caregivers for every elderly person.

Figure 15–5 The Shrinking Pool of Potential Caregivers.

for their very old and frail relatives or neighbors while also having the possibility of raising a second generation of children—their grandchildren.[1(pp10–11)]

Older people enter the care management purview because of social, medical, or financial need. The provision of services for any one of these needs can soon lead to the provision of services for the other needs.

Much geriatric care management has its roots in the social model. For example, a company already providing in-home care finds an increasingly frail customer in need of someone to pay the bills and someone else to monitor blood pressure. Geriatric care management began in the early 1980s as a unique new approach to a wide range of services, the original goal of which was to maintain the older client at home. Home nursing agencies experienced a similar push to broaden their operative range. Trust officers and certified public accountants (CPAs) began expanding their services.[4]

As noted earlier in the chapter, social workers and nurses are not the only professionals who provide geriatric care management services. In fact, there are more allied professionals entering the field each year. Accountants are the latest group to identify care management as a viable model of service delivery. They join the increasing numbers of insurance brokers, rehabilitation therapists, hospital discharge planners, psychologists, financial planners, trust officers, home health agency staff, and other business professionals entering the field.[5]

The care management profession needs to be inclusive rather than exclusive while maintaining high standards for its members. The focus should be on developing ways in which allied professionals can work together in a more integrated manner. GCMs can develop a multidisciplined professional cluster group. Each member can provide complementary services, enabling the cluster to comprehensively meet the service needs of older adults and their families. The professional cluster group may be composed of a select network of physicians, psychiatrists, attorneys, accountants, financial planners,

home health professionals, insurance brokers, caregiver providers, and allied therapists (physical, speech, occupational, psychiatric, art, music, etc.). In administering the cluster groups, the GCMs would coordinate and implement a shared marketing campaign to maximize advertising dollars. The cluster group creates a system in which consumers can enter the group from multiple access points. Using a profit-sharing model, one can create incentives for successful cross-referrals.[5]

Probably the most well-organized movement into the geriatric care management field by other professionals has involved the American Institute of Certified Public Accountants (AICPA). The AICPA has formed special committees on assurance services, and elder care is one of services recommended for accountants to specialize in. The AICPA Web site contains the following information:

> Elder care is the service designed to provide assurance to family members that care goals are achieved for older family members no longer able to be totally independent. The service will rely on the expertise of other professionals with the CPA serving as the eyes and ears of the family members of the responsible party. The purpose of the service is to provide assurance in a professional, independent and objective manner to third parties (children, family members or other concerned parties, or in some cases, the older persons themselves) that the needs of the older person to whom they are attached are being met. Or to put it in simpler terms: to provide the opportunity for older persons to live out their lives in their own homes with dignity and protection from predators who would take advantage of them.[6]

The accountants are exploring the elder care field and feel that their entry is needed because:

> One of the biggest problems facing relatives who must arrange for care for

an older relative is finding out whether home care is an option (as opposed to institutional care), what services are available in the community, and what to expect from the care providers. Often this information can only be obtained through care providers themselves or through word of mouth from other persons who have been faced with similar problems. The consulting services portion of elder care envisions the CPA as the focal point to assist family members in defining the standards of care needed and expected for the older person. This service could include providing the family members (the person responsible for care of an elderly person) with a listing of the services and options available in the community and working with them to establish goals for assistance; developing a customized delivery plan; indicating the types of service providers required to accomplish the care goals; and communicating expectations of required levels of performance to each service provider including the identification of criteria to be used to measure performance.[6]

The AICPA Eldercare Assurance Committee also suggests that the CPA might want to get into direct services.

In some instances either because of a lack of commercial providers in the community or because of the unique competencies of the CPA, the practitioner may be engaged to take a more active role in the management of elder care. This might include routine tasks that would normally be performed by the older person or a family member, tasks such as receipts deposit and accounting for income or making sure the expected revenues are received, supervision of investments and accounting for the estate, making arrangements for the appropriate level of care and periodically visiting the client to ensure care being received meets the standards set by family members. This might also include arranging transportation for clients, supervising household expenditures and making arrangements for unusual or unexpected requirements such as home maintenance repair and medical emergencies. Furthermore, this would include arranging for an assessment of the older person by a social worker, GCM or geropsychiatrist.[6]

The AICPA also suggests that assurance to the client from the CPA might be given on the following:

Review of routine financial transactions for reasonableness and adherence to criteria established for such transactions; investigating and providing information to family members for handling of unusual or unexpected situations such as home maintenance and repair or medical emergencies; inspection of logs, diaries, and other evidence (including direct observation) to determine whether the caregivers are meeting their performance criteria agreed upon with the client/family member; reporting to client or family members, as a part of any assurance engagement there should be a clear understanding as to whom reports are to be issued and in what frequency.[6]

For the CPA to get started in elder care, the AICPA says that the CPA:

will need to commit to providing staff and resources that will truly serve the purposes of the client. You will be at the hub of a wheel of providers conducting ongoing and objective reviews of the performance of each of the service providers. It may mean you are hiring permanent or on-call staff or developing a relationship with the geriatric care manager or other elder care professionals to assist in meeting the needs of elder care clients.[6]

The accounting professionals recognize that in order to best serve the clients some part of the elder care process must use professionals trained in geriatrics and familiar with the problems and resources of older persons.

As far as marketing and identifying potential customers for the CPA, the committee is fairly specific.

> The type of care envisioned in an elder care engagement will probably be more expensive than institutional care. Consequently, the services will be available to those able to pay the costs. Within your clientele, elder care clients will typically come from (1) older clients, many of whom may have been clients for tax preparation or estate planning purposes, and (2) clients who are responsible for the care of an aging relative. By making the client and the children aware of the elder care services you can offer during tax preparation or estate planning meetings you can position yourself to be of assistance as the needs arise.[6]

The committee even goes as far as suggesting information and documents that the CPA needs to get from the elder care client.

- name, address, telephone number, number of children, number of grandchildren, number of in-laws, the relationships between relatives, and whether there are any family conflicts or estrangements that could cause problems
- names and addresses of the client's attorney, accountant (if other than the CPA talking to the client), and primary care physician
- information pertaining to all real estate owned, including mortgage information or rental income, and copies of leases and fire and casualty insurance policies
- a personal financial statement that includes all retirement assets, investments, and liabilities

- an annual cash flow analysis, which would enable the CPA to determine that all income is being received and that expenditures are within reasonable limits
- copies of all personal documents, including wills, tax returns, trust instruments, guardian nominations, powers of attorney, care agreements and contracts, and long-term care insurance policies
- religious and other advance planning information as well as hospital preferences
- information about any Medicare benefits and prepaid medical transportation policies and preferences to hospitals
- an informal assessment by the older person (or responsible family member) of his or her assistance needs or, in some cases, a formal assessment by a GCM nurse or geropsychiatrist[6]

Essentially, the AICPA is suggesting that CPAs do a form of geriatric care management. Included in the plan is a provision for the possible employment of GCMs to do assessment and plans of care, along with other professionals such as elder-law attorneys. AICPA has held task force meetings on the subject and has developed a plan of required training for CPAs looking for certification. During 1998–1999, a series of task force meetings were held around the country, dealing with such issues as elder law, elder care in Canada, accreditation, advertising, and continuing professional education. CPAs are ready to approach this clientele and are doing so in many markets.

Hopefully, the allied professional fields targeting the elderly client will acknowledge the benefit of the care manager in the continuum of care. This entry of other nonmedical and nonsocial work professionals into the field of geriatric care management poses a significant challenge to the traditional GCM. Because of the entry into the elder care arena by those other professionals, the traditional GCM must be proactive in maintaining the valuable psycho-social model in the face of these increasing attempts at involvement by the other professions. The care management professional must be inclusive and develop ways for allied professionals to work together in a more integrated manner, providing complimentary services.[5]

To showcase how diverse professionals might deliver geriatric care management services, this section discusses a fictitious client, Mrs. Jones, an 85-year-old woman who has congestive heart failure. She lives alone and has three children who live around the country. She has chosen to live alone and her support system dwindles because as she gets older, less and less persons who are friends and serve as a support system are able to do so.

This client might have an attorney who serves as care manager. Most likely, the attorney would have done a power of attorney in case Mrs. Jones became frail; would have worked with her, perhaps once every 5 years, reviewing her will and her assets; would have recommended someone to have fiduciary responsibility for assets; and would have done a durable power of attorney. If Mrs. Jones had an acute episode of congestive heart failure and was taken to the emergency room, the attorney's role would be to, as soon as reasonable (probably the next morning), discuss the prognosis with the care providers. The attorney might monitor the client while she remained in the hospital, possibly visiting once or twice to assess her progress. When it was time for the client to leave the hospital, the attorney would talk with the discharge planner, a home health agency representative, or a GCM to try to assess the situation and make a recommendation as to what kind of care was needed. The attorney would then, after Mrs. Jones was transferred home or to a facility, remain involved, perhaps on a weekly basis, unless more was necessary, to monitor the situation and make sure that Mrs. Jones was progressing.

Or Mrs. Jones might have an accountant as her primary care manager. The accountant would have been involved with the client probably once a year to do tax returns and perhaps more often for estimated income tax filings. It would be possible that Mrs. Jones and the accountant never see each other, doing everything by mail. However, if the accountant wanted to get into the elder care assurance business, that accountant would probably ask the client for some face-to-face contact. When the acute episode described above occurred, the accountant, if listed as the person to call, would be notified. However, in most situations, that accountant would not be listed anywhere. An emergency call would go out to 911 and the accountant would not be notified until some other person, possibly a family member, came into town and notified that accountant. The accountant would have to figure out a way to ensure that he or she would be notified if there were problems. Upon the client's release from a facility, the accountant would have to call upon a GCM, a nurse practitioner, or someone in a home health agency to help make an assessment and to help with plans of care for the future. The accountant could help with estimating various costs for different services, but the accountant would probably not be the best person to do geriatric assessment and assess long-term care needs.

Historically, trust departments have been intricately involved with their clients' lives. Often, the client calls the trust department on a daily basis, checking on assets, and the trust administrator, the secretary, or another person who receives those phone calls becomes an intricate part of the older person's life. Mrs. Jones might be that trust officer's client. If she has congestive heart failure and that trust officer does not receive a call from Mrs. Jones for some time, then the trust officer will know something is wrong and try to find out where she is. Since the trust officer pays the bills, the trust officer will be involved in determining how much money will be spent for care and what type of care will be needed.

Many trust departments use the services of independent contractors who provide in-home care. The trust officers can oversee the care as a GCM would.

There are other opportunities within the services delivery system for the introduction of geriatric care management. "Primary health care for frail elders should be a coordinated, multidisciplinary process that reacts not only to medical conditions but also addresses underlying psychosocial, economic, family, community support, and home environment issues that affect the patient's health and their ability to function."[7(p3)] In 1992, the John A. Hartford Foundation funded a 5-year initiative designed to improve approaches to caring for the frail elderly. In eight geographically disbursed sites throughout the United States, physicians worked in tandem with other professionals (e.g., social workers, nurses, nurse practitioners, physician's assistants) who performed basic case management functions. At the ninth site, physicians served as their own case managers using self-reported assessment data. Project sites varied in setting, organization, allied personnel, methods of operation, and other factors. Each site represented an alternative model for enhancing the care of community-based older persons by primary physicians. Models of practice like these will continue to develop and give the GCM opportunities for the future.

The American Institute of Outcomes Case Management (AIOCM) is attempting to eliminate the excesses of traditional case management through the licensing of practitioners equipped to assess the bottom-line outcome of services. The organization's literature expresses doubt as to the efficacy of current "assessment, planning, coordination, intervention, monitoring, pre-authorization, and utilization management."[6] With projected tools providing data on service areas, the organization offers a multifaceted picture of all services provided, to "consumers, payers, providers, employers, regulators."[8] The AIOCM envisions including all health care professionals and some other professionals: physicians, executives, respiratory therapists, pharmacists, nurses, social workers, and more. The traditional "team" concept of geriatric care management is adhered to and enhanced by critical thinking, business acumen, financial management, and case management.

Other models of practice are being defined in professional organizations that service the case management industry. To identify oneself as case management certified (CMC), one must meet certain educational and experience requirements and pass an examination. The 2-hour examination covers outcomes case management, business, finance, general management, critical thinking, and other areas considered relevant. Fees are moderate, and ongoing membership in AIOCM is fortified by continued education. Members gain access to a job opportunity listing. A stringent code of ethics has been adopted.[8]

Recertification is required every 2 years. In the recertification process the outcomes-case manager demonstrates ongoing efforts to maintain and enhance the ability to perform in an informed and competitive manner. In addition to adhering to the code of ethics as defined by AIOCM, continuing education or professional service is required. To get recertified as a CMC, the case manager must

- take continuing education courses through approved educational entities, or
- publish relevant solely or jointly authored technical papers, case histories or opinion papers, books or chapters in books, or the AIOCM online journal, or
- serve as a faculty member in an approved continuing education institution, community college, university or graduate school, or
- serve as a peer reviewer for AIOCM.

The emphasis on outcomes data may limit the applicability of AIOCM principles to the traditional geriatric care management practice. Quality of life issues may not be easily measured. Hard-line economic outcomes may not reflect client comfort or happiness. Any effort to eliminate inefficiencies in case management is to be encouraged, but only the future will show the efficacy of this approach to managed care. Geriatric care management companies may include AIOCM professionals as one of many employees with different approaches.

So when does the GCM interface with these attorneys, accountants, trust officers, and diverse professionals who are delivering similar geriatric care management services? The GCM is usually trained and has many years of experience in working with the frail elderly. All the professionals need someone who understands geriatric assessment. As the demographics change and more and more people become frail elderly, the need for geriatric assessment and appropriate decisions based on that assessment will continue to grow. The future of geriatric care management in working with diverse professionals is unlimited. Because of the unique background and experience of the GCM, the GCM can position himself or herself with physicians, with attorneys who specialize in estates and trusts within trust departments, and with accounting firms that have decided to offer elder care assurance.

THE IMPACT OF CHANGES IN THE INSURANCE INDUSTRY: THE DEEP POCKETS OF THIRD-PARTY REIMBURSEMENT

Assuming the trend toward more disease-free or disease-delayed aging continues, the growth of the number of very old persons will clearly continue to boost demand for medical and long-term care services.[1] Between 1995 and 2010, the support ratio for the older population is projected to hold steady at 21 persons aged 65 and older per 100 persons aged 18 to 65. The ratio will rise 71% between 2010 and 2030, however, increasing to 36 older persons per 100 persons aged 18 to 65 (Figure 15–6). Moreover, of those 36 older persons, an increased proportion will be over 75 years of age, part of a group much more likely than the young elderly (aged 65 to 74) to experience health problems.[1]

> The next decade will bring a major shift in long term care emphasis toward home and community settings, a shift that will lay the groundwork for even more significant changes beyond 2010. The future infrastructure for home and community services will need to overcome a long term care system that is currently fragmented (i.e., without adequate transitions between acute and chronic care) and difficult to access. Truly integrated systems of care will need to include some combination of the following features: combined acute care and long term

care service (both financing and delivery) for the elderly; an organized continuum of services and providers; case management to assure care continuity across the acute care and long term care delivery systems; training for providers to promote awareness of patient focused care; and capitation and other financing incentives to contain costs.[1(p51)]

The book continues:

> Many such disease management strategies are already in evidence today for conditions such as congestive heart failure, chronic obstructive pulmonary disease and diabetes. Parallel, long term prevention oriented efforts are also being developed for the management of hospital and nursing home inpatients. In general, the strategy of disease management and efforts is to (1) identify the populations at risk, (2) establish and coordinate clinical information among primary care providers, specialists and ancillary care providers, and (3) develop and implement appropriate clinical treatment protocols. More widespread implementation of these programs will likely result in targeted, but expanded access to primary care, home health services and health education seminars and materials, all with the purpose of preventing avoidable health status deterioration and disability. This is in reference to establishing active chronic care management programs that are seen as a potential positive result with a new basis of competition for HMOs in the future.[1(p40)]

According to Chan et al.:

> The trend in health care has been toward consolidated delivery systems wherein multiple insurance lines, levels of care and populations are integrated into one system of care. As a

result, case managers who once dealt exclusively in either health care or disability case management have diversified into other "product lines." Clearly, there is a parallel in growth between health insurance costs and workers' compensation expenditures. Managed care programs are increasingly being used as a way to control these costs. As a result, there is a trend toward the use of integrated benefit systems (24-hour coverage) to link workers' compensation with traditional insurance, blurring the line between income security and treatment management issues. 24-hour medical coverage and team approaches in managing health care patients and/or industrially engineered workers will be the norm in the next century.[9(p27)]

These authors continue:

The movement from a provider driven health care system to a payer based system has now been completed. In the next decade we will move from a payer based system to a consumer driven system. The development of managed care has had the effect of shifting the competitive advantage of health care organizations from prestige to price and accelerating the conversion of health care entities from not-for-profit to for-profit structures. Managed care has cut the cost of health care services, eliminating excess capacity, and curtailed the demand for medical specialists. At the same time, managed care encourages risk based competition (designing plans to attract low risk populations), resulting in high risk groups (e.g., people with disabilities) being underserved, excluded or simply priced out of the market. The focus of some managed care organizations on profits has also compromised the quality of care in selected cases resulting in consumer complaints and increased attention from politicians. In a market based environment, consumer choice, consumer satisfaction and client health outcomes will drive the success of managed care organizations while the monitoring of quality will receive increased attention. Without doubt, case managers can play an important role in the managed care environment. The use of case managers for utilization management, intensive case management, health promotion and disability prevention can help control

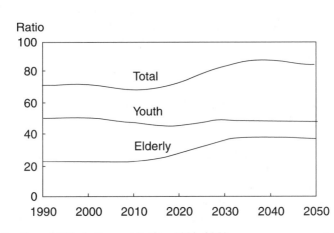

Figure 15–6 Total, Youth, and Elderly Support Ratios, 1990–2050.

health care and workers' compensation costs. Most important, the use of case managers as educators, patient advocates, problem solvers and negotiators will promote a better working relationship between patients and health care service providers that will prove vital as we move from a payer driven health care system to a consumer based managed care system. As expected, research/program evaluation, functional outcome measurement skills and conflict resolution/people skills are emerging from this study as important to case management practice.[9(p30)]

As geriatric care management becomes more mainstream and diverse professionals, often working with GCMs, continue delivering geriatric care management services, changes in the insurance industry will also greatly affect geriatric care management. GCMs traditionally have been paid privately, usually by trust departments or by family members and rarely by the people who are receiving the services. As the population ages and the system for delivering services to older persons remains diverse and fragmented, the need for someone to understand the different service levels and their costs will become greater. The insurance industry right now, under managed care, pays for certain services at a certain rate. Putting the frail older person into that system without any type of assessment, follow-up, or recommendations is bound to be more expensive for the managed care organization than reimbursing a GCM to keep the frail older person from returning to a nursing home or being hospitalized.

As the insurance industry looks at a growing older population, long-term care insurance will become a factor in more and more cases. The biggest question in long-term care insurance is what level of care is needed. It is much less expensive for the insurance company to have a home health agency check on an older person than it is to have the older person in a hospital. It is probably less expensive to have 24-hour care for a person in a home setting than it is for that person to be in a hospital. It is less expensive for the person to be in a nursing home than receive 24-hour personal care at home, but the nursing home scenarios are still expensive for the long-term care industry. So why would the long-term care industry be willing to pay for geriatric care management? Having a GCM assess, follow up, monitor, make recommendations, and coordinate the services of the diverse professionals involved in an older person's care would end up saving the insurance company money because of lack of reinstitutionalization and use of a less severely restricted setting with less services. The GCM can recommend services based upon what that frail older person actually needs.

Where will the insurance industry be in 2010? In 2030? How will third-party reimbursement affect the growth of the geriatric care management business? These are hard questions to answer. One can only assume that as the population ages and becomes more frail, the services provided by the GCM will become more valuable. If those services save the insurance industry money, then one can bet that the GCM will be reimbursed.

INTEGRATING TECHNOLOGY INTO IN-HOME MONITORING: 21ST-CENTURY CHANGES

At a speech on September 16, 1999, to the Rotary Club of Louisville, Patrick Mulloy, past President of Atria Communities, talked about the future use of technology to communicate with patients' families. He envisioned e-mailing clinical and progress reports to the families. He envisioned the family being able to log onto their Web site and monitor the activities in the community via a videocamera. He envisioned a very interactive communication via the Web so long-distance families could communicate with their loved ones as well as the facility staff.

No doubt, integrating technology into in-home monitoring will affect the future of geriatric care management. It is harder and harder to find qualified, caring, dependable, and mature persons to go into private homes and provide care. Most older persons want to remain in their own homes.

Right now the telephone is the most easily accessible safety device that most persons have. Almost everyone can afford to have a telephone, but there are problems with a frail older person having a telephone. Older persons are often tricked by callers into purchasing things or investing in things or contributing to causes. Screening incoming calls with caller ID is a perfect, simple, inexpensive way to use the telephone as a safety device and to protect the older person. Adding an answering machine to screen calls is also another way to protect that person. Getting call blocking mechanisms so the telephone company would actually only let calls through that come from family members or friends is another way to protect the older person. With large-button telephones and speed dialing in case of an emergency, family members can make sure that their loved one is safe. Blocking of long-distance calls to prevent unauthorized use of long-distance services by an aide or someone else who might be in the home is another protective mechanism. Another way to enhance use of the telephone by older persons is to annually update a list of drugstores, grocery stores, podiatrists, and durable medical equipment suppliers that deliver at home. This list can be useful when the frail older person does need help.

Most people have televisions in their home as well as telephone lines. There is a fairly new device called Web TV that is perfect for an older person who lives at home but does not want to learn how to use a computer. Web TV has its own Internet service. The home page has e-mail, a list of favorites, and search engines just like on a computer, and one can attach a printer to the Web TV unit so letters can be saved. The Web TV keyboard is just like a computer keyboard, but there are additional buttons that correspond to directions on the screen and are labeled. Web TV is a remote system with no cords. To activate the unit, the older person must point the remote keyboard toward the Web TV console (which looks like a VCR). Using Web TV, an older person can easily see the Web pages because he or she is using a regular television set with a large

screen. The print on the screen can be set to be large or small so everything is very easy to read and see. Wherever older persons normally watch television, they can access the Web and receive e-mail. The only negative to Web TV is that while the person is on-line, the telephone line is busy. Using Web TV, a frail older person can have a Web communication center at home, inexpensively.

The number of seniors who are signing up for computer classes and who are accessing the Internet is astounding. Using Web TV, an older person can e-mail and communicate easily with people all over the world.

How could communicating on the Web, either through Web TV or through a computer, affect geriatric care management in the future? As a long distance communications tool, e-mail is incredibly easy. It is less expensive than telephoning, less hassle than writing a letter and mailing it, and it can be done at any time of the day or night. One can access e-mail in public libraries or office computers or home computers. GCMs could correspond with clients and colleagues all over the country. They could use e-mail to respond or report to family members easily and at a very low cost. If the client did not respond to e-mail or communicate a problem, the GCM could respond or react. Clients could readily access information of all kinds. They could take self-tests, they could access information on all types of living situations, and they could fill a void in their social life by getting into interest groups and talking with persons from other interest groups so their circle of friends widens. This access would give more older persons more access to positive experiences and to interests that would keep them active and engaged.

The other type of monitoring that is developing now and shows great promise for the future is the videoconferencing products that are used with clients at home by some home health agencies and hospices. These telehealth units monitor all kinds of things. Depending on the unit, one can monitor blood pressure and vital signs and help people with procedures like bandaging wounds. These units can remind clients to take medication. They can also allow for two-way communications between a central setting like a physician's office or home health agency and the person at home. There are illnesses that can really benefit from the use of in-home video monitoring. Persons with chronic obstructive pulmonary disorder, diabetes, and congestive heart failure, for instance, are really helped by in-home video monitoring, which keeps recidivism and rehospitalization down.

If the in-home client can have a service provider actually see him or her via a videocamera, the service provider can make a determination if the person needs to go back to the hospital or just needs to take some medication or perhaps lie down. Units that can check vital signs and blood pressure also allow the medical personnel to make determinations as to whether the person needs an increase in medication, needs food, or needs an insulin dosage change. In-home monitoring is an incredible time and money saver for the client. The client does not have to continue to go back into emergency room settings or physician's office settings and can be effectively monitored at home. These units do not completely replace home visits, but they do take the place of having someone there 24 hours a day. They provide 24-hour medical monitoring so that the person with mild trouble can fix the problem before it becomes severe and the person has to go to a hospital or physician's office.

Most of these units work fairly easily, using the television and the phone wires. The monitoring is actually done by a video camera that sits on top of the home television set. The frail older person looks at the television set and can see the person who is talking, while that person can see the older person in their own home. The monitoring unit resides in a business that may monitor many frail older persons at home. There is always someone on duty to provide the monitoring service so the access to help via the home monitoring system is 24/7.

What clients would not be appropriate for telehealth? Persons who refuse to have equipment in their homes, persons who are not coherent, persons who are not motivated to participate in self-care, persons with a physical or cognitive impairment that prevents them from operating the equipment, and persons who need a lot of hands-on care would probably not be appropriate telehealth clients.

A less complicated type of telemonitoring equipment is the emergency medical alert system. The emergency medical alert system works with a pendant or a bracelet that the homebound person wears. The pendant or bracelet sends a signal to a unit in the home that is connected to the telephone and a monitoring station that can be local or far away. The phone call contacts a 24-hour monitoring service. As soon as the phone call is received, the system calls the frail older person back, and then, if there is a problem, summons help. The help can be whoever the client designates: it can be emergency medical services, a neighbor or a family member, or someone who has been predesignated to respond when help is called. This system also could be used as a safety mechanism for an older person, similar to a home alarm system. If the person thinks an intruder is in the house or the person is afraid of being home alone, he or she can activate the system and someone will call to talk.

ENSURING FUTURE SUCCESS IN GERIATRIC CARE MANAGEMENT: THINKING AHEAD

How will GCMs ensure their future success? According to Jeanne Boling:

Who wins in today's economic climate, the entity that can provide the lowest price or the best total outcome? The answer is not easily determined. The measure, though, must be taken while considering several facts about the economic trend. Who has not become aware of the uncertain future of the government sponsored health care programs. We are told the Medicare trust fund is approaching insolvency but the date is a moving target. The average growth in Medicaid demands is 12% each year and the trend is not voted particularly well for future recipients. There is a 23% increase per year in the population over age 85, which will serve to strain the system even more. The health care industry strives to do its part to manage a nation of increasing dependents with increased capitation and risk sharing mergers and acquisitions. Specialized geriatric case managers will no doubt grow in numbers as the medically complex elderly increase and as Medicare and Medicaid programs increasingly incorporate case management strategies.[10(p12)]

She continues:

> Where will case management find itself in the future under such circumstances? The costs of delivering case management is rising with its popularity. The case management is also uniquely tailored to work within the economy that is projected for the future. Inherently flexible, the case management industry is designed to operate within an integrated delivery system, a system which, by all measures, seems to be here to stay. By the year 2005, 93% of the U.S. economy is projected to be service oriented. Case management fits smoothly into this scenario.[10(p12)]

Boling explains GCMs' future role in cost containment and medically complex cases:

> By 2010, the population over 65 will increase by 25% and those over 85 will increase by 88%. This dramatic rise in life expectancy will mean more medically complex cases. Those insured by Medicare/Medicaid will double, increasing the numbers of patients requiring case management. Various institutions in the health care system will turn to case managers to address these complex issues. Case managers must be prepared to answer the concerns over cost containment, rationing medical necessity and fiduciary responsibility.[10(pp12–13)]

What changes is U.S. society experiencing that demand immediate forward-looking adaptations by the GCM, whether a solo practitioner or part of a company? How will it profit the GCM to modify operations between 2000 and 2010 to prepare for the 2010–2050 influx of clients? Forward-looking changes in one geriatric care practice include the following:

- compensation that is incentive based
- benefits for employees
- employee leasing
- use of professional marketing services
- collaboration with nonprofits
- more professional education
- a broadened scope, beyond traditional medical and social work services
- participation in managed care demonstration projects
- openness to opportunities to diversify the business
- service repackaging
- rewards for staff who have a leadership role in the local community
- participation in long-term care insurance projects
- participation in professional cluster networks[5]

In addition, geriatric care management is taking many organizational forms, ranging from "mom and pop" agencies to large companies to multiple franchises. The upcoming swell of clients challenges every type of geriatric care management organization.

Today's average geriatric care management client is a frail woman 85 years or older living in her home environment.[1] She needs help with at least some activities of daily living. In 2010, the average client will be older and therefore frailer. She will retain her determination to remain independent at home.[1] Home maintenance and adaptation for senior occupancy will be needed. Housecleaning, shopping, and personal care will also be necessary because the client's son or daughter, who would otherwise provide these services, is employed, living in another city, or limited in his or her own activities due to age.[1]

Food preparation will emphasize maintenance of a healthful diet. There will also be an emphasis on appropriate physical activity to prevent disability. Health care will be provided through a Medigap health maintenance organization policy. Managed care will factor into all dealings related to health and may result in a lack of referrals to private geriatric care management companies for help with cost and organizational considerations. GCMs will need to market their services accordingly. GCMs will stress the uniqueness of their services and the ultimate cost reduction to the managed care company.

The busy or distant family will depend on the GCM to locate senior social activities in the community. Accustomed to prompt and efficient services from other providers, family members will demand accelerated services from the GCM, who doubtless will already have available resources amassed in a computer directory.[10] The client's socialization with family and friends will increase through e-mail or Web TV. Libraries, universities, and social agencies have begun providing these communication services to older people.

In 2010 the GCM will make full use of electronic devices in the home to monitor the client and caregivers; to communicate via home computer or Web TV; to establish interaction with professionals, family members, or caregivers; and even to submit invoices. While electronic devices may simplify some operations, the need for personal attendants, housekeeping, home maintenance, and transportation will remain, calling for hands-on, face-to-face assessment and service delivery.

Transition to another level of care (at an assisted living facility or nursing home) will be deferred as long as possible because of the inflated cost. Long-term care insurance will provide some freedom of choice between home care and institutionalization, but the cost of the insurance will have deterred many clients from purchasing it.[11] At the present time 75% of the long-term care policies are handled by a small group of insurance companies, which have diversified policies to cover in-home care and assisted living, to delay or render unnecessary nursing home care. Opportunities exist for the GCM to contract with long-term care insurers to do in-home assessments of applicants and insured persons submitting claims.[11] Currently there is no built-in role for the GCM in the distribution of long-term care funds, but the forward-looking professional will attempt to sell his or her services to the insurer, noting that GCM services will help minimize insurance company expenses.[11]

The health status of seniors in 2010 should be both better and worse than in 2000 (Figure 15–7). A major goal of geriatric care management will be to avoid costly institutionalization. Preventive health maintenance, via diet and exercise, as well as proactive health care by geriatric specialists should begin to pay off as seniors become more active and vital. As noted above, there is some evidence that the number of older persons suffering disabling chronic conditions will decline by 2010.[12] Environmental and lifestyle factors seem to outweigh genetic ones as a person ages.[1]

The reverse side of the coin, however, is the chronic health conditions of the "old old," the sector of the aging population 85 and over, which will increase dramatically by 2010.[1] Some scholars are predicting a compression of these chronic conditions into a few years at the end of life, after an active old age.[1] Technology doubtless will provide the health care practitioner with the means of checking blood pressure, temperature, and other basic conditions, leading to diagnosis, appointments, and billing without the client leaving home. In the immediate future, children of geriatric care management clients will be baby boomers, who have already transformed finance and retail companies to a customer-friendly modality. Their impact on the geriatric care industry will show itself as GCMs respond to demanding questions asked by well-informed customers. These customers will look elsewhere for service when not satisfied. Communication is vital in these circumstances.[12] The health care system does not show signs of vertically integrating but rather of horizontal consolidation of service delivery (Figure 15–8). The GCM will need increasingly to coordinate ser-

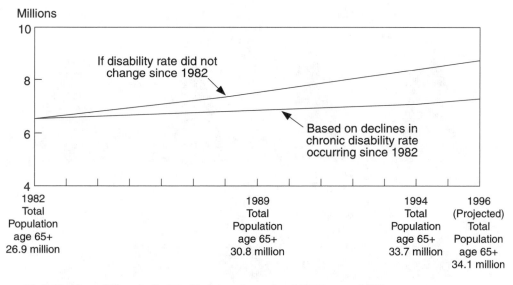

Figure 15–7 Number of Chronically Disabled Americans Aged 65 Years and Older.

vices from disparate sources in order to ensure seamless interface with the patient. The importance of these skills cannot be overemphasized.[12]

With the increased older population, the augmented intensity of need for care, and the skyrocketing cost of institutional care, the need for geriatric care management will grow. Whether this will be provided by the giant Medicare-Medicaid complex necessary to administer health care or will still exist among independent contractors is yet to be seen. Cost factors will also lead to an increase in Medicare health maintenance organizations, which may have in-house GCMs or contract with GCMs.[11]

By 2010, the GCM should be able to carry out all financial services needed by clients via computer. Many financial services are already in place, and the GCM will only need to adopt new instrumentalities as they are made available. While capitation, payment in advance for medical care, is not growing rampantly, it is one of a variety of funding sources. Several forms of fee for service, including traditional Medicare, will continue to exist and be joined by episodic prepayment and increasingly by performance-based payment (Figure 15–9).[12] One seeming certainty of the financial picture for senior adults in the

decades to come is larger inequity in income.[1] However, while poverty will inch up among aging baby boomers, there will always be persons able to afford the services of a private GCM. Whether they will choose the private over the publicly provided equivalent is not clear. The aging population in general will be better off, but problems will grow out of the combination of early retirement and longer life.[1] The factors calling for increased expenditures, public and private, on behalf of older persons are longer life expectancies and a higher number of chronic health problems resulting from the increase in age. These conditions will compel government to preserve the three benefits, Social Security, Medicare, and Medicaid, and will force the application of cost control.

The prospective combination of poverty, great age, and chronic illness segues the discussion into the problem of long-term care. Two out of five persons over 65 have at least one chronic condition requiring assistance in activities of daily living. In 1990, 6.5 million persons needed help in at least one field of care, compared with an estimated 10 million in 2010. Seventy percent of these persons relies on a family member for help.[1] Traditionally, the nursing home has been

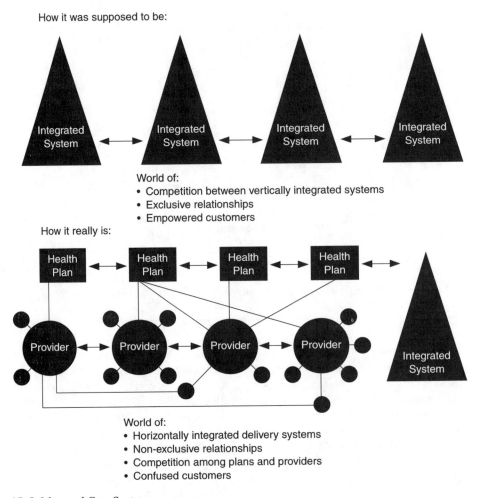

How it was supposed to be:

World of:
- Competition between vertically integrated systems
- Exclusive relationships
- Empowered customers

How it really is:

World of:
- Horizontally integrated delivery systems
- Non-exclusive relationships
- Competition among plans and providers
- Confused customers

Figure 15–8 Managed Care System.

the answer in this country when older persons need long-term care and the family cannot provide it. As mentioned earlier in the chapter, there are fewer family caregivers available. The huge cost of institutionalization is driving private insurers and the government toward using in-home care. By 2010, the preference for home care over institutionalization will force private insurers and state Medicaid programs to adopt some form of home care, with the maintenance of the quality of care an issue.[1] Again, the greater need for geriatric care management is evident.

Dementia is an unknown variable in these equations. Great age is a factor in increasing de-

mentia, but there is hope that enhanced quality of life and improved medications will lower the current rate of Alzheimer's disease and other dementias.[1]

Demands for community care with lower costs and higher quality will lead to the proliferation of care management services in the next 10 years. Given the fact that there are persons who cannot afford private geriatric care management, it is projected that the government will be forced to integrate geriatric care management into the Medicare-Medicaid system of care.[1] Can the government deny a service needed by all but affordable to only a few? Taking that into

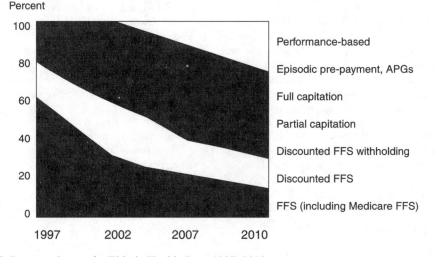

Figure 15–9 Payment Source for Elderly Health Care, 1997–2010.

consideration, can GCMs be anything but ready to market their profession?

CONCLUSION

So there are many possibilities for the future of geriatric care management. New technology could allow the GCM to be physically located anywhere in the country but part of a consortium of care managers so that assessments, information, and resources are accessed in a central location while each GCM is responsible for his or her geographic area and updating the local resource information. To be a mainstream business, geriatric care management will have to become a household word, so that when a frail older person has a problem, the first call would be to a GCM to help that person decide what types of care that person would need for the future and what the next move should be. There will still be some boutique geriatric care man-

agement practices in rural settings or settings where there are not population centers and persons are not moving. The GCM can either be a solo practitioner or have several people together that provide part-time services, combining, perhaps, the skills of social workers and nurses. There are also geriatric care management practices that will be associated with home care agencies and with hospitals so that there is someone providing that linkage between the home care agency, the hospital, and the client. Geriatric care management practice will be an extension of physician's offices, trust departments, and of accounting practices.

The time to plan is now. "It will be the post-2010 demographic title wave that challenges the nation to adjust its health and service systems but it will be the planning and policy work done pre-2010 that determines U.S. success, private, public and personal in meeting this challenge."[1(p7)]

NOTES

1. *Aging: 1998–2010.* Menlo Park, CA: Institute for the Future; 1998.

2. http://www.alz.org/research/current/stats.htm (22 March 2000). Accessed August 28, 2000.

3. Census Data Current Population Projections. 1970, 1990:25–1111; Kentucky Data Center, 1997.

4. Lewis GA, Sammons AE. "Assurance services: elder care." http://www.aicpa.org/pubs/tpcpa/jan98/elder.htm (January 1998). Accessed May 23, 1999.

5. Barlam S. Changes, fears, and opportunities: a survival guide for geriatric care managers. *GCM J.* 1998;8:4–9.

6. Lewis GA, Sammons AE. Developing an elder care practice. http://www.aicpa.org/pubs/tpcpa/jan98/elder. htm (January 1998). Accessed May 23, 1999.

7. Netting FE, Williams, FG. Geriatric case managers: integration into physician practices. *Care Manage J.* 1999;1:3–9.

8. AIOCM, http://www.aiocm.com/cmc%20certification. htm. Accessed June 1999.

9. Chan F, Leahy MJ, McMahon B, Mirch M, DeVinney D. Foundational knowledge and major practice domains of case management. *J Care Manage.* 1999;5:10–30.

10. Boling J. Creating the future of case management in a radically changing health care world. *GCM J.* 1998;8: 10–13.

11. O'Toole RE. Growth of private long-term-care insurance will expand the role of case management. *Inside Case Manage.* 1995;1:4–5.

12. Pascali M. Future trends in health care: implications for geriatric care managers. *GCM J.* 1998;8:24–28.

SUGGESTED READING

Crouch R. New demographics for the old ball game. *GCM J.* 1998; 14–16.

Contact Information

American Association of Retired Persons (AARP)
601 East Street NW
Washington, DC 20049
Telephone: (800) 424–3410
Fax: (202) 434–2588
Web site: http://www.aarp.com
E-mail: member@aarp.org

American Society on Aging (ASA)
833 Market Street, Suite 511
San Francisco, CA 94103–1824
Telephone: (415) 974–9600
Fax: (415) 974–0300
Web site: http://www.asaging.org
E-mail: info@asaging.org

Case Management Society of America (CMSA)
8201 Cantrell Road
Suite 230
Little Rock, AR 72227
Telephone: (501) 225–2229
Fax: (501) 221–9068
Web site: http://www.cmsa.org
E-mail: cmsa@cmsa.org

Internal Revenue Service (IRS)
1111 Constitution Avenue NW
Washington, DC 20224
Telephone: (202) 622–5000
Web site: http://www.irs.ustreas.gov

National Association of Elder Law Attorneys (NAELA)
1604 North Country Club Road
Tucson, AZ 85716–3102
Telephone: (502) 881–4005
Fax: (520) 325–7925
Web site: http://www.naela.org
E-mail: info@naela.com

National Association of Professional Geriatric Care Managers (NAPGCM)
1604 North Country Club Road
Tucson, AZ 85716–3102
Telephone: (520) 881–8008
Fax: (520) 325–7925
Web site: http://www.caremanager.org
E-mail: info@caremanager.org

National Association of Social Workers (NASW)
750 First Street NE, Suite 700
Washington, DC 20002-4241
Telephone: (202) 408–8600, (800) 638–8799
Web site: http://www.naswdc.org
E-mail: info@naswdc.org

National Council on Aging (NCOA)
409 Third Street SW
Washington, DC 20024
Telephone: (202) 479–6991
Fax: (202) 479–0735
Web site: http://www.ncoa.org
E-mail: info@ncoa.org

National Gerontological Society of America (GSA)
1030 15th Street NW, Suite 250
Washington, DC 20005
Telephone: (202) 842–1275
Fax: (202) 842–1150
Web site: http://www.geron.org
E-mail: webmaster@geron.org

Senior Care Review
P.O. Box 9506
Laguna Beach, CA 92652–7705
Telephone: (949) 489–8601
Fax: (801) 729–6091
Web site: http://www.seniorcarereview.com
E-mail: consult@seniorcarereview.com

Service Corps of Retired Executives
409 3rd Street SW, 6th Floor
Wahsington, DC 20024
Telephone: (800) 634–0245
Fax: (202) 205–7636
Web site: http://www.score.org

Small Business Administration (SBA)
Telephone: (800) 827–5722
Web site: http://www.sba.gov

US Chamber of Commerce
1615 H Street NW
Washington, DC 20062
Telephone: (202) 659–6000
Fax: (202) 463–3164
Web site: http://www.uschamber.com
E-mail: custvc@uschamber.com

Assessments

SOCIAL WORK ASSESSMENT

Date _____ Completed By _____

Patient Name _____

Address _____

City _____ State _____ Zip _____

Can the Patient Manage Finances without Assistance? _____ Yes _____ No

If no, give reason _____

Does Patient Have Someone Assisting with Finances? _____ Yes _____ No

Name_____ Telephone _____

Address _____

City _____ State _____ Zip _____

Is There a Substitute Payee, Guardian Conservator of Estate, or Power of Attorney?

(If so, please indicate which) _____

If so, please indicate

Address _____

Telephone Number(s) _____

If so, Date Established _____

Reason Established _____

Is There a Conservatorship of Person or D.P.O.A. for H.C. Established? _____

If so, Who Is the Designated Agent(s)? _____

Agent(s) Phone _____

Address _____

City _____ State _____ Zip _____

Residence/Has Patient Had Any Change in Residence in the Past Year? _____ Yes _____ No

(If yes, where/why?) _____

_____

If Patient Was in an Institutional Setting, Why Was the Patient Moved? _____

_____

_____

_____

Date of Move _____

If Patient Currently in Institutional Setting, Does He or She Wish To Remain There? _____

_____

If Patient Is at Home, Does Anyone Else Reside in the Home? _____

_____

If Patient Is at Home, Does He or She Wish To Remain at Home? _____ Yes _____ No

Is the Care Provision in the Home Adequate? _____ Yes _____ No

Has There Been Any Significant Life Event or Trauma in the Last 12 Months? (i.e., Hospitalization, SNF, Falls—if so, give details and dates) _____

_____

_____

_____

_____

_____

_____

What Initiated Call to Agency? _____

_____

_____

_____

_____

_____

_____

Problem List:

Self Care Deficit _____ Impaired Mobility _____

Impaired Home Mgmt _____ Knowledge Deficit _____

Alterations in Nutrition _____ Alteration in Bowel Elim _____

Impaired Skin Integrity _____ Alteration in Urinary Elim _____

Pain _____ Other _____

PROBLEM LIST

How Participants Evaluate Problem _____

_____

_____

_____

_____

_____

_____

How Family, Friends, Board/Care, Nursing Home Evaluates Problem _____

_____

_____

_____

_____

_____

_____

Present Client Solutions to Problems _____

_____

_____

_____

_____

_____

Orientation:

Time _____ Yes _____ No

Place _____ Yes _____ No

Person _____ Yes _____ No

CARE PLAN

Diagnosis _____

_____

_____

_____

_____

_____

_____

Problems _____

Interventions _____

_____

_____

_____

_____

_____

_____

_____

If Additional Space is Needed, Please Use Space Provided Below _____

_____

_____

_____

_____

_____

_____

NURSING ASSESSMENT

Date_____ Nurses Name _____

Patient Name _____ Temp._____ Pulse___/___ ___/___ Resp. _____

Place of Visit: _____ apical radial

Chief Complaint _____ B/P ___/___ ___/___ ___/___ ___/___ ___/___

_____ left right lying sitting standing

_____ Weight_____Height _____

		Norm.	Abnm.	not exam.	Describe or measure
Skin	Color _____				
	Condition (Wound) _____				
	Temperature _____				
	Turgor _____				
Head	Hair _____				
	Scalp _____				
Eyes	Appearance _____				
	Vision _____				
	Pupils_____				
Ears	Hearing _____				
Nose					
Mouth	Teeth (Dentures) _____				
	Gums _____				
	Tongue _____				
	Throat _____				
Neck	Appearance _____				
	Mobility_____				
Cardiac/ Pulmonary	Shortness of Breath _____				
	Exercise Tolerance _____				
	Cough _____				
	Sputnum _____				
	Chest Configuration _____				
	Auscultation _____				
Breast					
Neurological	Pain _____				
	Tremor_____				
	Motor function _____				
	Sensory Function_____				
Musculo/ Skeletal	Back _____				
	Extremities _____				
	Joints _____				
	Ambulation _____				

		Norm.	Abnm.	not exam.	Describe or measure
Gastro/ Intestinal	Shape _____				
	Palpitation _____				
	Girth Bowel Movements _____				
	Nausea/vomiting _____				
Peripheral/ Vascular	Puises _____				
	Temperature _____				
	Color _____				
Genitourinary	Continence _____				
	Signs/SX of Infect _____				
	Nocturia _____				
Nutrition	Diet _____				
	Fluids _____				
Mental/ Emotional	Orientation/MSQ _____				
	LOC _____				
	Communication _____				
	Behavior _____				
ADLs I = Independent A = Assist D = Depend	Feeding _____				
	Toileting _____				
	Personal Care _____				
	Household Activities _____				

Primary Diagnosis _____

Surgical Procedures/Incidents _____

Secondary _____

History _____

Medications _____

Diet _____ Allergies _____

Smokes _____ Alcohol _____

Social Language _____ Education _____

Social Activities _____ Interests _____

Family Structure _____ Past Occup. _____

Home Safety _____ Home Environment _____

Significant Others _____ Significant Life Events _____

Problem List:

Self Care Deficit _____Impaired Mobility _____

Impaired Home Mgmt _____Knowledge Deficit _____

Alterations in Nutrition_____Alteration in Bowel Elim _____

Impaired Skin Integrity_____Alteration in Urinary Elim

Pain _____Other_____

Care Plan	Intervention

Sources

CHAPTER 2

Exhibit 2–1 Reprinted with permission from Pledge of Ethics for Members of the National Association of Professional Geriatric Care Managers, *GCM Journal*, Vol. 9, No. 4, pp. 4–5, © 1999, National Association of Professional Geriatric Care Managers.

Exhibit 2–3 Reprinted with permission from Legal and Ethical Issues in Health Care of Older Adults, *GCM Journal*, Vol. 9, No. 4, p. 28, © 1999, National Association of Professional Geriatric Care Managers.

CHAPTER 5

Figure 5–1 Copyright © 1997, Lynn Hackstaff.

CHAPTER 10

Exhibit 10–1 Reprinted with permission from L. Teri, et al., Assessment of Behavioral Problems in Dementia: The Revised Memory and Behavior Problems Checklist, *Psychology and Aging*, Vol. 7, pp. 622–631, © 1992, Linda Teri, Ph.D.

CHAPTER 11

Exhibit 11–1 Republished with permission of the Gerontological Society of America, 1030 15th Street, NW, Suite 250, Washington, DC 20005. *Progress in the Development of the Index of ADL* (Tool), S. Katz, T.D. Downs, H.R. Cash, et al., *Gerontologist*, 1970, Vol. 1. Reproduced by permission of the publisher via Copyright Clearance Center, Inc.

Exhibit 11–2 Reprinted with permission from *Journal of the American Geriatric Society*, Vol. 20, pp. 318–382, © 1982, Lippincott, Williams & Wilkins.

Exhibit 11–3 Reprinted with permission from Tinetti Balance and Gait Evolution, *Journal of the American Geriatric Society*, Vol. 34, pp. 119–126, © 1986, Lippincott, Williams & Wilkins.

Exhibit 11–4 Republished with permission of the Gerontological Society of America, 1030 15th Street, NW, Suite 250, Washington, DC. *Assessment of Older People: Self-monitoring and Instrumental Activities of Daily Living* (Scale), M.P. Lawton and E.M. Brody, Gerontologist, 1969, Vol. 9. Reproduced by permission of the publisher via Copyright Clearance Center, Inc.

Exhibit 11–5 Reprinted with permission from E. Pfeiffer, A Short Portable Mental Status Questionnaire for the Assessment of Organic Brain Deficit in Elderly Patients, *Journal of the American Geriatric Society*, Vol. 23, pp. 433–441, © 1975, Lippincott, Williams & Wilkins.

Exhibit 11–6 From U.S. National Safety Council and American Association of Retired Persons, *Falling—The Unexpected Trip*, A Safety Program for Older Adults, Program Leader's Guide, © 1982. Reprinted with permission from the National Safety Council, 444 North Michigan Avenue, Chicago, IL 60611.

CHAPTER 12

Exhibit 12–1 Adapted with permission from G. McKhann, et al., Clinical Diagnosis of Alzheimer's Disease: Report of the NINCDS–ADRDA work group, *Neurology*, Vol. 34, pp. 939–944, © 1984, Lippincott, Williams & Wilkins.

Exhibit 12–2 Adapted with permission from G. McKhann, et al., Clinical Diagnosis of Alzheimer's Disease: Report of the NINCDS–ADRDA work group, *Neurology*, Vol. 34, pp. 939–944, © 1984, Lippincott, Williams & Wilkins.

Exhibit 12–3 Data from D. Geldmacher and P. Whitehouse, Evaluation of Dementia, *New England Journal of Medicine*, Vol. 335, No. 5, pp. 330–336, © 1996, Massachusetts Medical Society.

Exhibit 12–4 Reprinted with permission from M.F. Folstein, et al., "Mini-Mental State." A Practical Method for Grading the Cognitive State of Patients for the Clinician. *Journal of Psychiatric Research*, 12(3):189–198, © 1975, 1998 MiniMental LLC.

Exhibit 12–5 Adapted from *Journal of Psychiatric Research*, Vol. 17, J. Yesavage, Development and Validation of a Geriatric Depression Scale, A Preliminary Report, pp. 37–49, Copyright 1983, with permission from Elsevier Science.

Exhibit 12–6 Adapted with permission from D. Hanson, *User's Guide to the Goal Evaluation and Matrix Analysis, 4th Edition*, © 1998, Synergistic Psychology Associates, PA.

Exhibit 12–7 Adapted with permission from D. Hanson, *User's Guide to the Goal Evaluation and Matrix Analysis, 4th Edition*, © 1998, Synergistic Psychology Associates, PA.

Exhibit 12–9 Adapted with permission from D. Hanson, *User's Guide to the Goal Evaluation and Matrix Analysis, 4th Edition*, © 1998, Synergistic Psychology Associates, PA.

Exhibit 12–10 Adapted with permission from D. Hanson, *User's Guide to the Goal Evaluation and Matrix Analysis, 4th Edition*, © 1998, Synergistic Psychology Associates, PA.

Exhibit 12–11 Adapted with permission from D. Hanson, *User's Guide to the Goal Evaluation and Matrix Analysis, 4th Edition*, © 1998, Synergistic Psychology Associates, PA.

Figure 12–1 Copyright © 1999, Karen Knutson, Open Care, Inc.

Figure 12–3 Reprinted with permission from T. Sunderland, et al., Clock Drawing in Alzheimer's Disease, A Novel Measure of Dementia Severity, *Journal of the American Geriatric Society*, Vol. 37, pp. 725–729, © 1989, Trey Sunderland, MD.

Figure 12–4 Adapted with permission from D. Hanson, *User's Guide to the Goal Evaluation and Matrix Analysis, 4th Edition*, © 1998, Synergistic Psychology Associates, PA.

Figure 12–5 Adapted with permission from D. Hanson, *User's Guide to the Goal Evaluation and Matrix Analysis, 4th Edition*, © 1998, Synergistic Psychology Associates, PA.

Table 12–1 Adapted with permission from J. Corey-Bloom, et al., Diagnosis and Evaluation of Dementia, *Neurology*, Vol. 45, pp. 211–218, © 1995, Lippincott, Williams & Wilkins.

CHAPTER 14

Exhibit 14–1 Copyright © George Frichett.

Text (pp 283–284) Copyright © Amy Gottlieb

CHAPTER 15

Figure 15–1 Reprinted from *Population Projections of the United States by Age, Sex, Race and Hispanic Origin: 1993 to 2050*, Current Population Reports, Series P-25, No. 1130, U.S. Bureau of the Census, U.S. Government Printing Office, 1993.

Figure 15–2 Reprinted from General Population Characteristics, PC80–1-B1, U.S. Bureau of the Census, U.S. Government Printing Office, May 1963; 1990 Census of Population and Housing, CPH-L-74, *Modified and Actual Age, Sex, Race and Hispanic Origin Data: Population Projections of the United States by Age, Sex, Race and Hispanic Origin: 1995 to 2050*, Current Population Reports, Series P-25, No. 1130, U.S. Bureau of Census, U.S. Government Printing Office, 1993.

Figure 15–3 Reprinted from Office of Managed Care, Health Care Financing Administration, U.S. Department of Health and Human Services, 1995.

Figure 15–4 Reprinted from 1970 and 1990 Census Data, *Current Population Projections*, Kentucky State Data Center, 1997.

Figure 15–5 Reprinted with permission from *Chronic Care in America, A 21st Century Challenge*, © 1996, Robert Wood Johnson Foundation.

Figure 15–6 Reprinted from 1990 Census of Population and Housing, CPH-L-74, *Modified and Actual Age, Sex, Race and Hispanic Origin Data: Population Projections of the United States by Age, Sex, Race and Hispanic Origin: 1993 to 2050*, Current Population Reports, Series P-25, No. 1104, U.S. Bureau of the Census, U.S. Government Printing Office, 1993.

Figure 15–7 Reprinted with permission from K.G. Manton, L. Corder, and E. Stallard, Chronic Disability Trends in Eldery United States Populations: 1992–1994, *Proceedings of the National Academy of Sciences of the United States*, Vol. 94, pp. 2593–2598, © 1997, National Academy of Sciences.

Figure 15–8 Reprinted from Institute for the Future, for the Robert Wood Johnson Foundation. "Health and Health Care 2010: The Forecast, The Challenge," Jossey-Bass Publishers. © 2000 Institute for the Future, page 49.

Figure 15–9 Data from Institute for the Future, for the Robert Wood Johnson Foundation. "Health and Health Care 2010: The Forecast, The Challenge," Jossey-Bass Publishers. © 2000 Institute for the Future, page 56; Louis Harris & Associates; Interstudy; and American Medical Association.

Text (pp 295–297) From AICPA CPE *Course Assurance Services: Elder Care*. Copyright © 1998 by the American Institute of Certified Public Accountants, Inc. Reprinted with permission.

Index